Clinical Pathology of Pancreatic Disorders

PATHOLOGY AND LABORATORY MEDICINE

Series Editors: Stewart Sell and Alan Wu

2. Clinical Pathology of Pancreatic Disorders
edited by *John A. Lott*, 1997

1. Molecular Diagnostics: For the Clinical Laboratorian
edited by *William B. Coleman* and *Gregory J. Tsongalis,* 1997

PATHOLOGY AND LABORATORY MEDICINE

Clinical Pathology of Pancreatic Disorders

Edited by

John A. Lott

The Ohio State University, Columbus, OH

Humana Press ✳ Totowa, New Jersey

© 1997 Humana Press Inc.
999 Riverview Drive, Suite 208
Totowa, New Jersey 07512

All rights reserved. No part of this book may be reproduced, stored in a retrieval system, or transmitted in any form or by any means, electronic, mechanical, photocopying, microfilming, recording, or otherwise without written permission from the Publisher.

All authored papers, comments, opinions, conclusions, or recommendations are those of the author(s), and do not necessarily reflect the views of the publisher.

This publication is printed on acid-free paper. ∞
ANSI Z39.48-1984 (American Standards Institute) Permanence of Paper for Printed Library Materials.

Cover design by Patricia F. Cleary.

For additional copies, pricing for bulk purchases, and/or information about other Humana titles, contact Humana at the above address or at any of the following numbers: Tel.: 201-256-1699; Fax: 201-256-8341; E-mail: humana@mindspring.com; Website: http://humanapress.com

Photocopy Authorization Policy:
Authorization to photocopy items for internal or personal use, or the internal or personal use of specific clients, is granted by Humana Press Inc., provided that the base fee of US $8.00 per copy, plus US $00.25 per page, is paid directly to the Copyright Clearance Center at 222 Rosewood Drive, Danvers, MA 01923. For those organizations that have been granted a photocopy license from the CCC, a separate system of payment has been arranged and is acceptable to Humana Press Inc. The fee code for users of the Transactional Reporting Service is: [0-89603-475-5/97 $8.00 + $00.25].

Printed in the United States of America. 10 9 8 7 6 5 4 3 2 1

Preface

The pancreas is about the size and shape of the hand; the tail points to the spleen, and the head is nestled in a loop of the duodenum. Loss of the exocrine (digestive) functions commonly leads to severe gastrointestinal disturbances, malabsorption, a catabolic state, and weight loss in the face of an adequate diet. Loss of endocrine pancreatic function leads to a large spectrum of disorders associated with the loss of hormone secretions; the most common and most severe is diabetes mellitus. Loss of the entire pancreas owing to trauma, surgery, atherosclerosis, or other medical problems leaves the patient in a digestive and metabolic crisis.

The correct diagnosis of pancreatic disorders remains a challenge given the multifaceted function of the pancreas. The clinical laboratory plays an important role, and other tools such as CAT scans, ultrasound, radiographs, biopsies, and even surgery are used to make a diagnosis. The emphasis of *Clinical Pathology of Pancreatic Disorders* is on the clinical laboratory definition of pancreatic pathology.

Disorders of the endocrine pancreas can be highly complex, and sophisticated tests are needed to determine the nature of the disease, its prognosis, and its optimal treatment. Diabetes is the most common of the endocrine diseases; it presents in many ways, and has varied etiologies. We now know that the diabetes of childhood is usually an autoimmune disease, and this has a major effect on the treatment of these individuals.

The pancreas is easily inflamed in patients with chronic alcohol abuse, biliary tract diseases, a cyst or other inflammation in the abdomen, and a host of other miscellaneous causes including drug sensitivity. Pancreatitis can be mild and transient; severe disease also occurs, and hemorrhagic, necrotic pancreatitis has a near 100% mortality rate. The laboratory is important in the differential diagnosis of patients with an acute abdomen. Patients with pancreatitis are poor surgical risks, and often the laboratory studies can confirm the presence of pancreatitis. Chronic pancreatitis leads to loss of gland function and structure; with new bouts of pancreatitis, the patient may show trivial or no changes in the common laboratory tests.

Transplantation of the pancreas and simultaneous pancreas and kidney transplants are becoming more common, particularly in patients with diabetes and end-stage kidney disease. Often, euglycemia and normal kidney function can be restored by transplanting both organs. Many more transplants would be performed if suitable organs were available. Rejection and infections remain as the most serious problems. The ducting of the pancreatic juice into the urinary bladder creates problems, such as bladder inflammation and pain, in some patients. Nevertheless, this surgical technique is superior to other approaches in nearly all patients.

The exocrine disorders of the pancreas are fairly common; in children, cystic fibrosis usually leads to pancreatic insufficiency. In adults, repeated bouts of pancreatitis generally lead to exocrine pancreatic dysfunction after ~85% of the gland has been replaced by nonfunctioning tissue. An amazing fact about the pancreas is the reserve capacity for both endocrine and exocrine secretions. Extensive destruction of the pancreas must occur before pancreatic exocrine insufficiency is clinically evident.

Cancer of the endocrine or exocrine pancreas, particularly the latter, is usually a disaster for the patient. Adenocarcinoma of the pancreas is often silent until far advanced, and the prognosis is extremely poor. Death within 3–6 months after diagnosis is common. Early resection saves some patients, but the 5-year survival of pancreatic adenocarcinoma is still dismally low. The most common endocrine cancer affects the islet cells, and predominantly the beta cells. The laboratory's role here is pre-eminent in defining the stage and severity of the disease.

John A. Lott

Contents

Preface v

Contributors ix

1 Transplantation of the Pancreas or Pancreatic Islet Cells:
   A Clinical Laboratory Perspective
   John A. Lott *1*

2 Exocrine Disorders of the Pancreas
   Frederick Van Lente *27*

3 Biochemical Indicators of Acute Pancreatitis
   Steven C. Kamierczak *75*

4 Neoplastic Disorders of the Pancreas
   **Peter Muscarella II, William Fisher, Jerome A. Johnson,
   and W. Scott Melvin** *125*

5 Biochemistry, Pathogenesis, and Laboratory Diagnosis
   of Endocrine Disorders of the Pancreas
   Manjula K. Gupta *163*

Index *213*

Contributors

WILLIAM FISHER • *Department of Surgery, The Ohio State University Medical Center, Columbus, OH*

MANJULA K. GUPTA • *Department of Clinical Pathology, The Cleveland Clinic Foundation, Cleveland, OH*

JEROME A. JOHNSON • *Department of Surgery, The Ohio State University Medical Center, Columbus, OH*

STEVEN C. KAMIERCZAK • *Department of Pathology, East Carolina University School of Medicine, Greenville, NC*

JOHN A. LOTT • *Department of Pathology, The Ohio State University, Columbus, OH*

W. SCOTT MELVIN • *Department of Surgery, The Ohio State University Medical Center, Columbus, OH*

PETER MUSCARELLA II • *Department of Surgery, The Ohio State University Medical Center, Columbus, OH*

FREDERICK VAN LENTE • *Department of Clinical Pathology, The Cleveland Clinic Foundation, Cleveland, OH*

1
Transplantation of the Pancreas or Pancreatic Islet Cells
A Clinical Laboratory Perspective

John A. Lott

INTRODUCTION

Loss of the exocrine and endocrine pancreatic functions leaves the patient with serious digestive and metabolic problems. Causes of exocrine loss include cystic fibrosis, atrophic pancreatitis, chronic pancreatitis, infarction of the pancreas, surgical removal of the gland, atherosclerosis of the pancreas, pancreatic cysts, and other miscellaneous causes. More than about 85% of the acinar cells must be lost before abnormalities appear, indicating that the normal pancreas has tremendous exocrine reserves. Abdominal discomfort and abnormalities in digestion, including steatorrhea, weight loss, constipation or diarrhea, and flatulence, are typical findings.

Loss of the endocrine functions of the pancreatic islets is much more serious and common than loss of the exocrine function of the pancreas. Loss of the islet cells leads to profound disturbances of carbohydrate metabolism owing to the loss of insulin, glucagon, somatostatin, and other pancreatic hormone secretions; causes are varied and include autoimmune phenomena, infectious disorders, chronic pancreatitis, tumors, pancreatectomy, and others. The resulting insulin-dependent diabetes mellitus (IDDM) is a disease that afflicts an estimated 300,000–500,000 people in the United States. Although IDDM is observed in adults, approx 75% of cases diagnosed each year are individuals under 20 yr of age *(1)*.

IDDM has a worldwide distribution, although its incidence varies greatly from country to country; Finland and Greece show rates of 35.3 and 4.6/100,000 people/yr, respectively. Differences in diet, hygienic practices, exposure to viruses, and genetics may explain the different rates of development *(2)*. Constantly normal blood glucose concentrations, i.e., euglycemia, are impossible to maintain in patients with diabetes, even with intense glucose monitoring and insulin therapy, and essentially all diabetics develop secondary microaneurysms, retinopathy, nephropathy, neuropathy, and cardiovascular disease. An abnormally increased glycosylated hemoglobin is a common finding in diabetics and is the harbinger of long-term complications. Although mortality and complications of IDDM vary by country *(3)*, a study in Israel showed that overall mortality rates for diabetics are nearly the same as that of the general population for the first 15 yr, but by 20 yr of disease progression, the mortality rates accelerated by a factor of four *(4)*. Clearly, many patients with long-standing diabetes are good candidates for pancreas transplantation, the goal being the correction of glycemia to as close to normal as possible. Pancreas transplantation can prevent the inevitable complications of diabetes; however, existing complications cannot be reversed *(5)*. Transplantation of islet cells remains an experimental procedure. A brief review of the pathogenesis of diabetes follows. Knowledge of the pathogenesis of IDDM leads to a better understanding of the diagnosis and treatment with transplantation.

PATHOGENESIS OF DIABETES MELLITUS

IDDM has an autoimmune etiology in the great majority of cases *(6)*, but the current consensus is that it also includes a genetic and an environmental component. The major histocompatibility complex (MHC) on chromosome 6 is the primary gene associated with susceptibility to IDDM. This region encodes for the MHC class II molecules; human leukocyte antigen (HLA)-DR and HLA-DQ are two of the best studied of these. For example, the phenotypes HLA-DR3 and HLA-DR4 are strongly associated with an increased risk of developing IDDM *(7)*, whereas the phenotypes HLA-DR11 or HLA-DR15 correlate with a decreased risk of IDDM *(8)*. The genetic component is multifactorial. The presence of predisposing phenotypes is not sufficient to predict the development of IDDM; only 36% of identical twins of diabetic patients with the same HLA haplotypes develop IDDM *(9)*. Further, only about 10–15% of patients who develop IDDM have first-degree relatives with IDDM *(10)*.

Pancreatic islet cell destruction appears to follow more than one immune pathway, including destruction by cytolytic T-cells and autoantibody-mediated killing of islet cells *(11)*. In one proposed scenario, viral infection of the islets results in an inflammatory response that induces surface expression of HLA class II molecules on the β-cells, allowing them to present cell-specific antigens to CD4+ T-lymphocytes. Alternatively, soluble β-cell antigens released by islet cells damaged by nonspecific inflammatory reactions may be presented to CD4+ T-cells by professional antigen-presenting cells located within the inflammatory milieu. Either pathway occuring in genetically susceptible individuals who have lost tolerance to the presented self-antigens results in the activation of CD4+ T-lymphocytes with subsequent cytokine synthesis. Also, specific CD8+ cytolytic T-cells are generated that target β-cells through their expression of HLA class I surface molecules containing cell-specific peptides.

B-lymphocyte activation with maturation to plasma cells and production of autoantibodies to insulin, islet cells, or glutamic acid decarboxylase (GAD) may also occur in response to CD4+ T-cell activation. Although these autoantibodies may represent a nonfunctioning epiphenomenon, they bind to β-cells and mediate their killing through interactions with Fc-receptors present on neutrophils, macrophages, natural killer cells, or by complement activation. These antibodies are not found in all diabetics. Hence, they are not commonly used as diagnostic tools, but are currently being examined as possible predictors of diabetes *(12)*.

The presence of islet-cell antibodies in children without IDDM is a harbinger of the disease. Of the three autoantibodies, GAD is the best predictor for the development of IDDM. CD4+ T-cell-mediated immunity to GAD has a positive correlation with the development of IDDM *(13)*.

Environmental agents or certain foods may increase the risk of developing IDDM. Bovine serum albumin (BSA), a protein in cow's milk, has been implicated, because fewer children who are breast-fed develop IDDM compared to those given cow's milk from an early age *(14)*. The presence of antibodies to BSA in many diabetics remains puzzling, but a role for immune crossreaction with a self-antigen via molecular mimicry is theorized *(15)*.

Viruses including coxsackie A, coxsackie B, and ECHO virus have been implicated in inducing islet-cell autoimmunity because of antiviral antibodies detected in IDDM patients or because of coincident seasonal variances that parallel IDDM diagnoses *(16,17)*. Molecular mimicry occurs when a virus sharing an amino acid sequence with β-cell proteins infects a body cell. The antibodies developed against the virus attack the virus-infected cells, but they also crossreact with proteins in β-cells having similar amino acid sequences *(18)*.

Much of the actual destruction of the β-cells appears to be at least partly mediated by free radicals generated by activated lymphocytes *(19)*. The β-cells are particularly susceptible to damage by free radicals owing to the presence of lesser amounts of glutathione peroxidase and mangano-superoxide dismutase compared to other tissues *(20)*.

Although the triggering agent for IDDM remains uncertain, the consensus is that an early childhood exposure to the agent(s) is followed by a variable period of smoldering autoimmune activity during which many β-cells are destroyed. Because the endocrine pancreatic function is sufficient to maintain euglycemia until about 90% of the β-cell mass is destroyed, it is not until then that the classic signs of diabetes occur, i.e., hyperglycemia and (or) ketoacidosis *(21)*. Once these findings appear, the patient usually becomes insulin-dependent, with the exception of a possible honeymoon period. The diabetic honeymoon is a remission of variable length often occurring after the initial injection of insulin in newly diagnosed patients during which no insulin or a reduced amount of insulin is required for apparently normal glucose regulation *(22)*. The honeymoon invariably ends, followed by lifelong insulin dependency.

PANCREAS TRANSPLANTATION

Organ transplantation for the treatment of end-stage failure of the liver, kidneys, and pancreas is now well established. Pancreas transplantation has as its major goal the replacement of lost islet cell function in patients with diabetes and restoring euglycemia. Pancreas transplantation is commonly performed following kidney transplantation, or is done at the same time in patients with diabetes and diabetic renal disease. Unlike kidney transplantation, pancreas transplantation has not been standardized, and current alternative surgical techniques are described here briefly. Worldwide from the beginning of transplantation surgery up to approximately 1990, 3000 pancreas transplants have been performed. Many aspects of organ transplantation have been the subjects of reviews *(23–26)*. Reviews on other complications such as malignancy and the toxicity of immunosuppressive agents are available *(27–30)*. An extensive review exists of the organ distributions of cyclosporin A (CSA) and its metabolites *(31)*. Recent reviews are available on the evolution of pancreas and islet-cell transplantation at one large institution *(32)*, on islet transplantation *(33–35)*, on the artificial pancreas (trapped islet cells) in dogs *(36)*, on the isolation and purification of pancreatic islets

(30), and on alternate surgical techniques for pancreas transplantation *(37)*. With few exceptions, the discussion here is restricted to studies in humans.

The leading impediment of transplantation therapy is the shortage of suitable organs. Many patients die while awaiting a possibly live-saving organ transplantation. For kidneys in the United States in 1993, there were about 25,000 patients on the waiting list *(38)*. Roughly one-third of these had end-stage kidney disease as a complication of diabetes *(30)*. Unfortunately, only about 50% of families give consent for organ donation by their kin.

The major medical problems of patients having organ transplantation are acute and chronic rejection, and infections with bacterial, fungal, and viral agents, especially with cytomegalovirus (CMV). Other significant complications are leakages at anastomoses, thromboses, inflammation (e.g., pancreatitis), bleeding problems, and various malignancies, especially lymphoproliferative diseases. The dual goals of pancreas transplantation are to provide insulin independence and to halt the progression of diabetic complications affecting the kidneys, retinas, cardiovascular, and nervous systems.

Currently employed antirejection drugs are discussed. For some of these, the clinical laboratory plays a critical role because of the need to assay the blood concentrations of the parent drug and its active metabolites to assure adequate dosing, but to minimize overdosing and the attendant undesirable side effects. A new drug, tacrolimus (FK506), will likely also play an increasing role in delaying transplant rejection. Except for transplants between identical twins, and with very rare other exceptions, all patients receiving organ transplantation must take antirejection drugs for the rest of their lives.

This chapter considers the laboratory problems common to all transplantation, e.g., histocompatibility testing between donor and recipient, and then discusses laboratory issues that are pertinent for the support of patients having pancreas transplantation. Rejection, especially chronic rejection, is a common problem with transplantation, and tissue biopsy remains the "gold standard" for diagnosing rejection of solid-organ transplants.

Antirejection Drugs

Increasing success in the transplantation of solid organs is attributable in large part to the emergence of better immunosuppressive drugs; these include azathioprine, brequinar sodium, CSA, cyclosporin G, deoxyspergualine, rapamycin, glucocorticoids (e.g., prednisone), leflunomide, mizoribine (bredinin), mofetil (RS-61443), mycophenolic acid, and tacrolimus (FK506) *(39)*. Tacrolimus and rampamycin inhibit the phosphatase calcineurin and thereby inhibit transcriptional activation of the interleukin-2 gene. These drugs also inhibit the protein kinases that are important signaling mediators in CD4+ T-cell activation *(40)*. CSA is widely used, and tacrolimus is a new drug. Tacrolimus was discovered in 1984 in a fungus; it is a potent and selective anti-T-lymphocyte agent with actions similar to that of CSA. Unlike CSA, it has a hepatotrophic effect leading to active growth of normal liver tissue; this likely accounts for its success in liver allografts. Both are precursors of agents that become active only when bound to specific membranes of the cyclophilin or tacrolimus binding protein receptor complex; both are extremely potent inhibitors of T-lymphocyte activation *(41)*.

The primary action of rapamycin and leflunomide appears to be inhibition of the effects of cytokines and growth factors on B-, T-, and some nonimmune cells. B- and T-cells are more sensitive than somatic cells to the reduced concentration of purines and pyrimidines as caused by mizoribine, mycophenolic acid, and bequinar sodium. Note that nucleotide depletion causes a break in the synthesis of DNA and the glycosylation of adhesion molecules in the immune cells *(42)*.

Cell Chimerism

Evidence is accumulating that old and new immunosuppressive drugs permit the establishment of donor-derived multilineage cell chimerism following transplantation, i.e., the transplanted cells and the host cells exist compatibly without a rejection reaction. This phenomenon explains the rare patients who can wean themselves off all antirejection drugs without a rejection phenomenon. Fontes et al. *(43)* reported that in liver, kidney, and heart transplantation, tolerance to donor cells could be induced in 17 of 36 patients by the infusion of donor bone marrow, followed by conventional immunosuppression with tacrolimus and prednisone. This promising approach may improve survival of solid-organ transplants, including pancreas.

CLINICAL LABORATORY SUPPORT OF TRANSPLANTATION PROGRAMS

Transplant recipients need postoperative laboratory support to manage acute-care problems, such as fluid and electrolyte disturbances, acid-base abnormalities, bleeding and coagulation issues, and to test for organ function, infections, and rejection. Testing for infections caused by viral, fungal, and bacterial agents and for possible transplant rejection is a vital part of posttransplantation care; the two conditions have a similar clinical presentation: malaise, fever, and so forth The proper diagnosis of rejection or infection is a critical distinction for treatment. If rejection is suspected, then the regimen of antirejection drugs is usually stepped up, and new agents may be added. If, in fact, the patient has an infection rather than rejection, the increased antirejection therapy may exacerbate the infection and lead to graft and patient loss. The reverse case also applies: if infection is diagnosed, but the case is really rejection, reducing the antirejection drugs to fight the infection may also lead to graft loss.

Testing for CSA and Tacrolimus

Monitoring of serum concentrations of antirejection drugs, such as CSA and tacrolimus, is carried out to assure adequate serum concentrations and to avoid overdosing. Like CSA, tacrolimus is nephrotoxic, and careful blood concentration monitoring is necessary during its use *(44)*. The clinical response for both drugs does not correlate well with the administered dose; the concentrations in blood must be known to optimize treatment. Also, the range of drug concentrations is narrow to give adequate immunosuppression, yet minimize nephrotoxicity. The review on the monitoring of CSA and specific recommendations for the assay of the drug in whole blood by Shaw et al. is recommended *(45)*. Assays for CSA include monoclonal immunoassays *(46)*, radioimmunoassays, and high-pressure liquid chromatography. Fluorescence polarization immunoassay is the most widely used procedure for both CSA and tacrolimus.

HLA Compatibility Testing

The MHC, commonly called the HLA complex, is coded by the nucleotides on chromosome six. There are three classes of HLA antigens; when present, they occur on cell membranes: class I or HLA-A, HLA-B, and HLA-C; class II or HLA-DP, HLA-DQ, and HLA-DR; and class III, which contains proteins including those of the classic and alternate complement pathways, 21-hydroxylase, and tumor necrosis factor. The β-2 microglobulin gene is part of the class I-HLA complex on chromosome 15 *(47)*. HLA-class I antigens are expressed on all nucleated cells and platelets. The HLA-DR, HLA-DQ, and HLA-DP (class II) antigens are expressed on B-lymphocytes, monocyte macrophages, and dendritic cells *(48)*. Prior to assay, a concentration or isolation step of the B-cells is usually performed by using a nylon-wool column to retain the B-cells (class II MHC) and elute the T-cells (class I MHC); the B-cells are then brought out with another eluent to permit separate testing for class I and II antigens.

In typing for HLA compatibility, lymphocytes from the donor, serum from the recipient, and rabbit complement are used. Microlymphocytotoxicity is determined with and without complement by a technique described elsewhere *(49)*. With an HLA mismatch, lysis of the lymphocytes occurs. By staining the lymphocytes with vital dyes, the proportion of dead cells can be estimated by light microscopy. A positive mismatch is revealed by a large fraction of dead cells. The HLA crossmatch test can be made more sensitive by adding antihuman globulin to the incubation mixture. If the test is positive with antihuman globulin present, the likelihood of graft rejection is about 5% greater than if the test is negative. The evolving "gold standard" is molecular typing of the nucleotide sequences coding for the HLA class I and II antigens. With appropriate multiple primers and the polymerase chain reaction (PCR), the degree of compatibility of the host and graft can be determined.

Flow Cytometry

Flow cytometry makes possible the measurement of low concentrations of both complement-fixing and noncomplement-fixing antibodies. This technique is more sensitive than the standard lymphocyte cytotoxicity test in predicting graft rejection *(50–54)*.

Using flow cytometry, it is possible to identify, characterize, and separate cell populations based on the cell-membrane antigens. A tagged antibody, commonly a fluorescent tag, is bound to the cell antigen(s); only those cells having the specific cell-surface antigen will fluoresce. The cells are diluted, suspended, and passed through a fluorometer one at a time, and each fluorescing cell gives a signal or count, thereby giving an estimate of the proportion of the cells that carry the antigen in question. Modern flow cytometers can also sort cells based on the surface labels and allow the simultaneous detection of several fluorescent signals, each attached to a different cell-surface antigen.

Ogura et al. *(55)* showed that flow cytometry was clearly superior to a standard T-cell cytotoxicity test. Of 84 patients, 10 had a positive T-cell crossmatch and 20 of the 84 had a positive flow cytometry test. At 1 mo posttransplantation, 3 of 10 patients with a positive T-cell test lost their graft, whereas 17 of 74 with a negative

T-cell test had lost their graft, suggesting that the T-cell test gave some false-negative results. In an earlier report by the same group, they found that patients with a negative flow test had a 1-yr graft survival rate of 82 vs a 75% rate for those with a positive (abnormal) flow test. The patients with a positive lymphocyte cytotoxicity test also had a lower graft survival rate. It appears that patients with a negative flow test do better, and given the scarcity of suitable organs, preference should be given to patients with a negative flow test *(56)*. Others also reported that flow is superior to the cytotoxicity assay, and that flow cytometry alone is enough to make a go, no-go transplantation decision in about 80% of patients *(57)*.

The development of antibodies to the donor's T- and B-lymphocytes can be determined with a sensitive flow cytometric assay. These antibodies are harbingers of clinical kidney failure *(58)*, and most likely rejection of the graft as well. Of four patients with anti-B cell antibodies specific against the class II HLA antigens HLA-DR or HLA-DQ, three showed hyperacute rejection, and acute rejection was present in one *(59)*. Thus, a test for antibodies against donor B-cell class II HLA antigens should be part of a crossmatch test. Of considerable importance in the use of flow cytometry is the 97% sensitivity and 88% specificity in discriminating between patients with late (>2 yr) acute allograft rejection, and other causes of graft dysfunction, such as infection, immunosuppressant drug toxicity, arteriopathy, or chronic rejection. Flow analysis also has the advantage of predicting successful antirejection therapy within a few days, whereas the conventional T-cell test requires 1–3 wk *(60)*. Others also found that flow was more specific than the standard cytotoxicity techniques *(53)*, or was too sensitive and gave false-positive results *(61,62)*. Mahoney et al. *(54)* found that flow cytometric crossmatching was a better predictor of an allograft loss at <2 mo after surgery in patients receiving a first and especially for those receiving a second cadaveric organ who had a negative crossmatch by the standard complement-fixation cytotoxicity test. The general consensus is that flow analysis is more sensitive than the lymphocytotoxicity test, and that patients with a negative flow crossmatch do better and have a longer graft survival *(63)*. Most of these studies dealt with kidney transplantation; similar studies on pancreas transplantation would likely have the same outcome.

DNA Testing

Molecular techniques to compare the genotype of the donor and recipient are now being applied. Excellent reviews on molecular methods are by Eisenstein *(64)* and Housman *(65)*. Opelz et al. found that the graft survival rate was 87% when the recipient and donor were HLA-DR identical by both the cytotoxicity and DNA tests; graft survival decreased to 69% when the HLA-DR cytotoxicity test was negative, but the molecular test showed DNA inequalities between the donor and host *(66)*.

The HLA genes are highly polymorphic, and there are dozens of recognized HLA specificities. With the exception of identical twins, the likelihood of finding two immunogenetically identical individuals is essentially zero. The presence of donor-specific class I HLA antibodies in the recipient's serum effectively prohibits the use of an organ from that donor; 80–90% of those having such a positive test will have an acute or hyperacute transplant rejection *(67)*. Graft survival is inversely related to how many HLA mismatches are present. The current policy in many centers is that transplantation recipients must be phenotypically identical with the donor for the HLA-A, HLA-B, and HLA-DR antigens *(68)*.

The rejection phenomenon begins when the recipient's CD8+ T-lymphocyte precursors recognize HLA proteins that are expressed on the surface of the class I MHC antigen-presenting cells, i.e., on the graft; T-cell activation follows after recognition of donor antigens complexed with class I MHC. The recipient's activated cytotoxic CD8+ T-lymphocytes will then attack the cells of the transplanted organ. Rejection can be largely blunted with immunosuppressive drugs that inhibit cytotoxic T-cells; however, rejection is inevitable, and the greater the mismatch, the shorter the life of the transplanted organ. Late rejection may be caused by chronic obstructive endarteritis owing to complement-fixing antibodies. Investigators have found donor antigen-specific cytotoxic T-lymphocytes and antibodies to the donor HLA antigens during or just before an episode of clinically demonstrable rejection. HLA mismatch is the major cause of transplant rejection *(69)*. The mechanism of the antiallograft response of the host is described in detail elsewhere *(48)*.

Testing for CMV Infections

The most common and most serious posttransplantation infection is by CMV; it threatens the survival of both the graft and the patient. The general consensus is that a CMV infection alone does not lead to graft rejection. CMV infects the endothelium, the interface between the transplanted tissue and the recipient's immune system. Although expression of HLA class II antigens on endothelial cells is a hallmark of vascular rejection, CMV does not directly induce these antigens on infected endothelial cells; in fact, CMV renders endothelial cells refractory to HLA-DR induction by certain agents *(70)*. Sherlock et al. *(71)* made similar observations, and found active CMV infection in 11 of 18 patients who rejected their grafts and also in 13 of 18 patients who did not reject. Furthermore, an active CMV infection was found in 8 of 15 patients who developed antibodies to donor lymphocytes and also in 12 of 17 who did not develop such antibodies. In these patients, there was no statistically significant association between CMV infection and rejection, or between CMV infection and the development of antibodies to the donor's lymphocytes.

The most serious CMV infections are temporally associated with the most intense immunosuppression therapy that typically occurs within the first several months following transplantation. CMV infections present as a spectrum of disorders ranging from minimal disease, such as malaise, and fever to severe forms that include pancreatitis, hepatitis, gastrointestinal bleeding, multisystem organ failure, and death *(72)*. Our current knowledge of CMV has a number of unresolved issues. Many normal individuals harbor the CMV virus; it remains latent, and why transplantation and (or) antirejection drugs activate the virus is unknown. There is an important clinical difference between a serologically positive CMV test and overt CMV disease, and current laboratory testing technology cannot distinguish between the two. Also, better antiviral drugs are needed to treat a fulminant CMV infection, although gancyclovir is generally effective *(26)*.

It is not possible to diagnose a CMV infection based solely on clinical findings, because the signs and symptoms of organ rejection and CMV infection are similar.

Currently, the laboratory diagnosis of CMV relies primarily on the culture of the virus on fibroblasts by a shell vial procedure; the results are generally available in 24–48 h *(73)*. Other less widely used methods are the PCR to identify the presence of nucleotide sequences of the CMV genome in serum; the disadvantages of PCR are cost, complexity, long turnaround times, and difficulty in some cases of interpreting the results. The PCR test is nearly always positive if leukocytes are present, which does not necessarily mean that the patient is going to develop active CMV disease.

Serological tests for CMV-specific IgM or IgG antibodies have the disadvantages that the antibodies take at least 1–2 wk to appear after infection, and no antibody formation at all may occur in immunosuppressed patients. *In situ* hybridization with primers to CMV nucleotide sequences has been used to identify CMV infection in tissue biopsies *(74)*. Another test is the CMV-specific lymphocyte proliferation test *(75)*. The currently used standard test for CMV in tissue biopsies is an overlay with peroxidase-labeled antibodies to CMV that generates a chromophore followed by light or fluorescence microscopy.

Ideally, the test for CMV should be sensitive, specific, and available on a short turnaround time basis. Marsano et al. *(76)* compared the culture of the virus by a shell vial procedure to testing for IgM antibodies to CMV. Of 35 patients with active CMV infections, 31 showed positive viral cultures and 29 had detectable IgM antibodies to CMV. They claimed that after solid-organ transplantation, the determination of CMV with the viral culture technique can give a result earlier and with better accuracy. Others *(77)* described a rapid immunocytochemical test for CMV that is based on the reaction of CMV antigens in peripheral polymorphonuclear cells with a mixture of monoclonal antibodies (MAbs). The monoclonals react with the CMV immediate early antigen present on the leukocytes, and the results are available within 4 h. The test has excellent sensitivity, but almost no specificity for CMV disease, revealing one of the difficulties with CMV testing, i.e., patients may have viremia without obvious clinical infection. However, even asymptomatic patients with a strongly positive test for CMV may be candidates for CMV prophylaxis with an antiviral agent.

USE OF ORGANS FROM PATIENTS WITH HEPATITIS B (HBV) OR C (HCV)

HCV appears to be as important as HBV as a cause of chronic liver disease and hepatocellular cancer, especially in Japan, but most patients with chronic HCV have only mild symptoms, such as fatigue *(78)*. The transplantation of organs from donors having HBV to a recipient without the disease is clearly contraindicated; all patients become infected with HBV posttransplantation. Here, chronic active hepatitis is likely, and the chance of survival is reduced *(79,80)*. HCV-positive organs may be used in special circumstances. Most cases with "non-A non-B" hepatitis have HCV, and reasonably reliable tests now exist for HCV; the best test is PCR for part of the viral genome. An HCV infection of parenteral origin becomes chronic in 50–60% of patients, and cirrhosis develops in about 20% of these.

The first-generation enzyme-linked immunosorbent assay (ELISA) test for HCV detects antibodies to a recombinant HCV antigen (c100) from the nonstructural region of HCV *(81)*. We now know that this test has poor sensitivity. In the older literature, an HCV infection developing in a c100-negative patient has been attributed to unknown or sporadic causes of HCV *(82)*. A more likely explanation is that the test was falsely negative. The second-generation ELISA test detects antibody to recombinant HCV antigens from the c100, c200, and c20 sections of the nonstructural and core regions of the virus. A second-generation recombinant immunoblot assay (RIBA) detects antibody to four recombinant HCV antigens: 5-1-1, c100, c33, and c22, all from the nonstructural and core regions of HCV *(83)*. The detection of HCV RNA by PCR is currently the final arbiter for the presence of HCV antigens *(84)*. The details of the PCR assay are described elsewhere *(81)*. The PCR test is costly and time-consuming, and the diagnosis of HCV can be made in most patients with a positive RIBA test together with positive liver function tests and abnormal tissue pathology *(83)*.

Given the extreme shortage of transplantable organs, is it acceptable to perform transplants of an HCV-positive organ into an HCV-positive or HCV-negative recipient? For liver transplants, Shah et al. *(80)* concluded that the procedure is acceptable, and that there is "no increased risk for the development of HCV . . ." Obviously, patients should be told of this risk owing to the about 17% incidence of chronic liver disease associated with the transplantation of an HCV-seropositive kidney *(85)*. A similar situation likely applies to an HCV-seropositive pancreas, although the experience with pancreas transplantation is less than that with kidney.

There appears to be a trend toward a national organ procurement protocol much like that of the New England Organ Bank *(86)*. The evidence is clear that HCV can be transmitted by organ transplantation, sometimes with disastrous results *(87)*. Owing to the unacceptably high prevalence of liver disease in recipients of HCV-positive organs, such organs are used only for life-saving transplantation, i.e., heart, heart-lung, or liver, and they should not be used in kidney or pancreas transplants into HCV-negative recipients. Wherever possible, testing for HCV should be by PCR for the viral RNA owing to the superior sensitivity of PCR compared to the serological tests.

SURGICAL TECHNIQUES IN WHOLE-ORGAN PANCREAS TRANSPLANTATION

The surgical technique in widest use for whole-organ pancreas transplantation for replacement of the endocrine pancreatic function is pancreaticoduodenocystostomy, whereby the pancreatic exocrine duct is led into the urinary bladder via a small section of donor duodenum *(88)*. This eliminates exocrine function, but the endocrine functions are conserved. Earlier surgical techniques of performing pancreatic allografts included occluding the pancreatic duct with, e.g., latex, to cause atrophy of the acinar pancreas and thereby stop the exocrine secretions. This sought to avoid the problems of ducting the pancreatic juice to the small or large intestine, and the accompanying frequent bouts of pancreatitis owing to intestinal contents reaching the transplanted pancreas. These approaches have been replaced in most centers by urinary bladder drainage of pancreatic fluid owing to the better graft survival and a reduced incidence of acute pancreatitis *(89)*. Nevertheless, the routing of the exocrine flow or the obliteration of the exocrine pancreas is still under debate in the literature *(88,90)*. Some patients with urinary bladder drainage develop bladder irritation or cystitis. Pancreatic juice contains proteolytic enzymes that may or may not be catalytically active. Generally, the pancreatic fluids are led to the urinary bladder with a short section of duodenum; contact with a portion of duodenum probably leads to proteolytic

Table 1
Pros and Cons of Surgical Techniques Used to Divert Exocrine Secretions
in Pancreas Transplantation[a]

Technique	Pros	Cons	Detection of rejection with
Pancreatic duct occlusion by, e.g., injecting latex	Easy to perform	Pancreatitis in some, pancreatic fibrosis and (or) atrophy, loss of endocrine function	Glycemia, biopsy
Drainage into small intestine	Conservation of bicarbonate	Risk of enteric leak, pancreatitis, and infection of pancreas, peritonitis	Glycemia, biopsy
Drainage into urinary bladder	Reduced risk of pancreatic infection, pancreatitis	Irritation of bladder, cystitis, loss of bicarbonate, metabolic acidosis	Urinary amylase, glycemia, biopsy

[a]Adapted from ref. 37.

enzyme activation in some patients. Individuals who develop cystitis and related complications in the urinary bladder are generally converted to enteric drainage with good results (32).

Secchi et al. (91) occluded the pancreatic duct with neoprene in one patient to produce atrophy of the acinar pancreas and then transplanted a segment of the pancreas. They also transplanted the whole, unmodified pancreas into eight patients with ileal drainage of the pancreatic juice. Both techniques gave satisfactory results, although the patients receiving the entire gland had a better glucose tolerance.

Different surgical techniques have been used for the venous drainage of blood from the pancreas. Pancreas transplantation with systemic pancreatic venous or portal drainage of the pancreatic vein has been performed. The patients with systemic drainage showed higher insulin concentrations in blood, the consequences of which are unclear (92). Another group made similar observations: Pancreas transplantation with portal or systemic venous drainage showed higher insulin concentrations than did normals; the cause was ascribed to a possible side effect of the immunosuppression drugs (93). A summary of the pros and cons of pancreatic duct occlusion, enteric drainage, or urinary drainage is given in Table 1.

TESTS FOR REJECTION OF TRANSPLANTED PANCREAS

Pancreas transplant patients require close biochemical monitoring for possible transplant failures and for the metabolic disturbances owing to the profound loss of HCO_3^- in patients with urinary bladder drains of the exocrine secretions. If the patient's own kidney or renal allograft is functioning well, then the renal synthesis of HCO_3^- can usually keep up with the urinary loss. If the serum creatinine rises, the patient is then usually in a negative HCO_3^- balance and must receive about 25 g/d of HCO_3^- parenterally if the HCO_3^- falls below 16 mmol/L or about 3 g/d by mouth if the HCO_3^- is between 17 and 21 mmol/L. With renal dysfunction, hyperchloremic acidosis can be severe with Cl^- values of >110 mmol/L and HCO_3^- concentrations of <12 mmol/L (94).

The urine amylase test is useful in monitoring pancreas graft function. With a successful transplant, the urinary amylase rises steadily during the first 14–21 d to about 2000–6000 U/h *(95)* and then plateaus; testing should be on a daily basis on 24-h urine collections *(96–98)*. A postoperative delay or failure of the urinary amylase to increase, a marked drop in the urinary amylase value, hyperglycemic episodes, or increases in the serum amylase and lipase usually mean transplant dysfunction and possibly pancreatitis. Increases in serum amylase and (or) lipase are common in kidney and kidney-plus-pancreas transplant recipients; it does not necessarily mean that pancreatitis is present, but may reflect the general state of the patient and the likelihood of organ rejection *(99)*. Normally, amylase is excreted in urine, and lipase is catabolized by the renal tubules. The amylase content of urine depends on the patient's hydration, urinary dilution, and nutritional state. Small up or down changes in the urine amylase are meaningless, but long-term or persistent decreases signal rejection.

Glucose tolerance testing is helpful in estimating pancreatic endocrine function and can also signal rejection; however, reduction or loss of glycemic control generally occurs late in a rejection episode. Most patients with successful pancreas transplants and antirejection therapy nevertheless show slow and unrelenting declines in the urinary amylase excretion. With the improved surgical techniques and intensive clinical and biochemical monitoring, pancreas graft survival is approaching that of renal grafts. Once hyperglycemia returns, the loss of the pancreatic graft is generally complete. In our experience, the islets are more resistant to rejection than the acinar pancreas or kidney; in the usual picture of rejection of patients receiving both kidney and pancreas transplantation, the serum creatinine increases before glycemic control is lost. A summary of certain outcomes following pancreas kidney transplantation is given in Table 2 *(100–109)* (*see* pp. 14–15). Biochemical tests for diagnosing rejection of the transplanted pancreas are given in Table 3 *(110–121)* (*see* p. 16*)*.

TRANSPLANTATION OF PANCREATIC ISLETS

Pancreatic islet transplantation is still largely an experimental technique. The many issues in the procedure include isolation and purification of the islets, alternate routes of implantation, antirejection techniques, and possible immunomodulation of the islets. The current state of the art is summarized in Table 4 *(36,122–124)* (*see* p. 17). The measure of success is always the achievement of euglycemia and insulin independence. To date, very few patients have benefited from islet transplantation compared to whole-pancreas transplantation.

Islet-cell transplantation is certainly simpler to do than pancreas transplantation. There are no anastomoses, human islets are reasonably stable during cryopreservation, and there are no exocrine secretions to deal with. A multiauthored monograph on pancreatic islet transplantation appeared in 1992 *(125)*; most of the reports deal with islet-cell transplantation in animals.

Isolation of Islets

Peakman et al. *(126)* described a typical procedure for isolation of human islets. Their digesting medium contained collagenase, trypsin, DNase, ethylene diamine tetra-acetate (EDTA), and hyaluronidase for the isolation of islets from a pancreas obtained from a beating-heart donor. The use of ethylene glycol-bis(beta aminoethyl-ether) tetra-acetate (EGTA) gave a higher yield of monodispersed islet cells, but lower viability than did EDTA. The isolated cells showed an insulin secretory response to glucose and had surface class I MHC molecules immediately after digestion.

The degree of purification affects the yield of viable islets; the greater the purity, the lower the yield. Zeng et al. *(127)* confirmed this relationship using cadaveric pancreases. They named five factors that affect the yield, purity, and overall success of islet isolation: organ cold ischemia time, age of the donor, the donor's antemortem blood glucose, body weight, and cause of death. Islets from older (>55 yr) patients with hyperglycemia had impaired function in vitro and in vivo. Obese patients gave a lower yield of islets and a lower purity. A shorter (<8 h) cold ischemia time was associated with a better yield and purity of the islets. Other recommendations on islet-cell isolation were made by Robertson et al. *(128)*, who reported that cell swelling should be kept to a minimum during islet purification and a colloid should be present in the extracting medium owing to its protective affect on the islets.

Gores and Sutherland *(129)*, in their review, suggested that less-pure islet-cell preparations are satisfactory for allografts provided adequate immunosuppression is used. They cautioned, however, that lymphocyte contamination of the islets increases the immuongenicity of the allograft. Flushing of the pancreas prior to transplantation is recommended. The concept of "passenger lymphocytes" as initiators of an immune rejection response to grafts comes largely from studies in islet cell transplantation.

Route of Implantation

Several implant routes have been used: intraperitoneally, intramuscularly, under the kidney capsule, and intraportally *(30)*. Not surprisingly, rapid harvesting and infusion of islets is best, and all preservation techniques including cold storage, freezing, and culturing of cells result in a loss of islets. The more viable islets a patient receives, the greater the likelihood is of the patient becoming insulin-independent. Heparin is usually given to prevent coagulation disorders. With portal vein islet infusion, the cells populate the sinusoids of the liver. Some patients had transient increases in the transaminases probably indicating mild, reversible liver injury, and other patients had complications following intraportal islet autotransplantation *(130)*.

Antirejection Therapy After Islet Transplantation

In the absence of rejection, viable islet cells, if sufficient in number, can provide long-term insulin independence. Autografts do not require antirejection drugs. The problem here is often getting enough viable islets from a diseased and fibrotic pancreas. Prednisone, which is widely used as an antirejection agent, opposes the action of insulin and is a known cause of islet allograft failure *(131)*. Also, the use of CSA is limited because of its renal toxicity. The typical antirejection menu includes antilymphocyte globulin, CSA, azathioprine, and prednisone. Also commonly given is 15-deoxyspergualin, because it acts as an inhibitor of macrophage function, thus protecting the islets against early damage. Cigaret smoking and (or) alcohol abuse are detrimental to islet grafts *(132)*.

Table 2
Effects of Pancreas Transplants on Patients with Insulin-Dependent Diabetes (Type I)

Patient group(s)/procedure(s)	Pretransplant findings	Posttransplant findings	Conclusions	Ref.
Three patients, P and K Tx[a]	Defective glucose counterregulation and severe episodes of hypoglycemia, delayed or absent response to glucagon, growth hormone, epinephrine	Normalization or improvement in response to glucagon, growth hormone, epinephrine; normal glucose response after insulin infusion	P and K Tx corrects glucose counter-regulation defect	100
Nine patients, P and K Tx; 10 control patients with K TX only	Autonomic nephropathy judged from cardiovascular function tests	No improvement in findings in either Tx group	Change is irreversible owing to structural autonomic nerve damage	101
One hundred seventy-one patients, P and K Tx in 157, 129 segmental P Tx with neoprene occlusion, 14 duodenal drain, 25 bladder drain. P Tx only in 24	Typical picture of type I DM; abnormal OGTT, abnormal HbA1c, episodes of hyperglycemia and glycosuria	"Near-normal" glucose and "good" insulin release in most, 31 patients had abnormal OGTT at 1 yr, all were off insulin, had normal HbA1c	Whole-pancreas transplant gave better glucose control than injected segmental pancreas transplant	102
Thirty-seven patients P and K Tx, 12 segmental P grafts with duct occlusion, 25 bladder drainage	Typical picture of type I DM; abnormal lipid profiles	All had normal cholesterol, triglycerides, HbA1c, fat tolerance; C peptide increased in all	In patients with euglycemia, segmental and whole-pancreas transplant had same effect in correcting lipid abnormalities	103
Five patients with P after K Tx; 6 simultaneous P and K Tx, all with bladder drain	Typical picture of type I DM	Normalization of HbA1c; euglycemia in 6 patients and urine amylase >40,000 U/L	At 28 mo after surgery, 6 patients free of insulin need	104

Pancreas and Pancreatic Islet Transplantation

Patients	Clinical picture	Results	Ref.
Thirty-six patients; all P and K Tx with segmental graft and duct occlusion, systemic release of insulin	Typical picture of type I DM	100% normal glycemia, 54% normal IVGTT, 89% normal C-peptide, 54% normal HbA1c	105
Sixty-one patients, P Tx; 48 controls, no Tx	Neuropathy and typical picture to type I DM	Slight improvement in neuropathy in patients getting transplants with improvement in motor and sensory indexes; worsening in control group	Duct-occluded segmental pancreas transplant produced euglycemia, no exogenous insulin needed for up to 5 yr	106
Eight patients with P and K Tx, 4 lost graft, 4 grafts functional	Diabetic retinopathy with loss of visual acuity, macular edema, other eye pathologies	Functional grafts produced euglycemia, but no halting in progression of diabetic retinopathy	107
Eight patient with K and segmental P Tx	Typical picture of IDDM	Found reduced insulin sensitivity of recipients and impaired islet responsiveness	108
Eighteen patients P and K Tx; 18 with K Tx only as controls	Polyneuropathy with impaired nerve conduction	Euglycemia, normal HbA1c in all receiving K and P Tx, normalization of creatinine in both groups	109

Additional notes (column reorganized):
- Row 105: With successful P Tx, produce euglycemia and may halt progression of diabetic neuropathy
- Row 107: Patients with severe microangiopathy did not get improved vision following P Tx
- Row 108: The islet-cell function was not normal despite normal fasting glucose and HbA1c, had islet-cell hyperactivity owing to insulin resistance
- Row 109: Long-term improvement in nerve conduction in P and K Tx group, but not in K Tx only group; slight improvement of autonomic function in both groups

[a]Abbreviations: DM, diabetes mellitus; HbA1c, hemoglobin A1c; IVGTT, intravenous glucose tolerance test; K Tx, kidney transplant; OGTT, oral glucose tolerance test; P Tx, pancreas transplant; P and K Tx, simultaneous pancreas and kidney transplantation.

Table 3
Biochemical Tests for Rejection of Transplanted Pancreas

Test	Comment	Reference
Amylase (u),[a] ^{99m}Tc DTPA, glucose (s)	Both amylase and ^{99m}Tc DTPA decreased in rejection; latter is measure of pancreatic perfusion, if glucose > 180 mg/dL, suggests graft loss	110
Amylase (u)	Not a reliable marker of rejection	111
Amylase (u), anodal trypsinogen (s), creatinine (s)	Anodal trypsinogen more sensitive and specific than amylase; creatinine as good as trypsinogen for renal transplant rejection	112
Amylase (u)	A low-urine amylase was not always an indicator of poor endocrine function	113
Amylase (u), anodal trypsinogen (s)	Anodal trypsinogen is a graft-specific marker of rejection; amylase an insensitive test	114
Amylase (u), lipase (u), sIL-2R	Limited as biochemical markers; only decreases are meaningful; sIL-2R not useful	118
Amylase (u), glucose (s)	Amylase poor test; if glucose is increased, graft rejection nearly complete	117
Anionic trypsin (s), cationic trypsin (s), amylase (s), neopterin (s)	Neopterin and anionic trypsin look promising as tests for rejection whereas others did not	115
Anodal trypsinogen (s), creatinine (s), amylase (u)	Simultaneous K and P transplants; anodal trypsinogen increases because most of pancreas is acinar	119
C-peptide (s), insulin (s), neopterin (u)	Neopterin reliable marker of rejection; C-peptide and insulin of little value	99
Neopterin (u), neopterin in pancreatic juice	Neopterin increased in 19 of 24 patients with rejection and in 9 of 16 with infection; pancreatic juice neopterin increased in rejection, but was normal in infection, sensitive, but nonspecific test	116
Pancreatic trypsin inhibitor	Test for pancreas rejection; high percentage of false (+) tests	120
Pancreatic specific protein	Insufficient sensitivity for pancreas rejection	121

[a]Abbreviations: DTPA, diethylenetriamine penta-acetic acid; (s), serum; (u), urine. *See* footnote to Table 2 for other abbreviations.

Immunoisolated Islet-Cell Transplantation

Much work has been performed on the transplantation of immune-protected islet cells; the allogenic or xenogeneic cells are isolated behind a permeable barrier that allows low-mol-wt substances through, such as glucose, other nutrients, and insulin, but blocks immunoglobulins and of course leukocytes *(36,121)*. The devices are not immunogenic or thrombotic, and antirejection drugs are not needed. Three configurations of isolated islet have been described recently: microcapsules, diffusion chambers, and a device termed the "artificial pancreas," which relies on blood flow through it; the cells are isolated from the blood by a membrane barrier *(133)* (*see* Fig. 1 *[36]*). Most of the studies have been in animals, but a few reports of human trials are beginning to appear.

Table 4
Summary of Islet Cell Transplantation

Source of islets	Human	Porcine	Human	Canine allogenic and (porcine) xenogeneic
No. of patients	6	10	1	0 (dogs)
Implantation technique	Intraportal	Intraportal or under renal capsule	Portal vein	Injected intraperitoneally and surgically placed
Encapsulation of islets	No	No	No	Yes, microcapsules, diffusion devices, perfusion device
Immunosuppression therapy	Yes	Yes	Antilymphocyte globulin, cyclosporin A	No
Immunomodulation therapy	No	No	No	No
Period of insulin independence	15 d to 12 mo	Four patients produced "small amounts of C-peptide in urine"	None, but better control of glycemia in first 22 d; hyperglycemia after 25 d	about 100 d
Islet purification	NS	Yes	"95%" pure	Yes
Islet preservation	No	NS	NS	NS
Comments	Islets given with or after kidney transplant	All patient showed xenoantibody response	Islets from 1.4 cadaverics pancrease	Novel encapsulation techniques
Refs.	*124*	*123*	*122*	*36*

NS: Not stated

Microcapsules contain single or groups of islets with a permeable gel membrane; the typical placement is in the peritoneal cavity. Xenogeneic islets can be used; however, inflammation, membrane breakdown, and a steady loss of islet function remain as challenges. Soon-Shiong et al. *(134)* injected 10,000 encapsulated islets/kg into the peritoneal cavity of a patient and reduced the insulin need by 65%. A second injection of 5000 encapsulated islets eliminated the need for insulin. The authors did not report the functional life of the islets. Diffusion chambers use the same principle, but more islet cells are trapped inside a permeable membrane or permeable tube with closed ends. The need for insulin was abolished in three pancreatectomized dogs for 46–86 d. At autopsy, most of the permeable tubes were fractured.

The third type, or artificial pancreas, is quite large, and abdominal surgery for placement is necessary. The device requires the shunting of arterial blood through it, and attachment of veins and arteries. It has the advantage of easy retrievability and sturdiness. The surgical challenges of implantation are vessel anastomoses, the possible thrombotic events, and the increased heart load caused by the arterial-venous

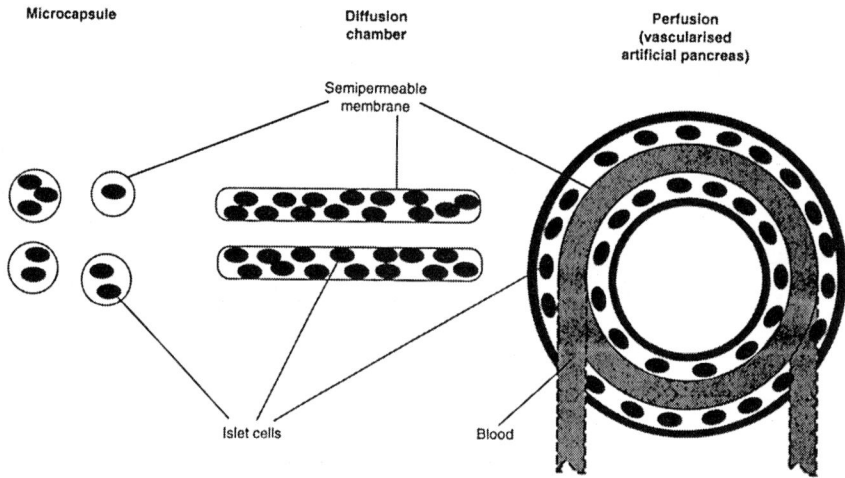

Fig. 1. Three typical isolation devices for pancreatic islet cells. The microcapsules are 500–800 μm in diameter, and contain one or more islets. Diffusion chambers are suitable for large animals and consist of 2-cm-long tubular membranes of 5–6 mm inner diameter. The ends are sealed. A prototype diffusion devised is shown on the right; it has an outer housing of 9 cm in diameter and 2 cm in height, and weighs 50 g. Islets in both diffusion chambers and perfusion devices are usually immobilized in agar or alginate to prevent settling and provide uniform distribution. From ref. *36* with permission.

shunt. Aspirin and low-dose warfarin are possible solutions for the thrombotic complications. The functional life to the artificial pancreas was about 1 yr in dogs. This device has a future once some of the technical problems are overcome. Major advantages are the ability to use easily available xenogeneic islets and the potential euglycemic control.

Islet-cell transplantation in humans has made major advances in the last 10 yr *(135)*. The rejection process is better understood, as are the predictors of rejection. It is now know that the islets are more sensitive to rejection than the whole pancreas, making the task of islet transplantation more difficult. The most promising areas for the future appear to be better and less toxic antirejection drugs, microencapsulated xenografts, immunomodulation of islet-cell membranes, and new implantation techniques. Based on what we have learned in the past, the future for pancreas and islet-cell transplantation looks bright indeed *(136)*.

SUMMARY

Whole pancreas transplantation is performed almost exclusively in patients with diabetes mellitus in an attempt to restore normal glucose metabolism and halt the progression of secondary complications. When kidney failure is also present, simultaneous kidney and pancreas transplantation is common. The current, widely used surgical technique is to place the organs into the peritoneal cavity, and anastomose the ureter and pancreatic duct to the urinary bladder. The exocrine secretions of the pancreas are voided, and in all patients, oral or iv bicarbonate replacement therapy is given. The two major problems following transplantation of organs are rejection and infection, especially with CMV. CSA and tacrolimus have had a major salutary impact on the success of transplantation. Perfect HLA matches between donors and recipients do not occur, with the exception of identical twins, and the chance of rejection of a transplant increases as the number of HLA mismatches increase.

All patients who are transplant candidates require HLA compatibility testing, and those receiving transplanted organs require laboratory support for the determination of plasma concentrations of antirejection drugs, for markers of rejection, such as urinary amylase, serum bicarbonate, glucose, insulin, c-peptide, and routine tests for management of specific problems. Testing for infections, especially by CMV, is important, because CMV infections can lead to graft and patient loss.

Islet cell transplantation is still an experimental technique, although much more is known about isolation of the islets from a donor, implantation techniques, immunomodulation strategies, and the use of encapsulated xenografts. The supply of human organs is greatly limited, but islet xenografts, hidden from the body's immune system by a suitable barrier, provide a challenge and a possible opportunity for treating diabetes. Much has been learned about islet transplantation, but significant barriers remain before it can be used routinely in patients with diabetes mellitus.

ACKNOWLEDGMENT

I am deeply grateful to Daniel D. Sedmak, Stephen C. Koesters, and Gloria Blair for their help in preparing the manuscript.

REFERENCES

1. Libman I, Songer T, LaPorte R (1993) How many people in the U.S. have IDDM? Diabetes Care 5:841, 842.
2. Karvonen M, Toumilehto J, Libman I, LaPorte R (1993) A review of the recent epidemiological data on the worldwide incidence of Type 1 (insulin-dependent) diabetes mellitus. Diabetologia 36:883–892.
3. Tajima N, Matsushima M (1994) Complications and prognosis of children with IDDM. Diabetes Res Clin Pract 24 Suppl:S165–S170.
4. Modan M, Karp M, Bauman B, Gordon O, Danon YL, Laron Z (1991) Mortality in Israeli Jewish patients with type 1 (insulin-dependent) diabetes mellitus diagnosed prior to 18 years of age: a population-based study. Diabetologia 34:515–520.
5. Malone JI (1994) Understanding diabetes in children. Adv Pediatr 41:33–52.
6. Eisenbarth GS (1986) Type 1 diabetes mellitus: a chronic autoimmune disease. N Engl J Med 314:1360–1368.
7. Todd JA, Bain SC (1992) A practical approach to identification of susceptibility genes for IDDM. Diabetes 41:1029–1034.
8. Maclaren N, Riley W, Skordis N, Atkinson M, Spillar R, Silverstein J, et al. (1988) Inherited susceptibility to insulin-dependent diabetes is associated with HLA-DR1, while DR5 is protective. Autoimmunity 1:197–205.
9. Olmos P, A'Hern R, Heaton DA, Millward BA, Risley D, Pyke DA, et al. (1988) The significance of the concordance rate for type I (insulin-dependent) diabetes mellitus in identical twins. Diabetologia 31:747–750.
10. Winter WE, Takeshi C, Schatz D (1993) The genetics of autoimmune diabetes. Am J Dis Child 147:1282–1290.
11. Abbas AK, Lichtman AH, Pober JS (1994) Self-tolerance and autoimmunity. In: Cellular and molecular immunology, 2nd ed., Philadelphia, Saunders Co., pp. 376–392.

12. Hagopian WA, Sanjeefi CB, Kockum I, Landin-Olsson M, Karlsen AE, Sundkvist G, et al. (1995) Glutamate decarboxylase-, insulin-, and islet cell-antibodies and HLA typing to detect diabetes in a general population-based study of Swedish children. J Clin Invest 95:1505–1511.
13. Crawford JM, Cotran RS (1994) The pancreas. In: Robbins pathologic basis of disease, 5th ed., Cotran RS, Kumar V, Robbins SL, Schoen FJ, eds. Philadelphia, W. B. Saunders Co., pp. 897–925.
14. Verge CF, Howard NJ, Irwig L, Simpson JM, Mackerras D, Silink M (1994) Environmental factors in childhood IDDM. Diabetes Care 17:1381–1389.
15. Karjalainen J, Martin JM, Knip M, Ilonen J, Robinson BH, Savilahti E, et al. (1992) A bovine albumin peptide as a possible trigger of insulin-dependent diabetes mellitus. N Engl J Med 327:302–307.
16. Federlin K, Otten A, Helmke K (1987) Islet cell antibodies and viral infections. Exp Clin Endocrinol 89:368–374.
17. Frisk G, Nilsson E, Tuvemo T, Friman G, Diderholm, H (1992) The possible role of Coxsackie A and ECHO viruses in the pathogenesis of type 1 diabetes mellitus studied by IgM analyses. J Infection 24:13–22.
18. Atkinson MA, Maclaren NK (1994) The pathogenesis of insulin-dependent diabetes mellitus. N Engl J Med 331:1428–1436.
19. Nerup J, Mandrup-Poulsen T, Helqvist S, Anderson HU, Podiot F, Reimers JI, et al. (1994) On the pathogenesis of IDDM. Diabetologia 37 Suppl 2:S82–S89.
20. Asayama K, Kooy NW, Burr IM (1986) Effect of vitamin E deficiency and selenium deficiency on insulin secretory reserve and free radical scavenging systems in islets; decrease of islet manganosuperoxide dismutase. J Lab Clin Med 1986;107:464–495.
21. Shah, SC, Malone JI, Simpson NE (1989) A randomized trial of intensive insulin therapy in newly diagnosed insulin-dependent diabetes mellitus. N Engl J Med 320:350–354.
22. Koivisto VA, Aro A, Cantell K (1984) Remissions in newly-diagnosed type 1 (insulin-dependent) diabetic patients: influence of interferon as an adjunct to insulin therapy. Diabetologia 27:193–7.
23. Green M, Michaels MG (1992) Infectious complications of solid-organ transplantation in children. Adv Pediatr Infect Dis 7:181–204.
24. Paya CV (1993) Fungal infections in solid-organ transplantation. Clin Infect Dis 16:677–688.
25. Dummer S, Kusne S (1993) Liver transplantation and related infections. Semin Respir Infect 8;191–198.
26. Stratta R (1993) J Clinical patterns and treatment of cytomegalovirus infection after solid-organ transplantation. Transplant Proc 25(5 Suppl 4):15–21.
27. Lu CY, Sicher SC, Vazques MA (1993) Prevention and treatment of renal allograft rejection: new therapeutic approaches and new insights into established therapies. J Am Soc Nephrol 4:1239–1256.
28. Vathsala A, Woo KT, Lim CH (1991) Pharmacokinetics and nephrotoxicity of cyclosporine. Ann Acad Med Singapore 20:507–512.
29. Distant DA, Gonwa TA (1993) The kidney in liver transplantation. J Am Soc Nephrol 4:129–136.
30. Marsh JW, Vehe KL, White HM (1992) Immunosuppressants. Gastroenterol Clin N Am 21:679–693.
31. Akagi H, Reynolds A, Hjelm M (1991) Cyclosporin A and its metabolites, distribution in blood and tissues. J Int Med Res 19:1–18.
32. Sutherland DER, Gores PF, Farney AC, Wahoff DC, Matas AJ, Dunn DL, et al. (1993) Evolution of kidney, pancreas, and islet transplantation of patients with diabetes at the University of Minnesota. Am J Surg 166:456–491.
33. Alejandro R (1995) Transplantation of islets of Langerhans in patients with insulin-dependent diabetes mellitus. Scan J Gastroenterol 30 Suppl 208:125–128.

34. Federlin KF (1993) The connection of experiment and clinic exemplified by the transplantation of islets of Langerhans. Exp Clin Endocrinol 101:334–345.
35. Hering BJ, Browatzki CC, Schultz A, Bretzel RG, Federlin KF (1993) Clinical islet transplantation—registry report, accomplishments in the past and future research needs. Cell Transplant 2:269–282.
36. Maki T, Mullon CJP, Solomon BA, Monaco AP (1995) Novel delivery of pancreatic islet cells to treat insulin-dependent diabetes mellitus. Clin Pharmacokinet 28:471–482.
37. London NJM, Donnelly PK (1994) Techniques of pancreas and islet transplantation. Baill Clin Gastroenterol 8:517–532.
38. Phillips MG, Ed., (1994) UNOS organ procurement, preservation, and distribution in transplantation. UNOS, Richmond, VA, 10:38–45.
39. Superdock KR, Helderman JH (1993) Immunosuppressive drugs and their effect. Sem Respir Infect 8:152–159.
40. Thomson AW, Starzl TE (1993) New immunosuppressive drugs: mechanistic insights and potential therapeutic advances. Immunol Rev 136:71–98.
41. Tocci MJ, Sigal NH (1992) Recent advances in the mechanism of action of cyclosporine and FK506. Curr Opinion Nephrol Hyperten 1:236–242.
42. Morris RE (1993) New small molecule immunosuppressants for transplantation: review of essential concepts. J Heart Lung Transplant 12:S275–S286.
43. Fontes P, Rao AS, Demetris AJ, Zeevi A, Trucco M, Carroll P, et al. (1994) Bone marrow augmentation of donor-cell chimerism in kidney, liver, and pancreas islet transplantation. Lancet 334:151–155.
44. Wallemacq PE, Reding R (1993) FK506 (tacrolimus) a novel immunosuppressant in organ transplantation: clinical, biomedical, and analytical aspects. Clin Chem 39:2219–2228.
45. Shaw LM, Bowers L, Demers L, Freeman D, Moyer T, Sanghvi A, et al. (1987) Critical issues in cyclosporine monitoring: report of the task force on cyclosporine monitoring. Clin Chem 33:1269–1288.
46. LeGatt DF, Coates JE, Simpson AI, Shalapay CE, Rintoul BJ, Yatscoff RW (1994) A comparison of cyclosporine assays using sequential samples from selected transplant patients. Clin Biochem 27:43–48.
47. Janeway CA Jr, Travers P (1994) Recognition of antigen. In: Immunobiology, The immune system in health and disease; Garland Publishing, pp. 4:18–4:30.
48. Suthanthiran M, Strom TB (1994) Renal transplantation. N Engl J Med 331:365–376.
49. Johnson AH, Hurley CK, Alper CA, Yunis EJ (1991) HLA: The major histocompatibility complex of man. In: Clinical diagnosis and management by laboratory methods, 18th ed., Philadelphia, W. B. Saunders Co., pp. 761–794.
50. Ogura K (1993) Sensitization, Clin Transplants 1992;357–359.
51. Shoskes DA, Wood KJ (1994) Indirect presentation of MHC antigens in transplantation. Immunol Today 15:32–38.
52. Miceli MC, Parnes JR (1991) The roles of CD4 and CD8 in T cell activation. Semin Immunol 3:133–141.
53. Karuppan SS, Lindholm A, Moller E (1992) Fewer acute rejection episodes and improved outcome in kidney-transplanted patients with selection criteria based on crossmatching. Transplantation 53:666–673.
54. Mahoney RJ, Ault KA, Given SR, Adams RJ, Breggia AC, Paris PA, et al. (1990) The flow cytometric crossmatch and early renal transplant loss. Transplantation 49:527–535.
55. Ogura K, Terasaki PI, Koyama H, Chia J, Imagawa DK, Busuttil RW (1994) High one-month liver graft failure rates in flow cytometry crossmatch-positive recipients. Clin Transplant 8:111–115.
56. Ogura K, Terasaki PI, Johnson C, Mendez R, Rosenthal JT, Ettenger R, et al. (1993) The significance of a positive flow cytometry crossmatch test in primary kidney transplantation. Transplantation 56:294–298.

57. Scornik JC, Brunson ME, Schaub B, Howard RJ, Pfaff WW (1994) The crossmatch in renal transplantation. Evaluation of flow cytometry as a replacement for standard cytotoxicity. Transplantation 57:621–625.
58. al Hussein KA, Shenton BK, Bell A, Talbot D, Clark KR, Rigg KM (1994) Characterization of donor-directed antibody class in the post-transplant period using flow cytometry in renal transplantation. Transplant Int 7:182–189.
59. Scornik JC, LeFor WM, Cicciarelli JC, Brunson ME, Bogaard T, Howard RJ, et al. (1992) Hyperacute and acute kidney graft rejection due to antibodies against B cells. Transplantation 54:61–64.
60. Reinke P, Fietze E, Docke WD, Kern F, Ewert R, Volk HD (1994) Late acute rejection in long-term renal allograft recipients. Diagnostic and predictive value of circulating activated T cells. Transplantation 58:35–41.
61. Garavoy MR, Reinschmidt MA, Bigos M, Perkins H, Colombe B, Feduska N, et al. (1983) Transplant Proc 15:1939–1944.
62. Wang GX, Terashita GY, Terasaki PI (1989) Platelet crossmatching for kidney transplants by flow cytometry. Transplantation 48:959–961.
63. Wahlberg J, Bengtsson M, Bergstrom C, Gannedahl G, Festin R, Lewen G, et al. (1994) Impact of flow cytometry cross-matching results on the outcome of cadaveric kidney transplantation. Transplant Proc 26:1752–1753.
64. Eisenstein BI (1990) The polymerase chain reaction. N Engl J Med 322:178–183.
65. Housman D (1995) Human DNA polymorphism. N Engl J Med 332:318–320.
66. Opelz G, Mytilineos J, Scherer S, Dunckley H, Trejaut J, Chapman J, et al. (1991) Lancet 338:461–463.
67. Williams GM, Hume DM, Hudson RP Jr, Morris PJ, Kano K, Milgrom F (1968) "Hyperacute" renal-homograft rejection in man. N Engl J Med 279:611–618.
68. Terasaki PI, Cecka JM, Lim E, Takemoto S, Cho Y, Gjentson D, et al. Clin Transplants 1991;409–430.
69. Squifflet JP, Moudry K, Sutherland DER (1988) Is HLA matching relevant in pancreas transplantation? Transplant Int 1:26–29.
70. Waldman WJ, Knight DA, Adams PW, Orosz CG, Sedmak DD (1993) In vitro induction of endothelial HLA class II antigen expression by cytomegalovirus-activated CD4+ T cells. Transplantation 56:1504–1512.
71. Sherlock CH, Denegri JF, Ashley RL (1991) Serological responses to cytomegalovirus during renal transplant rejection. Transplantation 52:272–275.
72. Dunn DL, Mayoral JL, Gillingham KJ, Loeffler CM, Brayman KL, Kramer MA, et al. (1991) Treatment of invasive cytomegalovirus disease in solid organ transplant patients with ganciclovir. Transplantation 51:98–106.
73. Wold AD (1992) Shell vial assay for the rapid detection of viral infections. In: Clinical microbiology procedures handbook, section 8.6; Isenbert HD., ed, Washington, DC, American Society for Microbiology. Vol 2, pp. 8.6.1–8.6.10.
74. Masih AS, Linder J, Shaw BW Jr, Wood RP, Donovan JP, White R, et al. (1988) Rapid identification of cytomegalovirus in liver allograft biopsies by in situ hybridization. Am J Surg Pathol 12:362–367.
75. Plotkin SA, Starr SE, Friedman HM, Brayman K, Harris S, Jackson S, et al. (1991) Effect of Towne live virus vaccine on cytomegalovirus disease after renal transplant. Ann Intern Med 114:525–531.
76. Marsano L, Perrillo RP, Flye MW, Hanto DW, Spitzer ED, Thomas JR, et al. (1990) Comparison of culture and serology for the diagnosis of cytomegalovirus infection in kidney and liver transplant recipients. J Infect Dis 161:454–461.
77. Halwachs G, Zach R, Pogglitsch H, Holzer H, Tiran A, Iberer F, et al. (1993) A rapid immunocytochemical assay for CMV detection in peripheral blood of organ-transplanted patients in clinical practice. Transplantation 56:338–342.

78. Sherlock DS (1994) Chronic hepatitis C. Dis Month 40:117–196.
79. Belli L, Dusheiko G, Rolles K, Burroughs AK (1991) Liver transplantation for chronic viral hepatitis. [Review] Ital J Gastroenterol 23:36–41.
80. Shah G, Demetris AJ, Irish W, Scheffel J, Mimms L, Van Thiel DH (1993) Frequency and severity of HCV infection following orthotopic liver transplantation. Effect of donor and recipient serology for HCV using a second generation ELISA test. J Hepatol 18:279–283.
81. Pereira BJ, Milford EL, Kirkman RL, Quan S, Sayre KR, Johnson PJ, et al. (1992) Prevalence of hepatitis C virus RNA in organ donors positive for hepatitis C antibody and in the recipients of their organs. N Engl J Med 327:910–915.
82. Martin P, Munoz SJ, Di Bisceglie AM, Rubin R, Waggoner JG, Armenti VT, et al. (1991) Recurrence of hepatitis C virus infection after orthotopic liver transplantation. Hepatology 13:719–721.
83. Rochlani M, Lewis JH, Ramsey GE, Bontempo FA, Shah G, Bowman RA, et al. (1992) Hepatitis C testing. Comparison of Ortho's EIA and RIBA II tests in 1 182 patients undergoing primary liver transplantation. Am J Clin Pathol 98:8–12.
84. Poterucha JJ, Rakela J, Lumeng L, Lee CH, Taswell HF, Wiesner RH (1992) Diagnosis of chronic hepatitis C after liver transplantation by the detection of viral sequences with polymerase chain reaction. Hepatology 15:42–45.
85. Rohr MS, Lesniewski RR, Rubin CA, Johnson RG, Heise ER, McDonald JC, et al. (1993) Risk of liver disease in HCV-seropositive kidney transplant recipients. Ann Surg 217:512–517.
86. Milfred SK, Lake KD, Anderson DJ, Hayney MS, Love KR, Emery RW, et al. (1994) Practices of cardiothoracic transplant centers regarding hepatitis C-seropositive candidates and donors. Transplantation 57:568–572.
87. Lim HL, Lau GK, Davis GL, Dolson DJ, Lau JY (1994) Cholestatic hepatitis leading to hepatic failure in a patient with organ-transmitted hepatitis C virus infection. Gastroenterology 106:248–551.
88. Hopt UT, Buesing M, Schareck WD, Becker HD (1992) Management der exokrinen Pancreassekretion-ein zentrales Problem der allogenen Pankreastransp!antation. Chirurg 63:186–192.
89. Sollinger HW, Belzer FO (1988) Pancreatic transplantation with urinary tract drainage. In: Pancreatic transplantation, Groth CG, ed. Philadelphia, W.B. Saunders Co., pp. 131–146.
90. Koenigsrainer A, Steurer W, Aichberger C, Gassner R, Schmid Th, Margreiter R (1991) Pancreatic transplantation with delayed duct occlusion versus bladder drainage: long-term results. Diabetologia 34 Suppl 1:S4–S7.
91. Secchi A, Dubernard JM, La Rocca E, LeFrancois N, Melandri M, Martin X, et al. (1991) Endocrinometabolic effects of whole versus segmental pancreas allotransplantation in diabetic patients- a two year follow-up. Transplantation 51:635–629.
92. Rosenlof LK, Earnhardt RC, Pruett TL, Stevenson W C, Douglas MT, Cornett GC, et al. (1992) Pancreas transplantation. An initial experience with systemic and portal drainage of pancreatic allografts. Ann Surg 215:586–597.
93. Esmatjes E, Fernandez-Cruz L, Ricart MJ, Casamitjana R, Lopez-Boado MA, Astudillo E (1991) Metabolic characteristics in patients with long-term pancreas graft with systemic or portal drainage. Diabetologia 34 Suppl 1:S40–S43.
94. Lott JA (1995) Enzyme tests in gastroenterology. In: Principles and practice of diagnostic enzymology, 2nd ed., Moss DW, Rosalki SB, eds, London, Edward Arnold Publishers, pp. 60–89.
95. Johnson & Johnson Company, Diagnostics Division, Rochester, NY 14650.
96. Stratta RJ, Sollinger HW, Perlman SB, D'Alessandro AM, Groshek M, Kalayoglu M, et al. (1989) Early detection of rejection in pancreas transplantation. Diabetes 38 Suppl 1:63–67.

97. Smith JL, Hunsicker LG, Yuh WT, Wright F H Jr, Van Voorhis L, Corry RJ (1989) Appearance of type II diabetes mellitus in type I diabetic recipients of pancreas allografts. Transplantation 47:304–311.
98. Steiner E, Klima G, Niederweiser D, Koenigsrainer A, Herold M, Margreiter R (1987) Monitoring of the pancreatic allograft by analysis of exocrine secretions. Transplant Proc 19:2336–2338.
99. Steiner E, Koller J, Geleff S, Dietze O, Koenigsrainer A, Margeiter R (1988) Viability of pancreatic transplants. Chirurg 59:469–471.
100. Bolinder J, Wahrenberg H, Persson A, Linde B, Tyden G, Groth CG, et al. (1991) Effect of pancreas transplantation on glucose counter-regulation in insulin-depended diabetic patients prone to severe hypoglycemia. J Intern Med 230:527–533.
101. Boucek P, Bartos V, Vanek I, Hyza Z, Skibova J (1991) Diabetic autonomic neuropathy after pancreas and kidney transplantation. Diabetologia 34 Suppl 1:S121–S124.
102. Caldara R, Martin X, Secchi A, Lefancois N, Touraine JL, Pozza G, et al. (1991) Metabolic control after kidney and pancreas transplantation: whole series results and effects of segmental duct obstruction versus whole pancreas with bladder diversion technique. Diabetologia 34 Suppl 1:S51–S52.
103. Drexel H, Palos G, Koenigsrainer A, Miesenboeck G, Aichberger C, Margreiter R, et al. (1991) Long-term follow-up of glycaemic control and parameters of lipid transport after pancreas transplantation. Diabetologia 34 Suppl 1:S47–S50.
104. Goldman J, Oh HK, Webb MG, Mozes M, Turza N, Kupin WL, et al. (1990) Allogenic whole pancreas transplantation in insulin-depended diabetes mellitus. Henry Ford Hosp Med J 38:246–251.
105. Holdaas H, Brekke IB, Hartmann A, Bentdal OH, Ganes T, Gjellestad A, et al. (1991) Long-term metabolic control in recipients of combined pancreas and kidney transplants. Diabetologia; 34 Suppl. 1:S68–S70.
106. Kennedy WR, Navarro X, Goetz FC, Sutherland DER, Najarian JS (1990) Effects of pancreatic transplantation on diabetic neuropathy. N Engl J Med 322:1031–1037.
107. Petersen MR, Vine AK (1990) Progression of diabetic retinopathy after pancreas transplantation. Ophthalmology 97:496–502.
108. Christiansen E, Andersen HB, Rasmussen K, Christensen NJ, Olgaard K, Kirkegaard P, et al. (1993) Pancreatic β-cell function and glucose metabolism in human segmental pancreas and kidney transplantation. Am J Physiol 264:E441–E449.
109. Solders G, Tyden G, Persson A, Groth CG (1992) Improvement of nerve conduction in diabetic neuropathy. Diabetes 41:946–951.
110. Stratta RJ, Perlman SB, Sollinger HW, Kalayoglu M, Belzer FO (1987) Early diagnosis of pancreas allograft rejection. Surg Forum 38:378–380.
111. Munn SR, Engen DE, Barr D, Carpenter HA, Perkins JD (1990) Differential diagnosis of hypoamylasuria in pancreas allograft recipients with urinary exocrine drainage. Transplantation 49:359–362.
112. Perkal M, Marsk C, Lorber MI, Markes WH (1992) A three-year experience with serum anodal trypsinogen as a biochemical marker for rejection in pancreatic allografts. Transplantation 53:415–419.
113. Moukarzel M, Benoit G, Charpentier B, Bouchard P, Bensadoun H, Verdelli G, et al. (1992) Is urinary amylase a reliable index for monitoring whole pancreas endocrine graft function? Transplant Proc 24:925–926.
114. Marks WH, Borgstrom A, Sollinger H, Marks C (1990) Serum immunoreactive anodal trypsinogen and urinary amylase as biochemical markers for rejection of clinical whole-organ pancreas allografts having exocrine drainage into the urinary bladder. Transplantation 49:112–115.
115. Brattstrom C, Tyden G, Reinholt FP, Bohman SO, Borgstrom A, Backman L, et al. (1989) Markers for pancreas-graft rejection in humans. Diabetes 38 Suppl 1:57–62.

116. Koenigsrainer A, Tilg H, Reibnegger G, Steurer W, Schmid T, Wachter H, Margreiter R (1992) Pancreatic juice neopterin excretion-a reliable marker of pancreas allograft rejection. Transplant Proc 24:907, 908.
117. Margreiter R, Ofner D, Reinl J, Koenigsreiter A (1992) Pancreas transplantation—a critical appraisal. Transplant Proc 24:2383–2386.
118. Abendroth D, Capalbo M, Illner WD, Landgraf R, Land W (1992) Critical analysis of rejection markers sIL-2R, urinary amylase, and lipase in whole-organ pancreas transplantation with exocrine bladder drainage. Transplant Proc 24:786–787.
119. Pleog RJ, D'Alessandro AM, Groshek M, Gange SJ, Knechtle SJ, Stegall MD, et al. (1994) Efficacy of human anodal trypsinogen for detection of rejection in clinical pancreas transplantation. Transplant Proc 26:531–533.
120. Ogawa M, Matsusda K, Shibata T, Matsuda Y, Ukai T, Ohta M, et al. (1985) Elevation of serum pancreatic secretory trypsin inhibitor (PSTI) in patients with serious injury. Res Commun Chem Pathol Pharmacol 50:259–266.
121. Nyberg G, Olausson M, Norden G, Mjornsted L, Blohme I, Hedman L (1991) Pancreas specific protein (PASP) monitoring in pancreas transplantation. Transplant Proc 23:1604, 1605.
122. Scharp DW, Laci PE, Santiago JV, McCullough CS, Weide LG, Falqui L, et al. (1990) Insulin independence after islet transplantation into type I diabetic patient. Diabetes 39:515–518.
123. Groth CG, Orsgren O, Tibell A, Tollemar J, Moeller E, Bolinder J, et al. (1994) Transplantation of porcine fetal pancreas to diabetic patients. Lancet 344:1402–1404.
124. Socci C, Falqui L, Davalli A. M, Ricordi C, Braghi S, Bertuzzi F, et al. (1991) Fresh human islet transplantation to replace pancreatic endocrine function in type 1 diabetic patients. Report of six cases. Acta Diabet 28:151–157.
125. Ricordi, C, ed. (1992) Pancreatic islet cell transplantation. Austin, RG Landes Company.
126. Peakman M, McNab GL, Heaton ND, Tan KC, Vergani D (1994) Development of techniques for obtaining monodispersed human islet cells. Transplantation 57:384–393.
127. Zeng Y, Torre MA, Karrison T, Thistlewaite JR (1994) The correlation between donor characteristics and the success of human islet isolation. Transplantation 57:954–958.
128. Robertson GSM, Chadwick DR, Davies J, Rose S, Contractor H, James RFL, et al. (1994) The effectiveness of components of University of Wisconsin solution in improving human pancreatic islet purification. Transplantation 57:346–354.
129. Gores PF, Sutherland DER (1993) Pancreatic islet transplantation: is purification necessary? Am J Surg 166:538–542.
130. Farney AC, Sutherland DER (1993) Pancreas and islet transplantation. In: Go VLW, ed., (1993) The pancreas: biology, pathobiology, and disease, 2nd ed. New York: Raven, pp. 815–835.
131. Morel P, Kaufman DB, Field MJ, Lloveras JK, Matas AJ, Sutherland DER (1991) Detrimental effect of prednisone on canine islet autograft function. Transplant Proc 24: 1048–1050.
132. Popkin MK, Callies AL, Colon EA, Lentz RD, Sutherland DER (1993) Psychiatric diagnosis and the surgical outcome of pancreas transplantation in patients with type I diabetes mellitus. Psychosomatics 34:251–258.
133. Colton CK, Avgoustiniatos ES (1991) Bioengineering in development of the hybrid artificial pancreas. J Biomech Eng 113:152–170.
134. Soon-Shiong P, Heintz RE, Merideth N, et al. (1994) Insulin independence in a type I diabetic patient after encapsulated islet transplantation. Lancet 343:950–951.
135. Federlin KF, Bretzel RG, Hering BJ (1992) Islet transplant registry. In Pancreatic islet cell transplantation, Ricordi, C, ed., Austin, RG Landes Company, pp. 463–472.
136. Hering BJ, Browatzki CC, Schultz A, Bretzel RG, Federlin KF (1993) Clinical islet transplantation—registry report, accomplishments in the past and future research needs. Cell Transplant 2:269–282.

2
Exocrine Disorders of the Pancreas

Frederick Van Lente

PANCREATIC EXOCRINE FUNCTION

The pancreas is an organ that lies parallel to and beneath the stomach and that is a major contributor to the overall digestive process. The pancreas has both endocrine and exocrine functions. The exocrine portion of the pancreas consists of clusters of cells known as acini that make up lobules separated by connective tissue. These cells constitute almost 80% of the organ. An acinus consists of up to 50 cells that have a common orientation toward a central lumen. Each acinus is drained by a ductule.

The pancreas secretes a large amount of bicarbonate (HCO_3^-) rich fluid containing a myriad of enzymes originating in the acinar cells and flowing through small ductules to the main pancreatic duct, and thence to the duodenum via the sphincter of Oddi (1). The flow of pancreatic exocrine secretions is controlled by both hormonal and neurological signals. During the gastric portion of the digestive process, parasympathetic nerve impules are transmitted via the vagus nerves directly to the pancreas, causing release of acetylcholine followed by release of pancreatic enzymes without significant generation of pancreatic fluid. Cholinergic stimulation of pancreatic enzyme release may also occur owing to stimulation of osmoreceptors in the duodenum.

Hormonal Control of Pancreatic Excretions

Pancreatic excretion is controlled by three endocrine hormones: secretin, cholecystokinin, and gastrin. Secretin, a polypeptide hormone of 27 amino acids, is released by the S-cells of the upper small intestine in response to gastric acid. Secretin stimulates pancreatic secretion of fluid rich in water and electrolyte that occurs when the duodenal pH is about 4.5 (2). Secretin release increases as the pH decreases toward 3.0. In response to secretin, the pancreas releases fluid with a bicarbonate concentration of up to 145 mmol/L. Bicarbonate reacts with gastric HCl in the following manner: $HCl + NaHCO_3 \rightarrow NaCl + H_2CO_3$. The carbonic acid formed ultimately dissociates into carbon dioxide and water. The carbon dioxide is absorbed into the blood and expired via the lungs leaving a more neutral solution of NaCl in the duodenum. Additionally, bicarbonate neutralization of gastric acid adjusts the intestinal pH to the range (pH ~8.0) that is optimal for the activity of pancreatic enzymes and prevents acidic damage to the intestinal mucosa.

From: Clinical Pathology of Pancreatic Disorders *Edited by: J. A. Lott Humana Press Inc., Totowa, NJ*

The presence of ingested food material in the upper duodenum stimulates the mucosal cells to release cholecystokinin (CCK), a polypeptide hormone of 33 amino acids. This release is potentiated by the partial protein degradation products resulting from gastric enzymatic action and by long-chain fatty acids *(1)*. CCK passes by way of the circulation to the pancreas in a manner similar to secretin; however, CCK provokes the release of enzymes and proenzymes from the acinar calls, rather than an electrolyte solution. These enzymes are an essential part of pancreatic exocrine function and will be discussed extensively. The degree of enzyme secretion observed after exogenous CCK infusion is similar to that seen postprandially *(3)*.

Gastrin, the gastric hormone secreted by gastric G-cells and the proximal glands of the duodenum, also has a moderate effect on the pancreatic acinar cells, resulting in additional stimulation of enzyme release. This occurs during the gastric phase of gastric secretion and is owing to the amino acid sequence homology between gastrin and CCK. Both hormones possess the same five N-terminal amino acids in this biologically active portion of the polypeptide *(4)*.

The various factors affecting pancreatic exocrine function are coordinated to an extent that the appropriate fluid, electrolyte, and enzymatic components are delivered to the duodenum in response to a given ingested food load. The major protein and lipid digestive processes are allowed to proceed without injury normally to either the pancreas or the intestinal mucosa. Approximately 1000–1500 mL of pancreatic fluid is secreted each day *(1)*.

Pancreatic Secretions

The pancreas secretes ions, water, and digestive enzymes. Bicarbonate anions and water are secreted primarily by the pancreatic epithelial cells that are located in the small ductules draining the acini. The concentration of bicarbonate in the final pancreatic fluid (145 mmol/L) is about five times the concentration found in the blood; obviously, there must be a physiological means to achieve this concentration. In brief, carbon dioxide enters the cell and forms carbonic acid in the presence of carbonic anhydrase and water. Carbonic acid dissociates into bicarbonate and hydrogen ion. Bicarbonate is then actively transported through the luminal border of the cell into the lumen of the ductule. The hydrogen ions produced are exchanged for sodium ions from the circulation that subsequently accompany the bicarbonate anion into the ductule. The net movement of sodium bicarbonate into the pancreatic ductules generates an osmotic gradient that also draws water into the ductule to form the final pancreatic fluid.

As the pancreatic output of HCO_3^- increases toward maximal rate, the corresponding chloride concentration falls with the sodium concentration remaining constant *(1)*. Therefore, the sum of the HCO_3^- and CL^- concentrations remains constant and about equal to the sum of the Na^+ and K^+ concentrations. Pancreatic fluid also contains about 1 mmol/L of calcium ion and trace amounts of magnesium, zinc, phosphate, and sulfate.

The carbohydrates, lipids and proteins in the human diet are digested by the process of hydrolysis, that is, the chemical bonds holding the monomeric units of these macromolecular fragments are broken by the net insertion of a water molecules. These reactions are catalyzed by the hydrolases secreted by the pancreas. These enzymes are produced in the pancreas by the exocrine acinar cells, which are almost entirely filled with rough-surfaced endoplasmic reticulum. The protein-synthesizing apparatus generates the various enzymes and proenzymes that are subsequently collected in condensing vacuoles that form mature zymogen granules in the cell. (Zymogen is an obsolete term for proenzyme.) These granules are released by the cell by exocytosis into the ductules in response to the stimuli already discussed. Malfunction of this impressive enzyme-producing apparatus has serious consequences.

The enzymatic constituents of pancreatic secretions are listed in Table 1. The enzymes represent the ability to catalyze the hydrolysis of the macromolecules of the major food sources, reducing these complex compounds to their monomeric components, such as amino acids, monosaccharides, and fatty acids, that can be absorbed by the intestinal mucosa. The environment created by the arrival of pancreatic fluid in the duodenum is optimized to allow these reactions to proceed. The pH is adjusted to that optimal for the enzymes, and bile salts and colipase are present to allow hydrolysis of fats at the phase interface.

The enzymatic components of pancreatic secretions are potentially damaging to both the pancreas and its associated network of ducts and vessels. Therefore, the pancreas produces both inactive precursor forms of the hydrolytic enzymes as well as protease inhibitors in order to prevent autodigestion. As shown in Table 2, the proteolytic enzymes trypsin, chymotrypsin, and carboxypeptidase are secreted as trypsinogen, chymotrypsinogen, and procarboxypeptidase, respectively. These precursors are somewhat larger than the active enzyme, since several amino acids are removed at specific sites during their activation by other proteolytic enzymes. Trypsinogen is activated by enterokinase (enteropeptidase), a special proteolytic enzyme secreted by the intestinal cells that hydrolyzes the peptide bond between Lys8 and Ile9 *(5)*. Free trypsin can subsequently activate itself by specific removal of a hexapeptide from the amino-terminal end of the precursor polypeptide; however, the rate of autoactivation is 2000 times slower than the reaction with enteropeptidase. Trypsin, once activated, also activates chymotrypsin by excision of two dipeptides from chymotrypsinogen. In a similar manner, trypsin cleaves activation peptides from the precursors of carboxypeptidase A, carboxypeptidase B, phosphilipase A2, colipase, and elastase. These reactions are catalyzed by enteropeptidase and proceed at a rate several orders of magnitude faster than trypsin autoactivation. This series of peptide bond cleavages should best be viewed as a classic activation "cascade" as outlined in Fig. 1. These particular enzymes may also act on each other at a slow rate *(6)*. It should be mentioned that there is some evidence that activated enzymes may participate in negative feedback regulation of pancreatic secretion *(7)*.

In addition to the production of digestive enzymes in inactive forms, the pancreas also synthesizes and secretes a trypsin inhibitor that is stored in the acinar cytoplasm surrounding the zymogen granules. This added protection prevents intracellular and extracellular activation of trypsin within the pancreas and its ducts. The inhibitor is secreted concurrently with the secretion of proenzymes, is a relatively small protein of 6000-Da mol wt, and is present in quantities sufficient to inhibit up to 20% of the potentially releasable trypsin *(8,9)*. The disruption of this important control is a major step in the evolution of acute pancreatitis with its autodigestion of the pancreatic parenchyma *(7)*. It has been shown, however, that small amounts of trypsin activity

Table 1
Enzymes Secreted by the Pancreas

Proeolytic enzymes	Amyolytic enzymes	Lipolytic enzymes	Nucleases
Trypsin(ogen)	Amylase	Lipase/colipase	Deoxyribonuclease
Chymotrypsin(ogen)		Phospholipase A2	Ribonuclease
(Pro) Carboxy- peptidase A		Carboxyl ester hydrolase	
(Pro) Carboxy- peptidase A			
Kallikrein			

Table 2
Precursor Forms of Pancreatic Enzymes

Precursor	Mol wt, Dalton	Active enzyme	Mol wt, Dalton
Trypsinogen	25,000	Trypsin	23,000
Chymotrypsinogen	24,000	Chymotrypsin	23,500
Procarboxypeptidase	47,000	Carboxypeptidase	35,500

can persist in the presence of this inhibitor. The plasma also contains protease inhibitors that bind all major classes of proteases, including those that are secreted by the pancreas; these proteins constitute almost 10% of the total protein in human plasma, and they prevent proteolytic activity under normal conditions (9).

Protein digestion initiates in the stomach with the action of pepsin, a gastric enzyme that reacts with all the major dietary proteins, including collagen. The latter reaction is essential for the efficient digestion of meats by the entire enzyme cascade. Pepsin accounts for about 10% of protein digestion; the remaining reactions are catalyzed by pancreatic enzymes (4). The partial protein breakdown products are further reduced in size by the endopeptidases trypsin and chymotrypsin. This action is complemented by the exopeptidases carboxypeptidase A and B, which remove individual amino acids from the carboxy-terminal ends of the peptides, a process that is completed by the action of peptidases located in the brush-border cells of the intestinal mucosa. The array of enzymes that participate in the overall digestion of proteins have a variety of active site specificities that allow hydrolysis of the spectrum of peptide linkages found in proteins.

The human diet contains three major sources of carbohydrates; these are sucrose, lactose, and starches. Starches are complex polysaccharides present in many food groups, particularly grains. Minor ingested carbohydrates include glycols, ethanol, pectins, and extrins. Cellulose, the major plant polysaccharide, cannot be broken down by human digestive enzymes. The pancreas secretes several enzymes to complete the digestion of carbohydrates, a process that begins with the action of salivary amylase. Chyme, or partly digested food, passing from the stomach to the duodenum contains a mixture of degraded starches. Amylase secreted by the pancreas reduces these compounds to maltose; in turn, maltose and other disaccharides, including lac-

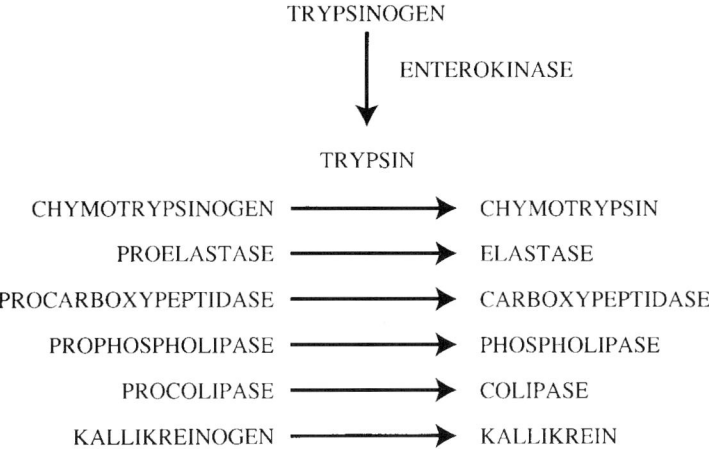

Fig. 1. The pancreatic enzyme activation cascade.

tose and sucrose, are split into their constituent monosaccharides by the enzymes maltase, lactase, and sucrase, respectively, that are located in the brush-border cells lining the lumen of the intestine.

The usual human diet contains a majority of neutral fats in the form of triglycerides, along with portions of phospholipids, cholesterol, and cholesterol esters. The digestion of fats, primarily existing as suspensions of insoluble particles, begins with emulsification by exposure to bile salts. Fat globules exist primarily as micelles with the polar portion of a triglyceride on the exterior and the nonpolar side chains on the interior. Pancreatic lipase cannot act effectively at the interface between the aqueous milieu and the fat globule without the emulsifying action of bile salts. As the emulsification process proceeds, the surface area available for lipase action increases significantly by a factor of up to 1000. Lipase acts in the presence of colipase at the surface of the lipid particle to hydrolyze the fatty acid-glycerol ester to free fatty acids and 2-monoglycerides. Bile salts also prevent the reversibility of this reaction by coordinating the formation of micelles containing the reaction products. This, in the net, forces the equilibrium of the reaction to the right or to complete hydrolysis, a process that also serves as a means to transport the reaction products to the brush-border cells for absorption. Cholesterol esters and phospholipids are hydrolyzed by cholesterol ester hydrolase and phospholipase A2, respectively. Bile salts, once again, serve a transport function, assisting the absorption of free cholesterol and free fatty acids.

PANCREATIC-SECRETED ENZYMES

Trypsin

Trypsin is a protease of the serine class; these enzymes are characterized by a catalytic "triad" of serine, histidine, and aspartate residues in the active site that are required for catalysis. Trypsin affects the hydrolysis of peptide bonds whose carbonyl group is contributed by either lysine or arginine, an action that does not occur at either the amino- or carboxy-terminal ends of the polypeptide chain; therefore, trypsin is known as an endopeptidase. It accounts for about 20% of the protein present in pancreatic fluid *(5)*.

As has already been described, trypsin is released from trypsinogen by cleavage of an "activation peptide" by enterokinase. Trypsinogen is synthesized by pancreatic ribosomes, and there is cotranslational removal of the initiator methionine. A transport peptide is then removed, and trypsinogen begins to accumulate in immature secretory vesicles that continue to concentrate protein until mature zymogen granules are formed. Trypsinogen is released into pancreatic fluid by exocytosis of these vesicles, which fuse only with the apical area of the cell membrane *(10)*. This is the general pattern of release for most pancreatic enzymes.

Two major and one minor form of trypsinogens have been isolated from human pancreatic fluid, and these can be separated by electrophoresis, ion-exchange chromatography, and gel filtration *(11)*. The so-called cationic form (trypsinogen 1) is present in an abundance of about three times that of the "anionic" form (trypsinogen 2). The amino acid compositions and molecular weights of these two forms are similar, 23,400 and 25,000 for trypsinogens 1 and 2, respectively. The terminology used to describe these isoforms can be confusing. The current, widely used terminology refers to the anionic form as trypsinogen-2 and the cationic form as trypsinogen-1 *(12,13)*. The sequences of the first nine N-terminal amino acids are identical, and the same activation peptide is cleaved from each protein by enteropeptidase. There is a minor trypsinogen component with a similar molecular weight (25,000 Da) and substrate specificity. It migrates between the two major forms on polyacrylamide gel electrophoresis and, therefore, was originally designated trypsinogen 2. This component appears to be a serine protease, but it is immunologically distinct from the other two isoforms. Its physiological role remains unclear. Synthesis of trypsinogen cDNA from human sources has allowed Southern blot analysis of genomic DNA using this material as a probe revealing the presence of a 10-member, trypsin-like multigene family *(14)*.

The study of trypsinogen cDNA has also provided insight into its mechanism of catalytic action. As mentioned previously, the triad of serine, histidine, and aspartate residues is essential for enzymatic activity, but this may be unrelated to those aspects of structure that determine substrate specificity. Through induced-mutation structural analysis, it has been determined that Asp 102 is critical for activity and that Asp 189 accounts for the specificity for positively charged amino acids *(15,16)*. Gly216 and Gly226 appear to dictate substrate binding *(17)*. Further investigation should delineate the remaining determinants of trypsin specificity.

Chymotrypsin

Chymotrypsin, in addition to being a major pancreas-derived protease, is one of the most thoroughly characterized proteins. Its three-dimensional structure was among the first characterized. It is also a serine protease, requiring the catalytic triad of Ser-His-Asp for activity. Two isoforms of chymotrypsinogen have been isolated from human pancreatic fluid *(18)*; however, the minor form represents only 7% of the total enzyme present and could be only a minor product of the activation reaction *(5)*. Chymotrypsinogen is activated by trypsin via a bond cleavage between Arg15 and Ile16 with the resulting polypeptides remaining attached by disulfide bridge *(5)*. It is worth noting that the activation cleavage(s) of the precursor forms of pancreatic enzymes does result in conformational changes in the protein. This process allows the appropriate juxtapositioning of the groups responsible for enzyme action. Chymotrypsin exhibits a substrate specificity different from that of trypsin; it hydrolyzes preferentially peptide bonds whose carbonyl groups are contributed by tyrosine, phenylalanine, and tryptophan (aromatic side groups).

Elastase

Elastase is found in two isoforms in pancreatic secretions. Elastase 2 is the major isoform and has a mol wt of 26,600 Dalton. Elastase is activated by trypsin; the cleaved activation peptide remains attached to the active protein via a disulfide bridge. Elastase is also a serine protease and has a relatively nonselective specificity, but will act preferentially at bonds of amino acids with aliphatic side chains. The reaction rate is affected by residues within five positions of the cleavage site, indicating a significant amount of interaction with the substrate *(5)*. Elastase 1 has a mol wt of 33,000 Dalton and is less abundant than elastase 2. The precursor form of elastase 2 contains 269 amino acids, and the cDNA sequence coding for this protein includes a 16 amino acid signal peptide that precedes the 12 amino acid activation peptide *(5,19)*.

Elastase is particularly effective in the breakdown of elastin, a major structural protein in connective tissue, including blood vessels. Elastase is produced by cells other than the pancreas, and neutrophil elastase has been implicated strongly in the pathogenesis of emphysema and adult respiratory distress syndrome (ARS) *(20)*. The role of pancreatic elastase in systemic disease is less certain, but may be a factor.

Carboxypeptidase

Carboxypeptidases are metalloproteins that require zinc for enzymatic activity. A single zinc ion is coordinated by Glu72, His69, and His196 *(21)*. These enzymes cleave the carboxy-terminal amino acids from proteins. As might be anticipated, the mechanism of bond cleavage is different from that found with the serine proteases. Two principal forms of carboxypeptidase are designated, carboxypeptidase A and carboxypeptidase B, and each of these exhibits multiple isoforms. Chromatographic separation of these isoforms from pancreatic fluid demonstrated three isoforms of procarboxypeptidase A (mol wt: 44.5–47 kDa) and two isoforms of procarboxypeptidase B, both with a mol wt of 47.3 kDa *(5)*. The molecular weight of these zymogens decreases to 35.5 kDa after activation. Interestingly, the activation peptide, once it has been cleaved from the precursor of carboyxpeptidase A, inhibits enzymatic activity until it is further degraded by proteolytic action *(22)*. Carboxypeptidase A is relatively nonselective with regard to substrate, but carboxypeptidase B cleaves preferentially terminal peptide bonds after Arg or Lys amino acid residues.

Kallikrein

Kallikrein represents a minor portion of the overall enzymatic content of pancreatic fluid, accounting for only 0.4% of total protein *(5)*. It is a glycoprotein of mol wt 48 kDa *(23)*. Another serine protease, the physiologic function of pancreas-derived kallikrein, is unknown in this setting. Its catalytic action results in the release of kinins from kininogens. Serum kinins activated in tissue function as mediators of inflammation.

Amylase

Amylase represents about 5% of the pancreatic fluid protein (4). It is a single-chain glycoprotein with a mol wt of 57 kDa; a precursor form of this enzyme has not been identified. It hydrolyzes the α-1,4-glycoside bonds in polysaccharides producing glucose, maltose, and a resistant portion of the macromolecule known as limit dextrins, that contains 1,6-glycosidic bonds at "branch points" not cleaved by this enzyme. The subsequent action of glucosidase is required to degrade dextrins further. Enzymatic activity is dependent on calcium ion, and is activated by chloride and other anions. The structure of this enzyme is organized into three domains, and there appear to be multiple substrate binding sites and a catalytic site (24). The mechanism of catalytic action has not been completely elucidated.

Lipase and Colipase

Pancreatic lipase, when purified from pancreatic fluid, exhibits a mol wt of 48 kDa (5). The cDNA for this glycoprotein indicates the presence of a signal peptide; however, there is no precursor form (25). Site-specific mutagenesis has demonstrated that lipase apparently possesses the same serine, histidine, and aspartic acid triad of catalytic amino acids as do the serine proteases. Lipase acts preferentially on insoluble micelles or emulsions of triglycerides, hydrolyzing the glycerol-fatty acid ester, and yielding free fatty acids and monoglycerides. Loops overlay the catalytic site that prevent binding of substrate (5). Movement of these loop domains during binding to a lipid–water interface may activate lipase activity. Lipase activity is diminished when acting on soluble substrates including carboxyl esters. Bile salts in concentrations found in the duodenum have been demonstrated to inhibit lipase activity, but the activity is restored in the presence of another protein, colipase.

Colipase has a mol wt of 10 kDa, and two forms have been isolated from pancreatic fluid. In apparent contrast to both amylase and lipase, colipase is secreted in a precursor form, which is activated by removal of a pentapeptide by trypsin. Because colipase limits the rate of lipid hydrolysis, lipase activity may be regulated by the degree of activation of procolipase. Colipase binds to pancreatic lipase in a equimolar ratio and also binds to the bile site–triglyceride interface (25). This protein has no apparent enzymatic activity. The structure of the lipase–colipase complex has been studied, and there is definite contact between procolipase and the carboxyl-terminal domain of human lipase (26). Salt bridges are formed between specific amino acid residues on each protein. As expected, colipase has also been shown to have lipid binding domains, but these have not been definitely located in the structure.

Carboxyl Ester Hydrolase

There are other enzyme activities similar to that exhibited by pancreatic lipase that have confounded clinical assays for serum lipase. One of these is pancreatic carboxyl ester hydrolase (cholesterol esterase). The enzyme is also lipolytic, and it represents about 4% of the protein in pancreatic fluid (5). It is a glycosylated protein with a mol wt of 100 kDa. cDNA analysis indicates the presence of a signal peptide, but not an activation peptide (27). This enzyme demonstrates activity toward a variety of substrates, and these include soluble esters, triglycerides, vitamin esters, and cholesterol esters. The action of this enzyme releases free cholesterol (for example) and a free fatty acid. This activity requires the presence of bile salts, which may prevent inappropriate activation in the pancreas. The amino acid sequence around the catalytic serine residue is highly homologous to that in serine proteases, and it may represent another member of this group of important enzymes. Site-specific mutagenesis has confirmed that Ser194 is required for activity *(27)*.

Phospholipase A2

Phospholipase A2 catalyzes the hydrolysis of the 2-acyl ester bond of phosphoglycerides. The reaction requires calcium ion, which is chelated by Tyr52, Tyr73, and Asp99 *(5)*. Enzymatic activity requires His48. The enzyme has a single polypeptide chain and is secreted as a larger precursor form of 14-kDa mol wt. It is activated by removal of a N-terminal heptapeptide by trypsin. Phospholipase A2, like pancreatic lipase, is an "interfacial" enzyme that acts at the organized interface of a lipid aggregate *(28)*. The catalytic site of these enzymes has been found to be analogous to the serine proteases, with water serving as a substitute for serine in the triad *(28)*.

The enzymatic rate for reactions with water-soluble, short-chain phospholipids is significantly less than that seen for reactions with organized lipid micelles. The binding of the enzyme to lipid aggregates has now been shown to induce appropriate conformational changes in the protein *(30)*. The active site becomes fully functional only after these changes occur.

Pancreatic phospholipase A2 should be distinguished from that apparently derived from macrophages and other cell types *(30)*. This enzyme is intimately involved in the acute-phase response and prostaglandin metabolism.

Nucleases (DNase and RNase)

The pancreas also secretes enzymes to break down nucleic acid chains. Deoxyribonuclease I degrades double-stranded DNA, producing 5'-oligonucleotide fragments. It has been isolated and characterized from human pancreatic fluid, and has a mol wt of 30 kDa. As with DNase I from other sources, it requires divalent metal ions for activity and exhibits a preference for cleavage on the 5'-side of pyrimidines. The specificity apparently depends on the metal ion present *(5)*.

Ribonuclease (RNase) has been isolated from human pancreatic tissue. However, the amount present is substantially less than in other animals, particularly ruminants *(5)*. This enzyme is specific for ribose and cleaves preferentially after a pyrimidine residue. The human form of RNase has a mol wt of 15 kDa *(31)*. RNase activity, with preferences for both polycytidylic and total RNA substrates, has been detected in the sear of patients with pancreatitis *(32,33)*. This supports the notion that multiple forms of the enzyme exist.

PANCREATIC FUNCTION TESTS

Direct Enzyme Measurements

The enzymes normally secreted from the pancreas into the gastrointestinal tract are released into the peripheral circulation after parenchymal damage. Some of these enzymes have become the standard serum tests for pancreatic inflammation, and amylase and lipase are the most frequently performed assays. To a lesser extent, immunoreactive trypsin, chymotrypsin, elastase, and phospholipase A2 have been used for this purpose. These assays have been described in detail elsewhere in this volume, and they will be discussed here only in the context of pancreatic hypofunction.

Modern amylase and lipase assays utilize defined substrates that have provided a means to improve the consistency of test results, although significant variation persists. It is important to remember, however, that commercially available assays are designed primarily to have maximal linearity to accommodate the significantly increased activities encountered in the sera of patients with acute pancreatitis. Therefore, these assays are ill-suited for detection of decreased activities that can be present in pancreatic insufficiency (34). The enzymatic assays are essentially applicable only for the routine detection and monitoring of pancreatic inflammation. The performance of total serum or urine amylase activity may be improved by determination of amylase isoenzymes. Pancreatic amylase separated by electrophoresis has been shown to be decreased in sera of patients with chronic pancreatitis (35–38). For example, one study found only 34% of serum amylase values were subnormal in patients with chronic pancreatitis, whereas 95% of pancreatic-isoamylase values (electrophoresis) were below normal (38). In patients with pancreatic insufficiency, salivary isoamylase tends to be the predominant contributor to the total amylase activity in urine and serum (39). Serum lipase activity also tends to remain within the normal reference interval in the presence of pancreatic insufficiency (40,41).

Serum and urine assays for phospholipase A2 exhibit similar characteristic to amylase and lipase, and have not been found to be useful in assessing pancreatic hypofunction (42). In the case of carboxypeptidase, studies indicate the complete absence of carboxypeptidase activity in the sera of normal individuals, and this mitigates against its use to assess pancreatic insufficiency (43,44).

Immunoassays for trypsin in sera have been more successful in the assessment of pancreatic hypofunction. Most immunoassays utilize antibodies that recognize trypsinogen, trypsin, and the trypsin–α-1-antiprotease complex. Therefore, the term "immunoreactive trypsin" or "immunoreactive trypsinogen" is usually employed when referring to an immunoassay for trypsin. In this chapter, the designation "immunoreactive trypsin(ogen)" will be used to indicate that these assays will measure the multiple forms of this enzyme present in serum. The advantage of these assays are their analytical sensitivity and range of values found in serum in the presence of various pancreatic pathologies. The immunoassays do not necessarily detect all the trypsin bound to circulating inhibitor proteins, and this can contribute to interassay variability (45). In addition, assays for both trypsin(ogen)-1 and trypsin(ogen)-2 (cationic and anionic) have been developed (46). Normal subjects exhibit immunoreactive trypsin concentrations in the ranges reported in Table 3. Assays for trypsin(ogen)-1 (cationic) have been used more frequently in the past, but there is renewed interest in the assay of trypsin(ogen)-2 (anionic). The ratio of trypsin(ogen)-1 to trypsin(ogen)-2 in normal sera has been reported to be about 1.5:1 (46). The ratio in normal pancreatic fluid is about 2:1 (50). The initial assays for immunoreactive trypsin(ogen) employed radioimmunoassay techniques (47,51). However, time-resolved immunofluorometric and enzyme-linked immunosorbent assay (ELISA) techniques have also been used (46,52).

Table 3
Range of Immunoreactive Trypsin Concentrations in Normal Individuals and in Patients with Pancreatic Insufficiency

Reference interval	Range of values in chronic pancreatitis	Refs.
207–260 µg/L	33–76 µg/L	38
6.5–36.1 µg/L	ND	46
10–43 µg/L	<40 µg/L	47
19.6–52.0 µg/L	<32 µg/L	48
15.1–61.3 µg/L	ND[a]	49

[a]ND, not determined.

Immunoreactive trypsin(ogen) is absent in the sera of patients who have undergone total pancreatectomy (45). Serum concentrations of immunoreactive trypsin(ogen) also may be decreased in patients with pancreatic insufficiency, as can be seen from Table 3. The frequency of decreased values in several studies varies greatly. Presuming that decreased values are diagnostic of exocrine insufficiency, test sensitivities of only 30–70% have been reported. The diagnostic value of these tests can be compromised by concurrent acute inflammation and changes in normal values with age. In the former situation, increases in the circulating concentrations of antiprotease inhibitors occur. In addition, the concentration of serum immunoreactive trypsin in normal subjects decreases with age (53,54). At one time, there was interest in the changes in circulating immunoreactive trypsin after a meal challenge, but this approach did not gain wide application (45). An evocative response of serum immunoreactive trypsin(ogen) to bombesin infusion also failed to identify adequately individuals with pancreatic hypofunction (55). Decreased concentrations of immunoreactive trypsin in serum do not appear to be totally specific for pancreatic insufficiency. Up to 100% of patients with diabetes mellitus have been reported to exhibit decreased values (55,56).

Immunoassays for chymotrypsin have also been developed. Assays for chymotrypsin 2 crossreact with chymotrypsinogen 2, chymotrypsin 1, and chymotrypsinogen 1, because these two isoforms of chymotrypsin are immunologically indistinct. The complexes of both forms of chymotrypsin with α-1-antiprotease inhibitor also react in the immunoassay, but not the complexes with α-2-macroglobulin. An assay for immunoreactive chymotrypsin(ogen), therefore, represents the sum of the major forms of the enzyme that can be released into the circulation. It is unlikely that any free, active enzyme exists in blood. The clinical usefulness of measurement of immunoreactive chymotrypsin(ogen) in serum has not been extensively evaluated.

Immunoassays for elastase have also been described. Again, the immunoreactivity represents both free and complexed forms of the enzyme. Assays for elastase I have shown that immunoreactivity is increased to a greater extent than amylase and remains abnormal for a longer period than amylase in the presence of pancreatic inflammation. There is evidence that this assay is considerably more specific for pancreatic pathology than amylase. However, there are few reports regarding the efficacy of elastase measurement in the assessment of pancreatic exocrine hypofunction.

The use of immunoassay for the determination of pancreatic exocrine zymogens, enzymes, and inhibitors has progressed in a manner similar to other immunoassays developed for clinical use. That is, initial work in the past decade focused on radioimmunoassay as the method of choice. Almost all current assays employ ELISA or another nonradiometric immunoassay. Few of these immunoassays are available commercially in kit form in the US.

The direct assessment of pancreas-derived proteins in serum as a means to determine pancreatic exocrine function *per se* is fraught with difficulties. First, the decrease from the normal release of pancreatic markers to the circulation requires analytical sensitivity unavailable for some enzymes. Second, even under normal circumstances, some markers may not be released in measurable quantity. This is consistent with the overall system of physiological checks and balances that exists in order to prevent inappropriate activation of pancreatic digestive capacity. Third, renal insufficiency can cause significant increases in all serum pancreatic markers in the absence of detectable pancreatic disease, an increase that is owing to the failure of the normal renal clearance of these proteins. This reduction in renal clearance will potentially mask the decreased output of pancreatic markers owing to pancreatic insufficiency. In the case of total amylase activity in serum, the salivary isoenzyme may result in normal values even in severe pancreatic hypofunction.

Direct Enzyme Assays in Fluid and Stool

A time-honored clinical assay for pancreatic exocrine function is the measurement of trypsin activity in duodenal fluid and stool. In contrast to immunoreactivity assays, this approach has directly assessed trypsin activity by its action on macromolecular or synthetic substrates. The X-ray film test utilizes the gelatin contained in the film as a proteinaceous substrate. Suspensions of duodenal fluid or stool are prepared in a series of buffered dilutions, which are placed as individual drops on a piece of unexposed X-ray film. After incubation, the film is rinsed with water and examined for "clear" areas where the trypsin has hydrolyzed the gelatin substrate *(57)*. The highest dilution that resulted in a clear area is the estimation of the trypsin content of the fluid. This method is, at best, a semiquantitative measure and is not satisfactory in adults *(45)*.

A better approach to the estimation of trypsin activity is the use of synthetic substrates, which are patterned after the enzymatic specificity of trypsin, such that there is no reaction with the other pancreatic enzymes present in these fluids. In addition, these synthetic peptides contain only one hydrolyzable bond, which results in straightforward kinetics. The major difficulty in the use of some of these substrates is the absence of a convenient indicator reaction. For example, the action of trypsin on benzoyl-L-arginine ethyl ester (BAEE) yields benzoyl-L-arginine and ethanol. Although benzoyl arginine shows a greater absorbency than BAEE at 253 nm, this is an inconvenient wavelength, and colorimetric interference is common *(57)*. The carboxyl hydrogen ion produced can also be monitored, using a pH STAT technique, and this approach eliminates colorimetric interference. Several of the synthetic substrates for trypsin are chromogenic or fluorogenic, and these make monitoring of the reaction more straightforward. For example, benzoyl-L-arginine-*para*-nitroaniline (BAPNA) yields *para*-nitroanilide, which absorbs strongly at 410 nm.

Chymotrypsin activity can also be measured directly in intestinal fluids using synthetic substrates. It can act specifically on N-substituted tyrosine esters, amides, and peptides. Chymotrypsin action on *N*-acetyl-L-tyrosine ethyl ester yields *N*-acetyl-L-tyrosine and ethanol. A kinetic assay has been described using the synthetic peptide Succ-Ala-Ala-Pro-Phe-2-nitroanilide as substrate. Again, the rate of *p*-nitroaniline formation can be monitored at 410 nm. Chymotrypsin is more resistant than trypsin to degradation in the lower intestinal tract and, therefore, is thought to be the more useful measurement in stool. In fact, the use of stool trypsin measurement for estimating pancreatic function has been abandoned worldwide *(35)*. The amount of chymotrypsin found in the stool is only about 0.5% of that secreted by the pancreas. Nonetheless, fecal chymotrypsin measurements can detect 80–90% of patients with severe pancreatic insufficiency, although sensitivities overall are only 50% *(58–60)*. The specificity of fecal chymotrypsin is acceptable and reported to be >90%. False-positive results can be seen in patients with diarrhea, protein deficiency, celiac disease, and in obstructive jaundice. Falsely normal results are observed when monitoring patients on enzyme-replacement therapy, if therapy is not discontinued for an appropriate period prior to testing.

Pancreatic Provocative Tests

As discussed earlier, the primary pancreatic exocrine function is the production of an enzyme and bicarbonate-rich fluid that furthers the process of food digestion. This fluid is produced in amounts of up to 1500 mL daily. The direct assessment of pancreatic or duodenal fluid for enzyme content, enzyme secretion rates, pancreatic fluid volume, or bicarbonate production is often conducted after stimulation of pancreatic secretion. Samples are collected via duodenal intubation of the patient. This approach provides a means to determine directly pancreatic output under near-physiological conditions.

Lundh Meal

The Lundh Test Meal consists of 5% protein, 6% fat, 15% carbohydrate, and 74% inert fiber *(35)*. This approach to pancreatic stimulation has the obvious advantage of duplicating the normal process of eating and digestion. The test meal is administered as a 300-mL volume. The patient is then intubated and duodenal contents are aspirated either in a series or singly after 2 h. Trypsin is usually the enzyme measurement of choice in the aspirated fluid, but more than one enzyme measurement has been recommended. The Lundh Meal fails to provide adequate stimulation of pancreatic secretion, however, in the presence of diseases of the intestinal mucosa. This is because of the need for appropriate hormonal response to the test meal for pancreatic stimulation to occur. The response of CCK and secretion is impaired in celiac disease. In addition, if surgical procedures have altered the normal gastric and duodenal anatomy, the meal stimulation will be impeded by the lack of appropriate signaling. The determination of volume and pancreatic secretion is also not possible. The Lundh Meal may also be used as an adjunct for indirect tests of pancreatic function to be discussed later.

Secretin Test

Stimulation of pancreatic fluid and electrolyte output can be accomplished by direct infusion of secretin, which is administered at one clinical unit per kg body weight using a 10 clinical units per 10 mL physiological saline preparation. This test has been complicated historically by variations in the potency of various secretin preparations. However, the *1995 Physician's Desk Reference* (49th edition) lists only the product supplied by Ferring Laboratories (Suffern, NY), and it yields a 10 u/mL solution for administration. The secretin challenge test is administered to a patient in the fasting state. A gastroduodenal tube with two lumens is guided into the duodenum using fluoroscopy. The opening of the tube is placed beyond the ampulla of Vater. After clearing the system and administration of secretin, 3–8 specimens of fluid are collected at 10-min intervals. An abrupt change in pH of the fluid signals contamination with gastric fluid (decrease) or duodenal fluid (increase). The individual specimens are pooled and the bicarbonate concentration determined. The normal rate of fluid and bicarbonate secretion is given in Table 4 *(61)*.

The secretin test provides accurate assessment of the fluid and electrolyte output only. The pancreatic enzyme output has been found to be variable and even normal in patients with documented pancreatic insufficiency.

Secretin-CCK Test

Stimulation of the pancreas by both normal hormonal effectors, secretin, and CCK allows assessment of fluid, bicarbonate, and enzymatic output. The enzyme chosen for measurement varies, but trypsin, amylase, and lipase have been determined. In this test, a lower dose of secretin than is employed in the secretin test is administered followed by administration of a CCK preparation. Various preparations and protocols have been used for this challenge, and results vary accordingly. A typical regimen consists of administration of one clinical unit of secretin/kg/h followed by 50 ng cerulein/kg/h *(62)*. Cerulein is a decapeptide with a C-terminal amino acid sequence identical to the C-terminal octapeptide of CCK, except for one substitution. However, the *1995 Physician's Desk Reference* does not list any preparations that could be used as the CCK component of this test. It would appear that this test is no longer used in the US.

The lack of standardized stimulation as well as the lack of standardized analytical methods has hindered the establishment of consistent interpretative guidelines for the secretin-CCK test *(63)*. Nonetheless, the secretion of <20 U/20 min of trypsin in pancreatic fluid has been shown to be consistent with abnormal pancreatic pathology. The secretin-CCK test is often considered the "gold standard" test of pancreatic exocrine function. One of the initial salient studies of this test estimated an 8% false-positive rate and a 6% false-negative rate *(64)*. There is some question regarding the relative accuracy of this test when compared with imaging techniques. Some investigators claim that the secretin-CCK test identifies the presence of histology consistent with chronic pancreatitis better than ERCP *(65)*. A complicating factor in the measurement of amylase output in duodenal aspirates in provocative testing is the presence of salivary amylase. Depending on the methodology employed, salivary amylase may result in an apparently normal or increased amylase output.

Indirect Tests of Pancreatic Function

The direct assessment of pancreatic function by analysis of duodenal aspirates entails a reasonable degree of effort and significant discomfort for the patient. In

Table 4
Normal and Abnormal Pancreatic Fluid and Electrolyte
Output After Secretin Stimulation (61)

Analyte	Normal subjects	Chronic pancreatitis
Volume mL/kg/hr	2.0–5.2	ND[a]–2.3
HCO_3^- mol/L	74–154	5–137
HCO_3^- mmol/kg/hr	0.156–0.718	0–0.291

[a]ND, none detected.

addition, there was a perceived need to improve on the performance of the direct analysis of pancreatic enzymes in stool specimens. Therefore, there has been considerable effort put into the development of indirect tests of pancreatic function that involves more reliable analytical techniques using easily obtained body fluids. These tests involve the ingestion of a synthetic substrate that releases a product that is absorbed following action of a specific pancreatic enzyme and that can be subsequently measured in serum or urine. The only other significant indirect test for pancreatic function is the assessment of stool composition.

NBT-PABA Test

The synthetic chymotrypsin substrate, *N*-benzoyl-L-tyrosyl-*p*-aminobenzoic acid (NBT-BTP: bentiromide), is hydrolyzed by pancreatic chymotrypsin as shown in Fig. 2. The terminal peptide linkage is cleaved yielding *N*-benzoyl-L-tyrosine and *p*-aminobenzoic acid (PABA). When this substrate is administered orally with a Lundh Meal or amino acid challenge, chymotrypsin acts on the substrate in the duodenum, releasing PABA, which is absorbed by the intestinal mucosa. After absorption, PABA is subsequently conjugated by the liver, forming both PABA conjugates that are excreted by the kidneys into the urine. Therefore, the amount of PABA conjugates in the urine is dependent on the amount of chymotrypsin activity in the duodenum, assuming normal intestinal, liver, and renal function. PABA conjugates were measured initially in urine using the Bratton-Marshall reaction, which detects all arylamines; however, this lack of specificity was not considered a significant problem owing to the absence of these compounds in normal urine *(66,67)*. Nonetheless, a basal urine sample could be analyzed for arylamine content in order to correct for any background.

The PABA test is affected by coadministration of many medications, particularly those that generate arylamines in urine. These medications include various antibiotics, pain medications, and diuretics. Foods yielding arylamine urine metabolites, such as prunes, and food products containing benzoate preservative should also be avoided. It is recommended that these substances be avoided for 2–3 d prior to the administration of the test *(35)*. Obviously, the test will be affected by the presence of renal disease, and results should be interpreted with caution in patients with decreased glomerular filtration rate and decreased creatinine clearance.

Consistent with many of the tests already discussed, there is considerable variability in protocols for administering the PABA test. A range of test doses from 150–2000 mg

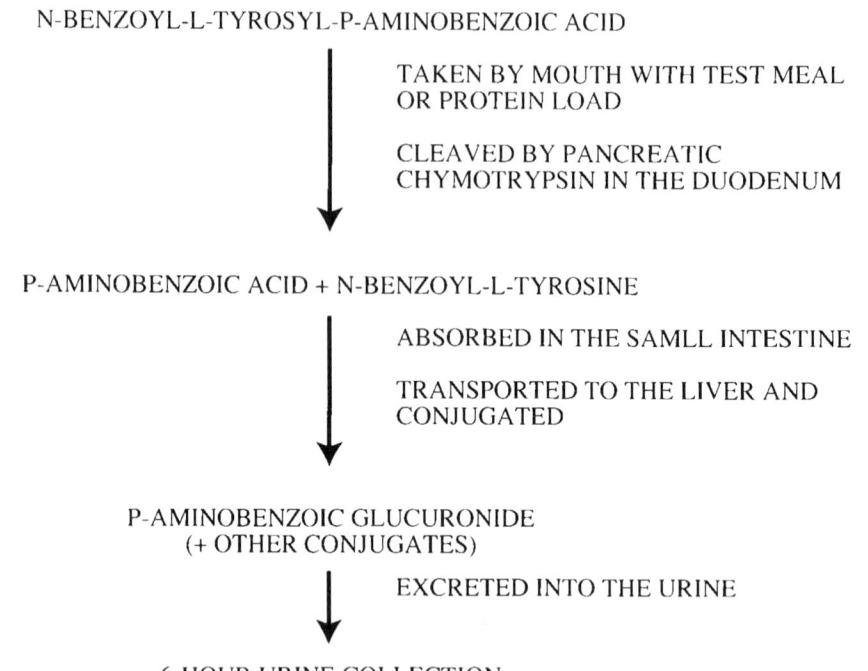

Fig. 2. The physiological basis for the NBT-PABA test. The test is dependent on intestinal, hepatic, and renal function.

has been reported with varying diagnostic results *(45,58,67)*. The dose of NBT-PABA used most frequently at this time is 500 mg *(58)*. Doses lower than 2000 mg have been shown not to compromise seriously the reliability of the test *(68)*. The meal challenge has also varied, and investigators have reported using the Lundh Meal, glucose solutions, "instant breakfast," normal meals, and bottle feeding *(69)*. Apparently, the composition of the meal or ingestion stimulus does not make a difference, but low diagnostic sensitivities have been reported if the test is administered without a meal *(69)*. Food ingestion during the course of the test is usually discouraged, but water intake is encouraged in order to generate sufficient urine. The urine collection interval varies up to 9 h, but 6 h are usually sufficient to obtain maximal diagnostic information from the test.

The percentage of the administered PABA equivalents recovered in the urine of normal individuals range from 47–80%, using a 6-h urine collection interval *(69)*. The low end of normal averaged 47% in a series of reports listed in a 1987 review *(69)*. Patients with pancreatic insufficiency tended to exhibit values <47%.

Some investigators have modified the original PABA test in order to correct for variations in intestinal, renal, and hepatic function. These modifications include two-stage tests using "free" PABA in order to determine a "PABA excretion index" *(70)*. The administration of PABA by itself presumably normalizes test results for individual absorption, metabolism, and excretion kinetics, allowing more specific assessment of pancreatic dysfunction. A shorter version of the "normalized" or "two-stage" NBT-PABA test has been described that uses coadministration of *p*-aminosalicylic acid

(PASA) *(71)*. As in the two-stage test, the PABA excretion index can be calculated by dividing the molar fraction of PABA excreted divided by the fraction of PASA excreted. Some investigators have advocated the measurement of serum PABA as a more convenient alternative to urine collection and measurement *(72–74)*. The blood specimen for PABA determination is usually obtained 3 h after the oral dose of NBT-PABA *(48)*; although others have sampled 90 min after the dosage *(75)*. The average normal response is a peak concentration of 0.04 mmol/L and values considerably less can be seen in pancreatic insufficiency *(58)*. There has been considerable debate regarding the relative value of serum vs urine measurements, but the convenience aspect cannot be discounted *(58,69)*.

The specificity of analytical methods for measurement of PABA in serum and urine has been improved significantly by the use of chromatographic techniques. Both gas-liquid chromatographic and high-performance liquid chromatographic (HPLC) methods have been developed *(76,77)*. These methods mitigate the effects of ingestion of interfering substances, such as benzoic acid food preservative.

The synthetic substrate NBT-PABA is relatively specific for chymotrypsin, but bacterial enzyme activity may cause hydrolysis. Falsely abnormal results can be seen secondary to gastric surgery *(68)*. Falsely normal results can be seen in patients on H-2 antagonists *(58)*. There is a large body of data regarding the sensitivity and specificity of the various modifications of the NBT-PABA test. Sensitivity has been reported to be from 39–100%, and reported specificities range from 76–100% *(69)*. Specificities are improved with use of the two-stage or "normalized" tests that calculated the PABA excretion index *(58)*.

The PABA test remains in active use in the European community, but the 1995 edition of the *Physician's Desk Reference* does not list the NBT-PABA substrate (Bentriomide) as a commercially available product. Therefore, it is not clear how frequently this test is performed in the United States.

Pancreolauryl Test

The pancreolauryl test is similar to the PABA test in principle. Fluorescein dilaurate is a water-insoluble ester that is hydrolyzed specifically in the gut by pancreatic arylesterases. When administered orally, this compound releases water-soluble fluorescein dye, which is quickly absorbed by the intestinal mucosa, partially conjugated by the liver, and excreted into the urine primarily as its glucuronide *(67,69)*. Fluorescein conjugate can be determined in urine by either spectrophotometry or fluorometry at alkaline pH *(67)*. The original laureate ester is colorless and does not interfere with this analysis. The concentration of fluorescein is usually determined in a 10-h urine collection, and the total amount of dye excreted during this period is calculated *(69)*.

The test is administered by having the patient consume a standard meal accompanied by 0.5 mmol of fluorescein dilaurate. The ingestion of fluids is encouraged during the collection period of the test. Certain medications are to be avoided prior to the test including sulfasalazine. As was described for the two-stage PABA test, a second stage of the test is administered over 24 h later using free fluorescein. This test corrects for variation in individual absorption, conjugation, and excretion kinetics. The fluorescein excreted after ester administration (E) and after free fluorescein administration (F) is calculated and expressed as a ratio (E/F). E/F ratios of >0.30 are found in individuals with normal pancreatic exocrine function. Ratios in the range 0.20–0.30 are considered equivocal or nondiagnostic, and these results should be confirmed by repeat testing *(69)*. Ratios <0.20 are considered consistent with abnormal pancreatic function.

A comparison with the PABA test is appropriate, because both tests have the same approach to pancreatic function assessment. The diagnostic sensitivity of the fluorescein laureate test has been reported to be between 60 and 100% compared to the secretin-CCK test as gold standard. It has been reported to have sensitivities that are up to 6% higher than the PABA test in comparative studies *(69)*. The specificity of the pancreolauryl test varies from 39–100% in published reports *(69)*. In comparison with the PABA test, the specificity of the pancreolauryl test is either 3–40% lower or 5–16% higher depending on the study *(69)*. Falsely abnormal values for the pancreolauryl test have been reported in patients with gastric surgery and celiac disease *(69)*. These conditions confound most pancreatic function tests. Bacterial overgrowth may also invalidate the test, because some species of bacteria, such as streptococci, are capable of hydrolyzing fluorescein dilaurate.

The pancreolauryl test has been shown to be relatively insensitive to alterations in renal function, although significant effects on recovery of PABA of altered renal function have been reported. It is possible that efficient hydrolysis of the laureate ester may require the presence of sufficient amounts of bile acids in the duodenum, a process unrelated to pancreatic function. There have been investigations into the determination of fluorescein in serum as an alternative to urine collection and analysis *(74,78)*. This approach would both shorten and simplify the administration of this test, particularly in the geriatric population. Fluorescein determinations in serum are conducted in a manner similar to those for urine, and the maximal concentrations are observed 4–6 h after ingestion. The use of the serum test after pancreatic stimulation with secretin or metoclopramide has also been reported *(79,80)*. Diagnostic sensitivity and specificity appear to be similar to those of the urine test. This would appear to be a more convenient means of administering this test.

Plasma Amino Acids

Pancreatic stimulation and fluid production are normally associated with a discernible drop in plasma amino acid concentrations. This change in plasma amino acid composition in response to pancreatic stimuli has been investigated as a potential indicator of pancreatic exocrine function. Total amino acid concentrations decreased maximally by 31 ± 19% in response to infusion of secretin (1 CU/kg/h) and CCK (1 U/kg/h), but only by 6.3 ± 19% in patients with pancreatic insufficiency *(81)*. The individual amino acids serine, valine, isoleucine, and histidine demonstrate better discrimination of pancreatic function than total concentrations *(81)*. These changes are also highly correlated with chymotrypsin output and demonstrate a sensitivity for moderate to severe pancreatic dysfunction of 100 and 91% sensitivity for all cases, including mild dysfunction at a cutoff of 12% or less reduction in amino acid concentration *(81)*. In a study utilizing secretin and cerulein stimulation, and a cutoff of 14% or less reduction in amino acid concentration, an overall sensitivity of 86.7% for pancreatic dysfunction was obtained *(82)*. In contrast, a sensitivity of just 64.2 and

66% was found for the pancreolauryl test and for stool chymotrypsin, respectively. There were no false positives.

CO₂ Breath Tests

Several procedures have been developed that involve the oral ingestion of triglycerides or cholesterol esters containing carbon-14-labeled fatty acids *(83,84)*. The radioactive isotope carbon-14 has been incorporated into the fatty acid component of triglycerides. It is assumed that the production of $^{14}CO_2$ is proportional to the rate of absorption of fatty acids released by pancreatic lipase and colipase in the presence of bile salts in the duodenum. The administration of labeled free fatty acids can also be used to distinguish the presence of fat malabsorption from pancreatic maldigestion. The carbon isotope (in CO_2) is determined by breath analysis. Carbon-13-labeled triglycerides have also been utilized for this purpose, and they have the advantage of being nonradioactive. $^{13}CO_2$ is measured in expired breath using a mass spectrometer *(85)*. A carbon-13 mixed triglyceride possessing a medium chain fatty acid in the 2-position has yielded breath $^{13}CO_2$ productions that correlate well with duodenal lipase output *(85)*. The cumulative $^{13}CO_2$ exhalation over a 6-h interval in both normal individuals demonstrated a sensitivity of 89% and a specificity of 81% *(85)*. The recovery of $^{13}CO_2$ from labeled trioctanoin in patients after pancreatoduodenectomy correlated significantly with duodenal output of lipase, amylase, and chymotrypsin *(86)*. These values were found to be just as sensitive as the direct secretin test *(86)*.

A breath test utilizing cholesterol [1-^{14}C] octanoate has also been developed *(87)*. The rate of appearance of $^{14}CO_2$ in breath is proportional to the rate of hydrolysis of the ester by pancreatic carboxyl ester hydrolase. This test also depends on relatively stable hepatic metabolism and functional intestinal absorption. The test compound is given as a gum emulsified in vegetable oil as part of a isotonic meal. In normal controls, breath isotope output peaked at 60–90 min, and this pattern was reproducible *(87)*. Patients with moderate to severe steatorrhea had an expiration rate of less than one-third of that of normal individuals *(87)*. Pancreatic enzyme supplementation increased the rate of breath isotope production in abnormal patients *(87)*.

Schilling Test

The use of the Schilling test to confirm the etiology of pernicious anemia is well established. The ability to absorb vitamin B_{12} administered orally with and without intrinsic factor and secrete into the urine cobalt-58 confirms any abnormality in intrinsic factor function. The ability to transfer cobalamin bound to gastric R protein to intrinsic factor is essential for proper absorption and is apparently bicarbonate-dependent. This transfer can be assessed by coadministration of cobalt-58 cobalamin bound to porcine R protein and cobalt-57 cobalamin bound to intrinsic factor *(88)*. The excretion ratio of [58Co]/[57Co] gives a relative indication of the efficiency of this transfer; the lower limit of normal was determined to be 0.68. This ratio correlated with the maximal bicarbonate concentration obtained in duodenal fluid. Relative to a direct test of pancreatic secretory capacity, the dual-label Schilling test exhibited a sensitivity of 65% in patients with mild to moderate pancreatic dysfunction; the specificity was 100%. Other reports have demonstrated lower sensitivity *(89)*. The major drawback of this procedure is that it has been evaluated in only small numbers of patients. The evaluation of alternative methods other than direct intubation collection and analysis of duodenal fluid requires comparison to these methods, and this renders any study difficult to conduct on large groups of patients with pancreatic disease.

Stool Lipids

Stool composition is dependent in part on pancreatic function. Any significant decrease in pancreatic function results in reduced absorption of starch, fat, and protein with a concurrent increase in the amount of these food substances in the stool. Under these conditions, stool contains undigested meat fibers (creatorrhea or azotorrhea), increased starch (amylorrhea), and increased fat (steatorrhea). The stool can become visibly abnormal in severe cases, and fat droplets may be grossly visible.

Normally, stool contains mono-, di-, and triglycerides as well as fatty acids, phospholipids, glycolipids, and cholesterol esters. Although most of this lipid material is derived from incompletely digested food material, a significant amount may be derived from intestinal sources *(67)*. The total lipid content is usually determined on a 72-h specimen. The patient should consume about 50–150 g of fat on each of 3 d prior to the collection period and during the collection period; furthermore, laxatives must be avoided. The stool specimen is collected in a 1-gal paint can. Collections for periods of <72 h are not recommended owing to presumed daily variability. The sample is weighed, homogenized, extracted, evaporated, and the residue weighed. Fecal fats have also been determined titrimetrically. The most common reference intervals applied to stool total lipids are <2 g/d for children and 2–6 g/d for adults. The excretion of stool fat can also be expressed as a percentage of fat intake, as a percentage of fecal dry weight or as a percentage of fecal wet weight *(67)*. For adults, the appropriate reference intervals are less than about 10, 15–25, and <2.5%, respectively *(67,90)*. Values significantly grater than the upper limit of normal are consistent with steatorrhea. Stool may also be examined microscopically after staining with Oil Red O or Sudan III to visualize fat droplets.

The efficacy of fecal lipid determination is compromised by difficulties in specimen collection, as well as by the fact that a considerable portion of stool lipids (up to 2 g/d) are not derived from the diet *(67,90)*. In addition, the microscopic evaluation of fat droplets is subject to observer variation owing to differences in training and interpretation criteria. Fecal microscopic examination is also often performed on random, not timed, stool specimens, so comparisons with quantitative determinations are problematical. However, some investigators have reported that appropriate microscopic examination may be of equal value to quantitative measurements *(91)*. In a manner analogous to the isotope breath tests, radioactive isotopes derived from triglyceride fatty acid may be measured in stool, but the correlation with titrimetric fecal lipid measurements is modest *(92)*. The measurement of hydrolyzed fats can help distinguish digestive from absorptive steatorrhea, although problems with postcollection changes are thought to occur *(67)*.

Near-infrared spectroscopy has also been used for analysis of stool analytes *(93)*, an approach that is based on the reflectance intensity observed on the surface of a stool sample at a specific wavelength proportional to the concentration of a specific component. Using this technique, the fecal dry weight, total fat, hydrolyzed fat, and total nitrogen content can be estimated. The correlation of these estimates with traditional measurement is 0.96–0.98 *(93)*. The relationship between estimations of total fat and hydrolyzed fat distinguishes pancreatic exocrine dysfunction from intestinal malabsorption. Those patients with malabsorption had a significantly higher (>70%) proportion of hydrolyzed fat compared with those with pancreatic insufficiency. This method has the distinct advantage of not requiring extraction and analysis, although homogenization is still necessary. There is also a report of the use of NMR spectroscopy for the estimation of total stool fat *(94)*.

Stool specimens can also be extracted and their individual lipid components quantified. Long-chain fatty acids, triglycerides, and cholesterol can be extracted from stool with detergents and analyzed enzymatically *(90)*. Further study should establish if this type of quantitative approach is superior to stool total lipids by gravimetric or titrimetric means as well as stool microscopy. It is interesting that most current reviews discount the use of 72-h fecal fat measurements, even though this test, in essence, defines the presence of steatorrhea in patients with chronic pancreatitis *(95)*. In patients without pancreatic steatorrhea, low fecal fat concentrations are expected, but the specificity of this finding is not complete. Decreased values can be found in patients with celiac disease *(96,97)*. Diarrhea has been shown to induce an apparently mild steatorrhea, and fecal fat values of up to 14 g/d can be observed *(98)*. A representative study reported sensitivities of 33 and 72.2% for fecal fat quantitation and Oil Red O stain microscopic examination, respectively *(99)*. Specificities of these two tests were 45.5 and 95.4%, respectively. The difficulty in assessing test performance is the lack of an independent standard for the diagnosis of fat malabsorption.

SPECIFIC DISEASES OF THE EXOCRINE PANCREAS

Diseases of the exocrine pancreas are defined by gastroenterologists as those diseases not hormonal in nature, and includes both acute and chronic conditions that are inflammatory and destructive in nature. As is usually the case, these conditions are either acute or chronic in nature and are viewed clinically in this manner. The dominant diseases involving the pancreas are acute and chronic pancreatitis, which are by far the most prevalent diseases affecting this organ. Acute inflammation of the pancreas, however, rarely affects the exocrine, digestive function of the pancreas in a significant way. The clinical pathology of these acute disorders is covered extensively elsewhere in this volume and will not be discussed here.

Repeated acute pancreatic insult, however, will lead to extensive and irreversible parenchymal damage; the loss of physiologically active tissue results ultimately in secretion failure and maldigestion, and is classified as chronic pancreatitis. Therefore, chronic pancreatitis will be discussed here as a major disease of pancreatic exocrine function rather than an extension of acute pancreatitis.

Diseases that are associated with maldigestion owing to pancreatic secretory insufficiency are listed in Table 5. This list is short by most standards, and cystic fibrosis and chronic pancreatitis are by far the most prevalent.

Table 5
Diseases of the Exocrine Pancreas

CF
Chronic pancreatitis
Abdominal surgeries
Hereditary disorders other than CF
Hereditary pancreatitis
α-1-antitrypsin deficiency (?)
Shwachman Syndrome
Johanson-Blizzard Syndrome
Inherited enzyme deficiencies

Cystic Fibrosis (CF)

CF was first identified as a specific disease 50 years ago. It is the most common inherited metabolic disorder, and affects about 1 in 1900–3700 Caucasians in the US. CF is a multifaceted disorder in which several organ systems are affected adversely by a single biochemical abnormality. The many clinical manifestations include respiratory failure, chronic sinusitis, pancreatic insufficiency, and infertility *(100,101)*, and result from a defect in epithelial chloride transport *(102)*.

Transport of chloride across epithelial membranes is part of the delicate water and electrolyte balance necessary for organ function. The cells possess regulated chloride channels in their membranes that allow chloride to move along an electrochemical gradient. These channels are opened by an increase in intracellular cAMP with resultant activation of protein tyrosine kinase A. In CF, the chloride channels are not responsive to opening signals *(103)*. An intense effort to identify and clone the gene responsible for CF has resulted in a major improvement in the understanding of this defect.

Molecular Biology

The gene associated with the inheritance of CF is located on chromosome 7 (band q31-32). It is 250 kilobases in length and contains 27 exons *(104,105)*. The gene has an associated messenger RNA (mRNA) that is 6.5 kilobases in length *(106)*. The gene product is a protein of 1480 amino acids and was named the CF transmembrane conductance regulator (CFTR) before its physiological function was completely determined in anticipation of this functionality being confirmed. In fact, the elucidation of the molecular biology of CFTR represents a major accomplishment of the practice of reverse genetics in which the biochemistry and biology are determined only after a gene is located and isolated.

The CFTR has been predicted to be a protein integral to the cell membrane with two portions containing a domain capable of spanning the membrane six times *(106)*. There is also a region thought to be a nucleotide binding domain associated with each transmembrane domain *(106)*. The two portions of the molecule are separated by a highly charged domain known as the regulatory (R) domain, which contains several possible phosphorylation sites. This part of the molecule may be crucial to the regulation of CFTR function. The nature of the structure of CFTR is analogous to members of the ATP binding cassette family of transmembrane transport proteins *(101)*.

CFRT expression is found predominantly is epithelial cells. High levels of expression are found in exocrine glands, including salivary, pancreatic, and sweat glands *(101)*. An exception to the association between CFTR expression and organs affected in clinical CF is the pulmonary epithelial cells, which exhibit minimal expression even though chloride transport is defective in the respiratory epithelium in CF *(107)*. These findings suggest that other factors are involved in the cellular manifestations of a defective CFTR protein. Investigations using recombinant CFTR have confirmed that this protein is, in fact, responsible for the CF phenotype and that it is a chloride channel protein *(101)*.

Mutations

As of 1992, 200 clinically relevant mutations in the CF (CFTR) gene had been identified *(101)*. Several types of mutations are included in this cohort, including frame shift, nonsense, missense, and RNA-splicing mutations. The most common mutation is a three-nucleotide deletion of a codon normally coding for a phenylalanine residue at amino acid position 508 *(108)*. In the standard designation, this mutation is known as ΔF508, and it occurs on about 70% of all CF alleles *(109)*. Approximately 91% of patients have at least one chromosome bearing this mutation *(101)*. Several other mutations account for most of the remaining patients, and the vast majority of mutations have been found in only one individual *(101)*. In North American Caucasians, ΔF508 is found on 60–75% of chromosomes of patients with CF *(109)*. ΔF508, G542X, G551D, R533X, W1282X, and N1303K mutations are present in almost 85% of North American Caucasians with the disease *(110)*. Mutations may result in defective plasma membrane chloride channel transport owing to decreased expression or defective processing and placement.

The most common CF alleles, such as ΔF508, are associated with pancreatic insufficiency. These mutations also tend to be associated with severe respiratory disease and increased sweat chloride concentrations (*see below*) *(111)*. In the group of patients with "severe" mutations, prognosis is difficult to judge because of a wide variation in the severity of respiratory complications *(101)*. A subset of alleles is associated with mild respiratory disease, female fertility, and normal sweat chloride concentrations *(112)*. Male infertility alone is apparently the mildest phenotypic manifestation of CF *(113)*.

Screening for CF

When considering screening for a disease, such as CF, several population categories can be considered: all newborns, the general population at risk for carrier status, pregnant women with or without a family history of CF, siblings of affected individuals, and other relatives of affected children at risk for carrier status *(114)*. Screening for CF is somewhat different than screening for phenylketonuria or hypothyroidism in that there is no strong evidence that improved outcomes are associated with neonatal diagnosis. As stated earlier, the disease is transmitted in an autosomal-recessive manner, and it is estimated that 5% of the general population may carry a defective gene *(114)*.

Several countries have adopted the use of immunoreactive trypsin assays for neonatal screening for CF. The immunoreactive trypsin concentration in blood is actually increased in newborns with CF, perhaps reflecting the pancreatic involvement in this disease *(49,115)*. The concentration of immunoreactive trypsin in normal infants decreases rapidly with age, but newborns with CF show higher values during the first several months of age *(49)*. These assays can be performed on the same type of dried blood spot used for phenylalanine and hypothyroidism screening programs. The immunoreactivity is lost more rapidly in dried blood than in frozen sera, but this loss was not considered of sufficient magnitude to prevent the use of this type of specimen *(115)*. The immunoreactive trypsin is extracted from a 3-mm disk of dried blood and the analysis subsequently performed by radioimmunoassay *(49,116)*.

In the salient US study, 279,400 newborns in the state of Colorado were screened for immunoreactive trypsin *(117)*. At an initial cutoff value of 140 µg/L, a false-positive rate of 92.2% and a false-negative rate of 4.9% were observed. This cutoff resulted in a recall rate of 3.2/1000 births. A cutoff of 80 µg/L for repeat testing appeared to yield a false-negative rate of <2% and a false-positive rate of 19.2%. This program identified 95% of newborns with CF who did not present with meconium ileus. The costs of this type of screening were estimated to be $8877 (1991) per child identified. Other programs have used an initial cutoff of 180 µg/L and a repeat cutoff of 75 µg/L, but have reported a higher false-negative rate that was deemed unacceptable *(118)*. The initial false-positive rate for immunoreactive trypsin in most studies is >90%. In addition to the lack of definitive benefit to early identification of patients with CF, the high false-positive rate will generate considerable anxiety and concern for the parents of many newborns.

The burgeoning knowledge of the genotypes of CF has led to much debate regarding the efficacy of screening for these mutations. The use of DNA analysis to aid in the detection of carrier status and diagnosis has been thoroughly evaluated in recent years. The 1990 Workshop of Population Screening for the Cystic Fibrosis Gene conducted by the National Institutes of Health recommended that screening for heterozygotes in the general population should not be considered until 95% of the mutations can be detected *(119)*. This would allow 90% of couples at risk to be detected by such a program. The 1991 Canadian Task Force on the Periodic Health Examination recommended that DNA analysis not be performed on newborns or the general population, and stated that the ΔF508 mutation detection would account for only 50% of individuals homozygous for CF and for about 70% of carriers *(114)*. They also recommended that first-degree relatives of children with CF should be tested by DNA analysis for carrier status and that siblings of children with CF should have a sweat test after 4–6 wk of age.

Laboratory Diagnosis

Most patients with CF exhibit the triad of chronic obstructive pulmonary disease, pancreatic exocrine deficiency, and an increased sweat chloride concentration. The latter two of these are amendable to detection by laboratory testing. The gold standard for the laboratory confirmation of CF remains the sweat chloride test. Patients with CF have a normal sweat rate; however, the fluid contains increased concentrations of sodium, chloride, and potassium. The most commonly employed electrolyte measurement is chloride, although sodium can also be determined either separately or in combination with chloride *(120)*. The sweat chloride concentration in conjunction with family history and clinical presentation provide the diagnosis of CF, which can be confirmed by DNA analysis.

The sweat test has a long history of variability and inaccuracy owing to the way it is administered and the analytical techniques employed *(121,122)*. The recommendations of the Cystic Fibrosis Foundation and the National Committee for Clinical Laboratory Standards are based on the use of the original Gibson and Cooke method of stimulated sweat collection followed by titrimetric determination of chloride concentrations *(123,124)*.

The collection of sweat is performed using pilocarpine iontophoresis where an electric potential is established in the skin so that ions can penetrate the surface in response to the applied potential. Pilocarpine nitrate (a cholinergic stimulant) is applied to a positive electrode and a potential of up to 15 V are established with a corresponding current of up to 4 mA for 5 min. Preweighed gauze or filter paper is then applied to the site, covered, and sweat is collected for at least 30 min. Reported minimal sample requirements vary, but usually 100 mg or 15 µL of sample are necessary for accurate testing *(123)*. The chloride can be measured in the sweat sample using titrimetric techniques. Sweat collection should be conducted when the patient is clinically stable, well hydrated, free of concurrent illness, and not receiving steroids. The definitive, recommended procedure for the sweat test is available from the Cystic Fibrosis Foundation.

Healthy individuals and healthy siblings of patients with CF exhibit sweat chloride concentrations that are usually <60 mmol/L *(124)*. There is an effect of patient age on the concentration of chloride in sweat. During the neonatal period, sweat chloride values may be transiently increased to >65 mmol/L in up to 25% of individuals *(125)*. Therefore, it is recommended that sweat testing be delayed until at least 48 h after birth if an adequate sample can be obtained; an adequate sample is more reliably obtained after 4 wk. The desire for early testing can be a result of the finding of meconium ileus at birth or prenatal familial risk. Sweat chloride values also increase with age in unaffected individuals, but this does not cause a problem in the interpretation of results. A sweat chloride concentration of >60 mmol/L is consistent with the diagnosis of CF. About 5% of sweat chloride results are in a borderline range of 40–60 mmol/L, and repeat testing is needed to confirm either positive or negative results *(126)*.

False-negative sweat chloride results are not common if the test is conducted correctly and repeat testing follows a borderline result. Reported causes of false-negative tests include hypoproteinemia and edema. Siblings have been described with mild pulmonary disease and normal sweat chloride concentrations that were found to have a homozygous glycine-to-serine substitution mutation at amino acid position 551 in CFTR *(112)*. This and other "mild" CFTR mutant alleles may require DNA analysis to confirm the presence of CF. A variety of other conditions are reported to cause false-positive results in the sweat chloride test, and these include adrenal insufficiency, hypothyroidism, and Klinefelter's Syndrome. However, these are not a major problem in the differential diagnosis, and DNA analysis might help confirm cases where indicated. There is no significant correlation of the sweat chloride concentrations and the degree of pancreatic insufficiency in patients with CF *(127)*.

About 20% of infants born with CF present with meconium ileus *(100)*. This condition is characterized by the failure of the newborn to excrete meconium, the viscous, greenish-brown intestinal contents of a neonate, within a few days of birth. This clinical findings should be confirmed by sweat testing and mutation analysis. It was found that the albumin content of meconium is increased in patients with CF *(128)*. Normal newborns exhibit a meconium albumin concentration of <50 mg/g of dry weight, but neonates with CF could exhibit concentrations of up to 400 mg/g *(100)*. A pH-effect test strip for screening meconium for albumin concentration was also developed. A report of the use of this strip on 28,000 samples revealed a sensitivity of 75% with a positive predictive value of only 4.0% *(129)*. The specificity was 99.7% with a negative predictive value approaching 100%. Serum activities of amylase and lipase are not helpful in the diagnosis of CF *(100)*.

Evaluation of Pancreatic Sufficiency

Patients with CF secrete an overly concentrated, very protein-rich pancreatic fluid that may contain all the pancreatic enzymes. However, with progression of the disease, secretions become inspissated and cause blockage of the pancreatic ducts with resultant cystic dilation or fibrosis *(130)*. Over 80% of CF patients exhibit pancreatic insufficiency. The most obvious evidence of significant pancreatic involvement in patients with CF is the presence of steatorrhea. However, in the case of more subtle manifestations, the full range of pancreatic function testing may be required to determine the degree of pancreatic functionality. In the subgroup of patients without overt pancreatic insufficiency, it has been determined that lipase and colipase secretion rates are as low as 1–2% of normal values *(131)*. These patients also exhibit milder pulmonary disease, lower mortality, and milder electrolyte and fluid deficits, although they are still identified by immunoreactive trypsin screening programs *(132)*. Patients with homozygous ΔF508 mutation alleles demonstrate pancreatic insufficiency in almost all cases (99%) *(127)*. In comparison, about three-quarters of patients heterozygous for the ΔF508 allele and another mutation and one-third of patients with other phenotypes develop pancreatic insufficiency. These proportions are based on an average of 10 yr of longitudinal study *(127)*.

The classification of pancreatic function in CF is somewhat arbitrary. The accepted criteria for establishing clinical pancreatic insufficiency are the presence of steatorrhea or an abnormal response to the secretin-CCK provocative test. Following intubation, pancreatic secretions are usually collected for 1 h using three 20-min collections. Determination of one of the salient pancreatic enzymes in the aspirated duodenal fluid completes the test. The threshold values are usually determined by comparison with normal controls. That is, for pancreatic colipase, an output of >120 U/kg of body wt/h indicates pancreatic sufficiency. Pancreatic sufficiency is also indicated by a fecal fat loss of <7% of dietary fat intake for children of age >6 mo *(127)*. Although these cutoffs just represent points on a continuum of pancreatic function, they are used as the primary indices for classifying CF patients. The only alternative, objective parameter for CF pancreatic function is the magnitude of enzyme replacement therapy required for adequate digestion *(133)*. The discussion that follows will focus on more convenient means to classify and assess CF pancreatic sufficiency.

Duodenal aspiration studies are unpleasant and challenging in children as well as being very time-consuming. Screening tests that are easier to perform obviate the need for more exhaustive workups in many cases. The determination of fecal chymotrypsin has been found to be a more reliable indicator in children than in adults *(45)*. Fecal chymotrypsin exhibits a reasonable correlation with the NBT-PABA test with values <135 µg/g stool corresponding to 6-h urine PABA recoveries of <60% *(134)*. A similar correlation with the pancreolauryl test has been reported. Fecal chymotrypsin is also reported to exhibit a 100% sensitivity and a 97% specificity for severe pancreatic insufficiency *(59)*. In normal children, fecal chymotrypsin values increased significantly during the first 2 yr of life from 73–567 µg/g *(59)*. This change clearly indicates the need for age-specific ranges during the first 2 yr of life. Nonetheless, the sensitivity of fecal chymotrypsin measurements drops significantly in patients with mild pancreatic insufficiency, and fewer than one-half of these patients have abnormal values *(135)*. The performance of the orally administered indirect tests as indicators of pancreatic insufficiency in patients with CF is shown in Table 6. The NBT-PABA test controlled with PASA demonstrates reasonable sensitivity and specificity with respect to abnormal fecal fat excretions. Complete sensitivity and specificity (100%) have been reported in a small study for the NBT-PABA/PASA test in patients with and without steatorrhea *(136)*. Although a similar sensitivity can be obtained in the single-stage NBT-PABA test using an appropriate cutoff, the specificity decreases to <50% *(136)*. In contrast, pancreatic amylase activity in serum demonstrates a 80% sensitivity and 100% specificity *(137)*. The reported specificity of these indirect tests is to a great extent dependent on the means for classifying the patient's pancreatic sufficiency.

The pancreolauryl (fluorescein dilaurate) test has also been evaluated in patients with CF; however, the accumulated experience with this indirect test over the past several decades is less than that for the NBT-PABA test. Some reports have claimed complete discrimination between CF patients with severe pancreatic insufficiency and their healthy siblings *(138)*. A random urine pancreolauryl test using mannitol as an ingested internal standard has been suggested as a test for use in infants *(139)*. The ratio of urinary fluorescein to mannitol exhibited a sensitivity of 96% and a specificity of 95% *(139)*. Similarly a dual-marker, 1-d pancreolauryl test also using mannitol as an internal marker has been developed *(140)*. There is a degree of variability in the dose of fluorescein dilaurate administered, a problem that confounds the standardization of these procedures *(141,142)*. The lack of a convenient dosage form is also a problem *(142)*.

The extent of pancreatic insufficiency worsens with time in patients with CF. Investigation of patients with pancreatic sufficiency has shown that about 13% of proven exocrine sufficient patients have become exocrine insufficient after 5 yr *(143)*. Pancreatic function testing is required to monitor these changes. Patients who retain pancreatic sufficiency also consistently exhibit significantly higher serum immunoreactive trypsin(ogen) concentrations *(144)*.

Pancreatic enzyme replacement is the usual therapeutic approach to exocrine insufficiency in CF. The effect of enzyme supplementation can be maximized by concurrent therapies, such as H_2 antagonists and antacids. Pancreatic function testing, including the NBT-PABA and increase in serum pancreatic polypeptide, correlates with the decrease in fecal fat excretion effected by enzyme supplementation *(145)*. Hyperuricemia secondary to the high purine content of commercially available enzyme supplements can occur in a minority of patients with CF *(130)*.

Table 6
Efficacy of NBT-PABA Test for Detection of Pancreatic Insufficiency in CF

Type	Sensitivity	Specificity	No. subjects	Refs.
One-stage (PASA)[a]	100%	100%	48	*136*
Two-stage[b]	71%	71%	21	*75*
Two-stage[b]	92%	78%	34	*137*

[a]Coadministration of NBT-PABA and PASA.
[b]Administration of NBT-PABA and urine collection followed by administration of free PABA and urine collection.

There is some disagreement among clinical investigators regarding the appropriate manner for evaluating CF patients for their pancreatic status. One definite point of view is evident from the following statement, "may I recommend a simple, cheap, sensitive, specific, and repeatable alternative for which patients are generally only too happy to provide specimens—fecal chymotrypsin measurement" *(146)*. This test represents the primary means to assess CF patients for pancreatic sufficiency. It is straightforward and does not involve the complications of even the indirect ingestion tests. However, others feel that other indirect tests are appropriate.

Chronic Pancreatitis

Historically, the classification of chronic pancreatitis has been confusing. The first attempt to standardize the diagnosis was the 1963 Marseilles conference on pancreatitis. The criteria established at that time were subsequently modified in two additional conferences held in 1983 and 1984. These criteria are focused on the difficult task of distinguishing recurrent acute pancreatitis from recurrent chronic pancreatitis. In addition, the classification of pancreatitis was grouped only into acute and chronic types *(147)*.

According to Marseilles convention, chronic pancreatitis is defined as an inflammatory disease of the pancreas characterized by persistent and progressive parchencymal damage. Acute pancreatitis, by contrast, is characterized by the resolution of organ damage on elimination of the cause. Chronic pancreatitis is further classified into calcifying and obstructive forms. All portions of the pancreatic lobule are affected. There is atrophy of the acini, fibrosis is present, the ducts are dilated and may contain plugs, and there are foci of calcification. In the obstructive form, the lesions are not lobular.

Autopsy studies have shown a prevalence of chronic pancreatitis that ranges from 0.04–5% *(147)*. Incidence rates have been reported to be from about 2–9 new cases/100,000 inhabitants in the US, Europe, Scandinavia, and Japan. The incidence rate of chronic pancreatitis is dependent on the rate of alcohol consumption.

The etiology of chronic pancreatitis is predominantly (70–80%) alcohol-related. At autopsy, alcoholics exhibit a rate of chronic pancreatitis that is up to 50 times that found in nonalcoholics. There does not appear to be a threshold level of chronic ingestion above which the risk for pancreatitis significantly increases, because abstainers have a lower risk than light drinkers (1–20 g ethanol/d). Therefore, it is difficult to distinguish idiopathic disease from that possibly caused by consistent light drinking.

The duration of drinking is also important and usually prolonged (>6 yr) intake is required for disease to appear *(148)*. Diets high in fat and protein potentiate the risk for chronic pancreatitis as occurs in animal models. The pathophysiological mechanism(s) by which chronic alcohol intake results in disease is not known. In the long term, alcohol may interfere with the careful orchestrated processing, secretion, and inhibition of pancreatic enzymes such that organ autodigestion occurs.

Chronic pancreatitis owing to nutritional causes is a major etiology of this disease worldwide. It occurs often in juveniles who are malnourished and show signs of kwashiorkor as well as nonketotic diabetes mellitus *(147)*. However, these individuals do not have a history of kwashiorkor at the time of presentation. Disseminated pancreatic calcification is often present. The important etiological factor in nutritional chronic pancreatitis may be the presence of severe trace metal deficiencies of copper, zinc, and selenium. These deficiencies result in significant decreases in antioxidant activities, and this, in turn, results in chronic free radical-induced organ injury *(149)*. Associated antioxidant enzymes include superoxide dismutase, catalase, and glutathione peroxidase. It is also likely that the important antioxidant vitamins, such as vitamin E (tocopherols), are also deficient.

Chronic pancreatitis is also associated with the inherited form of pancreatitis. This condition is inherited in an autosomal-dominant manner, and the incidence is about the same in both genders *(147)*. The defect in these individuals is unknown, although a defect in free radical scavenging has been proposed *(150)*.

Other causes of chronic pancreatitis include hyperparathyroidism, pancreatic duct obstruction, pancreatic trauma, pancreas divisum, and idiopathic pancreatitis. Pancreatic calcification occurs in untreated hyperparathyroidism presumably owing to hypercalcemia and its stimulative effect on acinar cells. With more than 20 years of routine biochemical screening for serum calcium concentrations, the incidence of this condition has decreased significantly. Obstruction of the pancreatic duct by tumors, scars, or pseudocysts can result in the distinctive form of chronic pancreatitis known as obstructive chronic pancreatitis, which is characterized by acinar atrophy, fibrosis, and ductal dilation without the findings of intraductal plugs or stones *(147)*. Pancreas divisum is a congenital abnormality of the pancreas in which the fusion of the dorsal and ventral pancreatic ducts does not occur completely and pancreatic drainage occurs via the minor papilla. It has been reported that the incidence of this condition in patients with chronic pancreatitis is about 6% *(151)*. Pancreas divisum may account for some cases of obstructive and idiopathic chronic pancreatitis; the latter accounts for 10–40% of nonalcoholic cases of this disease in North America and Europe *(147)*.

The clinical presentation of patients with chronic pancreatitis is dominated by the presence of abdominal pain. The pain is usually epigastric, dull, and constant. Radiation to the back is a salient feature, and is relieved by sitting in a forward position or lying prone. Lying in the supine position is most uncomfortable. Pain may be constant or intermittent over the course of several days. Ingestion of food results in an almost instantaneous exacerbation of pain; however, pain is absent in about 15% of patients who tend to have idiopathic disease *(147)*. Nausea, vomiting with associated anorexia, and weight loss are common. The pain in response to eating prevents patients from ingesting appropriate food. The presence of diabetes or malabsorption also contributes to weight loss, and clinical jaundice may be present if the common bile duct is compressed. The physical examination is of limited value in the diagnosis of chronic pancreatitis since the physical findings may be insignificant in relation to the magnitude of the patients' complaints.

Diarrhea, steatorrhea, and azotorrhea occur in patients whose pancreatic exocrine secretions have become insufficient for proper digestion. These manifestations occur late in the course of the disease, and signal massive loss (90%) of organ function. The differential diagnosis of pancreatic insufficiency will be discussed below.

Laboratory Diagnosis

Laboratory studies of blood are not particularly useful in the diagnosis of chronic pancreatitis, in sharp contrast to the diagnosis of acute pancreatitis. Leukocytosis may be present, although the nutritional anemias associated with intestinal disease are seldom present. The presence of common bile duct involvement can cause an increase in alkaline phosphatase activity, and evaluation of other abnormal liver function tests may be indicated if chronic pancreatitis is associated with alcoholic liver disease.

The serum activities of pancreatic enzymes are not markedly increased in contrast to acute pancreatitis, but they are usually slightly increased, normal, or decreased. This is true for amylase, lipase, immunoreactive trypsin (ogen), and phospholipase A2. In acute exacerbations of the disease, there is a greater likelihood that increased activities will be present. Patients with mild to moderate disease usually demonstrate normal serum enzyme activities. Decreased serum enzyme activities are generally thought to be solely associated with severe chronic pancreatitis *(147)*. Most of the pancreatic enzymes have been evaluated diagnostically in this context with the exception of total amylase. The latter activity usually remains in the reference interval regardless of the degree of pancreatic insufficiency because of the contribution of salivary amylase necessitating the determination of pancreatic amylase rather than total amylase.

Pancreatic amylase, lipase, immunoreactive trypsin(ogen), and elastase have been evaluated for the diagnosis of chronic pancreatitis. It should be mentioned that it is very difficult to determine the diagnostic accuracy of tests for chronic pancreatitis *per se*, because in the absence of definitive biopsy information, there is no "gold standard" for confirming the diagnosis. The presence of pancreatic insufficiency can be confirmed by provocative testing, but this represents just a portion of the spectrum of the disease. Therefore, there is an inherent insensitivity to this type of confirmation.

Decreased serum concentrations of immunoreactive trypsin(ogen) have been reported in an average of 85% of patients with severe chronic pancreatitis and in 30% (range 0–60%) of patients with mild to moderate disease *(see* Table 3). However, up to 100% of patients with diabetes mellitus exhibit decreased values as well *(56,152)*. A positive predictive value for cationic trypsin(ogen) of 82.7% has been reported for the presence of chronic pancreatic "disorders" *(153)*. These consisted of chronic pancreatitis (51.7%) or pancreatic cancer (31%). In another study of emergency medicine admissions, serum immunoreactive trypsin(ogen) demonstrated a positive predictive value of 70% *(48)*.

An attempt was made to increase the diagnostic usefulness of serum enzyme activities in the diagnosis of chronic pancreatitis by measuring activities after infusion of CCK as a provocative stimulus *(35)*. Specificities of 98.5 and 96.3% were observed for serum isoamylase and immunoreactive trypsin(ogen) after secretin-CCK stimulation *(35)*. However, sensitivity was low—45.1 and 41.5% for isoamylase and immunoreactive trypsin(ogen), respectively. Earlier work showed that this approach was not particularly accurate *(154)*. Urine pancreatic enzyme measurements do not add incremental information above that demonstrated by serum measurements.

A similar approach has been employed for the measurement of serum pancreatic polypeptide (PP) concentrations in serum. As was the case with serum enzymes, early clinical studies reported relative diagnostic success in measuring serum concentrations after stimulation *(155)*. One study reported a sensitivity of 90% and specificity of 91% for distinguishing pancreatic insufficiency from pancreatic sufficiency after secretin stimulation *(156)*. Subsequent studies have not consistently confirmed these values *(58)*. The sensitivity, specificity, negative predictive value, and positive predictive value for fasting PP concentrations were found to be 88, 67, 88, and 66%, respectively *(157)*. Patients with mild to moderate pancreatic dysfunction can exhibit normal PP responses *(146)*. The variability in the diagnostic performance of this assay is, in part, owing to the considerable variation in the type of pancreatic stimulation, if any, employed in the testing protocol. The fact remains that patients with end-stage chronic pancreatitis can be diagnosed clinically without great difficulty. However, detection of early disease by serum tests remains difficult.

Evaluation of Pancreatic Sufficiency

Pancreatic exocrine enzymatic capacity normally possesses a 10-fold reserve. That is, malabsorption occurs only after pancreatic enzyme secretion is reduced more than 90%. For example, Fig. 3 shows the relationship of pancreatic lipase production to fecal fat output. The one is directly related to the other, and the tremendous reduction of duodenal lipase activity required to increase the fecal fact content is obvious. This relationship is similar to that seen for serum creatinine concentration and glomerular filtration rate. Chronic pancreatitis is a long-term condition taking one or two decades for a significant decrease in pancreatic output to ensue. Apparently lipase output decreases before trypsin and other proteases; therefore, steatorrhea tends to occur before azotorrhea *(147)*. Clearly, the challenge for the laboratory detection of pancreatic insufficiency is to detect it before it becomes severe.

Although it can be argued that fecal fat measurement defines steatorrhea on a population normalcy basis, some authors consider this test obsolete. Nonetheless, fecal fat measurement using a 72-h collection establishes the presence of steatorrhea. Since this can occur in both pancreatic exocrine deficiency and intestinal disease, further evaluation is warranted. Fecal weight has been evaluated as a more straightforward assessment of fat output, but this parameter fails to correlate with quantitative fecal fat values in over a quarter of cases. Over 10% of patients with steatorrhea exhibit normal fecal weights.

The value of indirect pancreatic function tests for the evaluation of pancreatic sufficiency in patients with chronic pancreatitis has been extensively studied for almost two decades. A major survey of the diagnostic accuracy of these tests was conducted at an international symposia in 1986. The results of this survey are shown in Table 7. The most commonly employed tests are fecal chymotrypsin, the NBT-PABA test, and the pancreolauryl test. The sensitivity and specificity of these tests vary significantly.

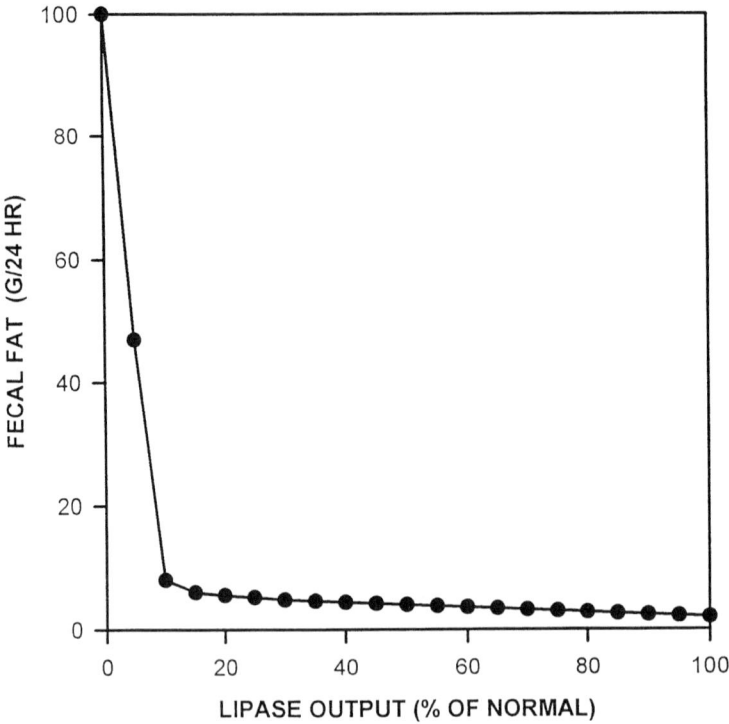

Fig. 3. The excretion of fat in stool as a function of pancreatic lipase output. Abnormal fecal fat values are >6 g/24 h.

Table 7
Sensitivity and Specificity of Indirect Pancreatic Function Tests for Pancreatic Exocrine Function—the Ulm Symposium (158)

Test	No. studies	No. subjects	Mean sensitivity	No. studies	No. subjects	Mean specificity
Fecal Chymotrypsin	4	256	84% range: 73–89%	10	361	78% range: 50–100%
NBT-PABA	2	384	87% range: 87–88%	3	255	87% range: 85–94%
Pancreolauryl	11	604	82% range: 39–100%	11	371	90% range: 55–100%

In addition to inherent differences in the diagnostic performance of these indirect tests, variations in patient selection, patient preparation, and analytical techniques introduce further differences in performance. Sensitivity and specificity alone do not demonstrate the performance of laboratory tests in the evaluation of individual patients. In particular, the tests can be dramatically different depending on the severity of pancreatic dysfunction.

The sensitivity of the NBT-PABA test, the pancreolauryl test, and fecal chymotrypsin can be related to results of duodenal aspiration analysis, the reference method for assessing residual pancreatic function. The NBT-PABA test exhibited a sensitivity of 79% when bicarbonate output was normal, but enzyme output was abnormally low and a sensitivity of 93% when both bicarbonate and enzyme output were subnormal *(159)*. The corresponding values for the pancreolauryl test were 75 and 98%, respectively; fecal chymotrypsin was abnormal 32 and 86%, respectively *(159)*. When the NBT-PABA test is compared to fecal fat output in addition to bicarbonate and enzyme output, the sensitivity increases to 97% when all three parameters are abnormal *(159)*. The pancreolauryl and fecal chymotrypsin tests sensitivities increase to 100 and 92%, respectively, when all three parameters are abnormal *(159)*. Generally, pancreatic insufficiency is graded as mild when only bicarbonate output is decreased, moderate when enzyme output is also decreased, and severe when fecal fat output is increased (steatorrhea). Indirect pancreatic function tests tend to lose sensitivity in mild disease as just illustrated.

The diagnostic performance of indirect tests must be assessed using appropriate negative patient groups. These groups should include comorbid diseases as well as patients with pancreatic disease without pancreatic insufficiency. These studies are not easy to perform, particularly if intubation analysis is employed as the reference standard. In a study of the NBT-PABA test on 72 patients with a clinical diagnosis of chronic pancreatitis, 353 patients without chronic pancreatitis were included *(160)*. The test exhibited a sensitivity of 86 and a specificity of 93% *(160)*. However, the predictive value of a positive result was 71% and the predictive value of a negative result was 97% *(160)*. That is, the NBT-PABA test tended to generate more false-positive than false-negative results. The pancreolauryl test demonstrated similar performance. By utilizing an appropriate cutoff, the pancreolauryl test has been reported to achieve 100% sensitivity, but with an accompanying 54% false-positive rate (46% positive predictive value) *(161)*. It should be mentioned that the false-positive rate is minimized by use of the multiple-stage modification of both the NBT-PABA and the pancreolauryl test. The inclusion of free PABA or PASA or fluorescein should be part of the standard test protocol to control for nonpancreatic alteration of the rate of substrate hydrolysis, metabolism, and excretion. If the indirect tests are used to "screen" patients with chronic pancreatitis for significant pancreatic insufficiency, the overall false-positive rate can be reduced by further diagnostic workup, including the secretin-CCK test.

The most promising new indirect tests for pancreatic insufficiency are carbon-isotope breath tests and the stimulated decrease in plasma amino acid concentrations. The 6-h cumulative CO_2 excretion rate after administration of a C_{13}-labeled mixed triglyceride exhibited a sensitivity for decreased lipase output of 83–89% for a lipase output of 100 and 90 kU/h, respectively *(85)*. For a lipase output of 90 kU/h, the CO_2 exhalation had a specificity of 81%, a positive predictive value of 63%, and a negative predictive value of 95%. As is the case with other indirect tests, there is a significant false-positive rate leading to a less-than-optimal predictive value of a positive result. Abnormalities have been observed in patients with diabetes mellitus and patients with chronic liver disease. The decrease in plasma amino acids after pancreatic stimulation has shown a sensitivity of 86.7% and a specificity of 100% in initial studies of patients with chronic pancreatitis *(82)*. It will be important to validate the performance of this test; it is simple to administer, and its initial diagnostic accuracy is impressive.

The radiological imaging of the pancreas is a major component of the diagnostic approach to chronic pancreatitis. The demonstration of diffuse calcification of the pancreas on a plain film of the abdomen is diagnostic (specificity = 100%), although quite insensitive (30–40%) *(147)*. Both ultrasound and CT scanning have also demonstrated adequate performance in distinguishing chronic pancreatitis from other pathologies, such as carcinoma of the head of the pancreas *(34,147)*. CT demonstrates a sensitivity of 80% and a specificity of about 90% for the diagnosis of chronic pancreatitis, whereas ultrasound has a sensitivity of 70% and specificity of also about 90% *(147)*. ERCP is now considered the "method of choice" or gold standard for confirming the diagnosis of chronic pancreatitis. The general consensus is that this technique has a sensitivity of 90% and a specificity of 100%, the latter finding necessary for a gold standard *(162)*. The reader is advised to consult radiological texts or appropriate reviews for the image findings considered diagnostic for chronic pancreatitis.

The imaging of the pancreas in patients with chronic pancreatitis may reveal areas of calcifications or cysts *(163)*. It is interesting that analysis of intraductal precipitates and calculi obtained from the pancreas in these conditions demonstrates significant amounts of immunoreactive trypsin(ogen), and this protein may contribute to the formation of pancreatic stones *(164)*.

It has been recommended that the clinical presentation of the patient with chronic pancreatitis guide the use of diagnostic laboratory tests in the evaluation of pancreatic insufficiency. If significant epigastric pain is present, ERCP can be performed prior to any laboratory testing *(35)*. However, if weight loss and diarrhea predominate, then fecal fat analysis should be performed to confirm the presence of steatorrhea, and indirect pancreatic function tests can also be preformed to assess pancreatic exocrine function before ERCP. If chronic pancreatitis is still suspected, after normal findings from an ERCP as well as from indirect function tests, then more direct evaluation using the secretin-CCK test is indicated *(35)*.

The major diagnostic dilemma concerning the evaluation of exocrine function in chronic pancreatitis is the detection of early changes in pancreatic sufficiency. In addition, there is a long period between the onset of symptoms and the diagnosis. The outcomes of early detection and treatment of pancreatic insufficiency in chronic pancreatitis are largely unknown. Nonetheless, it does not appear that laboratory tests are major indicators of minimal change disease at this point.

Patient Monitoring

The management of pancreatic insufficiency in chronic pancreatitis centers on enzyme replacement therapy. As has been mentioned, insufficiency is generally thought to occur only when pancreatic enzyme output reaches <10% of normal. The output of pancreatic lipase after a meal approaches 140,000 U/h for 4 h after a meal *(165)*. Ten percent of this output is 14,000 U/h for 4 h for a total of 56,000 U of lipase activity. Pancreatic enzyme supplement tablets contain about 2000–8000 U of lipase activity *(147)*. It is no surprise, therefore, that correction of steatorrhea is rarely accomplished since eight tablets would be required with every meal. Gastric pepsin activity can also inactivate pancreatic replacement enzymes. Duodenal sampling has shown that only 8–22% of ingested enzymes lipase and trypsin are recovered with intact activity *(147)*. This effect is apparently independent of the dosage schedule. The high dosage contributes to hyperuricemia (owing to their high purine content) and renal stone formation.

Because delivery of pancreatic lipase to the duodenum is very inefficient, the complete correction of steatorrhea is uncommon. However, most patients treated with sufficient amounts of replacement enzyme preparations become relatively asymptomatic, and the reduction of dietary fat has obvious advantages. The effective duodenal activities of amylase and lipase are increased if H_2 receptor antagonists are taken with enzyme supplements. The antagonists decrease acid production, which, in turn, decreases pepsin activity. However, this approach is recommended only if conventional supplementation is ineffective (147). The coating of pancreatic enzyme supplements with a pH-dependent coating that dissolves at pH > 5.0 has been shown to deliver enzymes to the upper small intestine intact by avoiding gastric inactivation if gastric pH does not rise above 5.0 during the postprandial period. Although several studies have failed to show a distinct advantage of enteric coating, it can still be effective in reducing steatorrhea in patients with sufficient acid secretion. If the treatment measures described are ineffective clinically, then tests of pancreatic function are indicated to assess the adequacy of replacement.

The usual approach to establish the efficacy of pancreatic supplement therapy is to determine the quantitative fecal fat output. Indirect tests can also be employed as a means of therapy assessment. However, it must be remembered that an indirect test will only assess one enzyme component of the enzyme supplement. For example, the NBT-PABA test will assess only chymotrypsin activity, and the cholesterol octanoate breath test will assess only cholesterol ester hydrolase activity. In the latter case, it has been shown that enzyme supplementation has a significant effect on $^{14}CO_2$ output (87). A ^{14}C-triolein breath test has also been used to monitor patients' response to enzyme replacement therapy (166).

Abdominal Surgeries

Surgery involving the stomach and the pancreatic–duodenal axis can disrupt the normal digestive signaling process. Although overt steatorrhea occurs in <20% of patients with chronic pancreatitis, some degree of fat malabsorption is present in at least two-thirds of these patients (167), so malabsorption can be unmasked by pancreatic surgery. Gross steatorrhea has been reported to develop in almost 40% of patients undergoing 80–90% subtotal pancreatectomy and only 20% of patients undergoing 40–80% distal pancreatectomies (168). Pancreaticojejunostomy also resulted in steatorrhea in 20% of patients after surgery. Gastric resection involving the pyloric and antrum anreas can also result in fat malabsorption owing to the loss of gastric function and presentation of appropriate chyme to the duodenum (169).

Pancreatic resections are performed to remove pancreatic islet cell tumors or cystic malignancies. The usual procedure is pancreaticoduodenectomy for removal of tumors at the head of the pancreas. This procedure also can induce functional pancreatic insufficiency, which is exacerbated by any gastric abnormalities created by operative procedures. The induction of pancreatic insufficiency can apparently occur even if the pancreas is not affected by the tumor or is otherwise normal. Pancreatic malignancies can cause pancreatic insufficiency prior to being removed. This can result from the direct obstruction of the pancreatic duct. However, it has been estimated that the proximal 40% of the pancreas is sufficient for appropriate enzyme secretions (170). Fewer than 5% of patients with pancreatic cancer exhibit pancreatic insufficiency (169).

There have been some studies to evaluate the usefulness of indirect pancreatic function tests in the assessment of pancreatic exocrine capacity after operations that significantly affect the pancreas. The ^{13}C-trioctanoin breath test has been shown to correlated with the duodenal outputs of lipase, amylase, and chymotrypsin in patients after pancreatoduodenectomy *(86)*. Sensitivities reported for the breath test, the NBT-PABA test, and fecal chymotrypsin were 93, 76, and 64%, respectively. To determine specificity of this type of testing, indirect pancreatic tests were performed on patients after undergoing gastrectomy. The specificity of the pancreolauryl test, the NBT-PABA test, plasma amino acid challenge test, and fecal chymotrypsin after gastrectomy were 10, 70, 100, and 70%, respectively *(171)*. It can be seen from these data that gastrectomy can have a significant effect on indirect tests of pancreatic function, apparently in the absence of impairment of pancreatic exocrine function.

Hereditary Pancreatitis and Inherited Enzyme Deficiencies

Several congenital causes of pancreatic dysfunction exist other than CF, all leading to pancreatic insufficiency. Hereditary pancreatitis is a known cause of chronic pancreatitis and may represent up to 10% of the incident cases of pancreatitis *(172)*. As previously discussed, the nature of the defect in hereditary pancreatitis is unknown; therefore, clinical–pathological correlations are not possible. The disease will progress to chronic pancreatitis and is treated in the manner appropriate for that condition.

There are indications that α-1-antitrypsin deficiency is associated with chronic pancreatitis and pancreatic insufficiency *(173)*. However, this association is not well established, and it remains to be definitively proven that decreased presence of this protease inhibitor can lead directly to pancreatic damage.

Shwachman Syndrome is the second most frequent cause of pancreatic hypofunction in children, and is characterized by pancreatic exocrine deficiency, neutropenia, metaphyseal dysotosis, short stature, and eczema *(172)*. The condition is relatively rate with an incidence estimated at 1 in 20,000 births, and is inherited in an autosomal-recessive manner. Infants present with failure to thrive and obvious steatorrhea. The pancreas is small and exhibits deficient secretion of enzymes even after stimulation. The pancreas also exhibits significant fatty infiltration. This syndrome should be suspected in any infant with steatorrhea without a confirmed diagnosis of CF. The diagnosis can be confirmed by a negative sweat chloride test and the presence of neutropenia. A particularly low serum immunoreactive trypsin(ogen) concentration has been described in infants with Shwachman Syndrome *(174)*. The indirect tests of pancreatic function are not well validated in these patients. The syndrome does maintain a higher level of pancreatic function than is the case in CF. The disease is treated with pancreatic enzyme replacement therapy and dietary management. Patients may improve with age, and in some, the pancreatic insufficiency may normalize.

The Johanson–Blizzard Syndrome consists of congenial malabsorption, deafness, hypothyroidism, and dwarfism. The disease is quite rate with only about 20 cases reported. The abnormalities of the pancreas are similar to those observed in Shwachman Syndrome *(172)*. Patients with Johanson-Blizzard Syndrome also exhibit decreased pancreatic secretion of trypsin, lipase/colipse, and low serum immunoreactive trypsin(ogen) concentrations *(175)*. Much of the normal pancreatic tissue is replaced by fat, and the disorder appears to be a result of improper acinar development *(176)*.

Inherited deficiency of pancreatic lipase has been described in several individuals *(177)*. These patients exhibit profound steatorrhea without creatorrhea and have greasy, foul-smelling stools *(172)*. Oil droplets are observed in the stool as well. These symptoms appear early in life, but significant nutritional deficiency is not observed. Alternative triglyceride hydrolase activities must provide sufficient lipid hydrolysis, such that fatty acid deficiencies severe enough to prevent growth do not occur. There is complete absence of immunoreactive lipase in the pancreas, and the diagnosis may be confirmed by demonstration of the absence of lipase with normal amounts of trypsin and amylase in duodenal fluid after cholecystokinin-secretin stimulation *(172,178)*. An inherited deficiency in colipase has also been reported. These individuals were found to have normal amounts of lipase, amylase, trypsin, and chymotrypsin activity in the duodenum. They also exhibited fat malabsorption that was corrected by the administration of purified colipase *(172)*.

An inherited deficiency of amylase only has also been reported *(179)*. However, some of the patients thought to have such a deficiency subsequently normalized their amylase activity *(179)*. It appears that amylase activity in children requires time to reach normal expression in some cases. Therefore, it is unclear if a true deficiency state exists. Congenital deficiency in trypsinogen has been described in several infants characterized by failure to thrive, hypoproteinemia, edema, and anemia *(180)*. However, the absence of enterokinase has the same consequences and this condition has also been reported *(181)*. Analysis of duodenal fluid reveals decreased trypsin activity, but normal amylase and lipase activities after stimulation. The diagnosis of enterokinase deficiency can be confirmed by addition of exogenous enterokinase *(172)*. Administration of pancreatic enzyme supplements obviates the need for enterokinase supplementation, because the former contain trypsin, not trypsinogen and do not require endogenous activation.

Intestinal Disease

It is obvious that pancreatic exocrine function is but one step in the overall process of the digestion and absorption of essential nutrients from ingested food. Therefore, in many cases, the failure to demonstrate adequate absorption may be owing to either pancreatic exocrine dysfunction or intestinal dysfunction. These causes are usually termed maldigestion and malabsorption in order to distinguish the nature of the problem. Patients with either of these conditions may present with generalized malnutrition and weight loss. There might be evidence of iron, folate, or vitamin deficiencies. These can lead to overt nutritional anemias or bleeding disorders. Depending on the degree of protein malnutrition, edema could be present. Electrolyte imbalance or dehydration can result in weakness or a decrease in mentation. Abdominal symptoms may be present, and these include diarrhea, flatus, and distention. When steatorrhea is present, stools may be loose, foul-smelling, and greasy. Presentation during the early course of these diseases is less obvious. Patients may exhibit only a mild weight loss accompanied by slight changes from normal stool consistency. Patients may be fatigued or have a changed attitude toward eating, but these symptoms are very nonspecific.

The intestinal diseases that may be confused with pancreatic exocrine insufficiency are listed in Table 8. Differentiating steatorrhea and malabsorption may require an

Table 8
Nonpancreatic Malabsorption Syndromes

Decreased intestine bile acid concentration
    Hepatic disease
    Bacterial overgrowth
    Ileal resection or inflammation
    Calcium carbonate
    Cholestryramine
    Intestinal resection or bypass
Lymphatic obstruction
    Primary mucosal defects
        Regional enteritis
        Eosinophilic enteritis
        Tropical sprue
        Infectious enteritis
        Collagenous sprue
        Celiac sprue
    Endocrine disorders
        Diabetes mellitus
        Hyperthyroidism
        Zollingen-Ellison Syndrome
        Carcinoid

assessment of pancreatic exocrine function using direct stimulation, indirect testing, and radiological examination of the pancreas.

Several approaches used to differentiate steatorrheas resulting from pancreatic insufficiency from those owing to intestinal disease have been described. The determination of fecal fat concentration has been advocated for this purpose. About 40% of patients with pancreatic exocrine hypofunction have fecal fat concentrations <10 g% *(96)*. However, most patients with nonpancreatic steatorrhea exhibited fecal fat concentrations from 8.3–9.5 g%, yielding a diagnostic sensitivity of no more than 60% at complete specificity (100%) for this test *(96)*. Other investigators have achieved similar results when comparing steatorrhea owing to pancreatic disease with that caused by celiac sprue *(182)*.

SUMMARY

Diseases of the exocrine pancreas result from the inability of this organ to produce and secrete sufficiently effective pancreatic fluid. Pancreatic exocrine cells produce a fluid rich in bicarbonate and digestive enzymes. This fluid is secreted in response to neurological and hormonal signals after the ingestion of food. The fluid enters the duodenum via the pancreatic duct where it contributes a vital role in the digestion of food. The bicarbonate-rich fluid adjusts the pH of the partially digested food or chyme arriving from the stomach, insuring an environment that is optimal for hydrolytic enzyme action.

Pancreatic enzymes include those that catalyze the cleavage of protein peptide bonds (trypsin, chymotrypsin, carboxypeptidase, and elastase), those that cleave lipid ester bonds (lipase, phospholipase, and carboxy ester hydrolase), those that cleave glycosidic bonds of polysaccharides (amylase), and those that cleave phosphodiester bonds of nucleic acids (nucleases).

Clinical laboratory tests that have been developed to diagnose pancreatic exocrine disease can be classified as either direct or indirect as well as either provocative or nonprovocative. Direct tests for pancreatic insufficiency measure pancreatic fluid and electrolyte output or pancreatic enzyme output. These tests are usually performed on pancreatic fluid aspirated from the duodenum after stimulation of the pancreas with a test meal or infusion of secretin and cholecystokinin. Measurement of amino acids in serum shows promise as a convenient test. Indirect tests include the NBT-PABA and Pancreolauryl tests that allow the measurement of cleavage products of ingested pancreatic enzyme substrates in urine. Breath tests have also been proposed but the indirect diagnostic standard for pancreatic insufficiency remains the measurement of fecal lipid excretion.

Diseases affecting pancreatic exocrine function include inherited conditions (cystic fibrosis, Shwachman Syndrome) and chronic pancreatitis. These conditions are characterized by abdominal pain and steatorrhea. The use of laboratory tests to evaluate pancreatic sufficiency is hampered by their poor sensitivity.

REFERENCES

1. Owyang C, Williams (1991) Pancreatic secretion. In: Textbook of gastroenterology, Yamada T, ed., Philadelphia, PA, J.B. Lippincott, pp. 294–314.
2. Fahrenkrug J, Schaffalitzky OB, Rune SJ (1978) pH threshold for release of secretin in normal subjects and in patients with duodenal ulcer and patients with chronic pancreatitis. Scand J Gastroenterol 13:177–183.
3. Beglinger C, Fried M, Whitehouse I (1984) Pancreatic enzyme responses to a liquid meal and to hormonal stimulation. J Clin Invest 75:1471–1474.
4. Guyton AC (1986) Textbook of medical physiology, Philadelphia, PA: W.B. Saunders, p. 777.
5. Lowe ME (1994) The structure and function of pancreatic enzymes. In: Physiology of the gastrointestinal tract, 3rd ed, Johnson LR, ed. New York: Raven, pp. 1531–1542.
6. Rovery M (1988) Limited proteolyses in pancreatic chymotrypsinogens and trypsinogens. Biochimie 70:1131–1135.
7. Owyang C, Louie DS, Tatum D (1986) Feedback regulation of pancreatic enzyme secretion in man: suppression of cholecystokinin release by trypsin. J Clin Invest 77: 2042–2047.
8. Rinderknecht H (1986) Activation of pancreatic zynogens. Dig Dis Sci 31:314–321.
9. Travis J, Salvesen GS (1983) Human plasma proteinase inhibitors. Annu Rev Biochem 52:655–709.
10. Alberts B, Bray D, Lewis J, Raff M, Roberts K, Watson JD (1989) Molecular biology of the cell, 2nd ed., New York: Garland, p. 411.
11. Guy O, Lombardo D, Bartalt D, Amic J, Figarella C (1978) Two human trypsinogens. Purification, molecular properties and N-terminal sequences. Biochemistry 9:1669–1679.
12. Itkonen O, Koivunan E, Hurme M, Alfthan H, Schroder T, Stenman U-H (1990) Time-resolved immunofluorometric assays for trypsinogen-1 and -2 in serum reveal preferential elevations of trypsinogen-2 in pancreatitis. J Lab Clin Med 115:712–718.
13. Figarella F, Amouric M, Carrere J, Miszczuk-Jamska B, Guy-Crotte O (1984) Pancreatic proteins in normal state and pancreatic diseases in pancreatic juice and blood. Ric Clin Lab 14:349–359.

14. Emi M, Nakamura Y, Ogawa M (1986) Cloning, characterization and nucleotide sequences of two c DNAs encoding pancreatic trypsinogens. Gene 41:305–310.
15. Craik CS, Roczniak S, Largman C, Rutter WJ (1987) The catalytic role of the active site aspartic acid in serine proteases. Science 237:909–913.
16. Graf L, Craik CS, Patthy A, Roczniak S, Fletterick RJ, Rutter WJ (1987) Selective alteration of substrate specificity by replacement of aspartate A with lysine in the binding pocket of trypsin. Biochemistry 26:2616–2623.
17. Craik CS, Largman C, Fletcher T, Roczniak S, Barr PJ, Fletteride R, Rutter WJ (1985) Redesigning trypsin: alteration of substrate specificity. Science 228:291–297.
18. DeCaro A, Figarella C, Guy O (1975) the two human chymotrypsinogens. Purification and characterization. Biochem Biophys Acta 379:431–441.
19. Fletcher TS, Wei-Fang S, Largman C (1987) Primary structure of human pancreatic elastase 2 determined by sequence analysis of the cloned mRNA. Biochemistry 26: 7256–7261.
20. Janoff A (1985) Elastase in tissue injury. Ann Rev Med 36:207–216.
21. Christianson DW, Lipscomb WN (1986) X-ray crystallographic investigation of substrate binding of carboxypeptidase A at subzero temperature. Biochemistry 83:7568–7572.
22. Pascual R, Burgos FJ, Salva M, Soriano F, Mendez E, Aviles FX (1989) Purification and properties of five different forms of human procarboxypeptidases. Eur J Biochem 179: 609–616.
23. Terashima H, Atomic Y, Ohnistic N (1989) Characterization of human pancreatic kallikrein. Adv Exp Med Biol 247B:177–182.
24. Seigner C, Prodanov E, Marchis-Mouren G (1987) The determination of substrate binding energies of porcine pancreatic α-amylase by comparing hydrolytic activity towards substrates. Biochem Biophys Acta 913:200–209.
25. Winkler FK, D'Arcy A, Hunziker W (1990) Structure of human pancreatic lipase. Nature 343:771–774.
26. Erlanson-Albertsson C (1992) Pancreatic colipase-structural and physiological aspects. Biochem Biophys Acta 1125:1–7.
27. Reue K, Zambaux J, Wong H. et al. (1991) cDNA cloning of carboxyl ester lipase from human pancreas reveals a unique proline-rich repeat unit. J Lipid Res 32:267–276.
28. Gelb MH, Jain MK, Hanel AM, Berg OG (1994) Interfacial enzymology of glycerolipid hydrolases: Lessons from secreted phospholipases A_2. Annu Rev Biochem 64:653–688.
29. van den Berg B, Tessari M, de Haas GH, Verheis HM, Boelens R, Kaptein R (1995) Solution structure of procine pancreatic phospholipase A_2. EMBO J 14:4123–4131.
30. Nevalainen TJ (1993) Serum phospholipase A_2 in inflammatory disease. Clin Chem 39: 2453–2459.
31. Weickmann JL, Elson M, Glitz DG (1981) Purification and characterization of human pancreatic ribonuclease. Biochemistry 20:1272–1278.
32. Celinski A, Naskalski JW, Sanajd J, Nowacki G (1990) Poly-C avid ribonuclease, but not RNA-avid ribonuclease increases in serum of patients with acute pancreatitis [Abstract]. Clin Chem 36:1143.
33. Naskalski JW, Sznajd J, Popiela T, Kedra B, Krzemien D (1990) Poly-C ribonuclease in detection of acute necrotizing pancreatitis [Abstract]. Clin Chem 36:114.
34. Green JA, Barkin JS (1994) The exocrine pancreas. Curr Gastroenterol 14:115–153.
35. Lankisch PG (1993) Function tests in the diagnosis of chronic pancreatitis. Int J Pancreatol 14:9–20.
36. Skude G (1977) On human amylase isoenzymes. Scand J Gastroenterol; Suppl 44:1–37.
37. Berk JE, Ayulo JA, Fridhandler L (1979) Value of pancreatic-type isoamylase assay as an index of pancreatic insufficiency. Dig Dis Sci 24:6–10.
38. Fahrenkrug J, Magid E (1980) Concentration of immunoreactive trypsin and activity of pancreatic isoamylase in serum compared in pancreatic disease. Clin Chem 26:1573–1576.

39. Bank S (1992) P amylase is always greater than S in spot urine of normal subjects: diagnostic implications. Int J Pancreatol 11:191–194.
40. Lott JA, Patel ST, Sawhney AK, Kazmierczak SC, Love JE Assays of serum lipase: analytical and clinical considerations. Clin Chem 32:1290–1302.
41. Gumaste V, Dave P, Sereny G (1992) Serum lipase: a better test to diagnose acute alcoholic pancreatitis. Am J Med 92:239–242.
42. Fabris C, Basso D, Panozzo MP, Del Favero G, Maggiato T, Plebani M, Ferrara C, Fogar P, Zaninotto M, Naccarato R (1992) Urinary phospholipase A2 excretion in chronic pancreatic diseases. Int J Pancreatol 11:179–184.
43. Brown KS, Kingsbury WD, Hall NM, Dunn GL, Gilvarg C (1987) Determination of carboxypeptidase A using N-Acetyl-phenylalanyl-3-thiaphenylalanine as substrate: application to a direct serum assay. Anal Biochem 161:219–225.
44. Kazmierczak SC, Van Lente F (1989) Measuring carboxypeptidase A activity with a centrifugal analyzer: analytical and clinical considerations. Clin Chem 35:251–255.
45. Goldberg DM (1983) Enzymes and isoenzymes in the evaluation of diseases of the pancreas. In: Clinical and analytical concepts in enzymology, Homburger HA, ed., Skokie, IL: College of American Pathologists; pp. 31–56.
46. Kimland M, Russick C, Marks WH, Bortstrom A (1989) Immunoreactive anionic and cationic trypsin in human serum. Clin Chim Acta 184:31–46.
47. Andriulli A, Masoero G, Felder M, Vantini I, Petrillo M, Caballini G, Bianchi PG, Dobrilla G, Verme G (1981) Circulating trypsin-like immunoreactivity in chronic pancreatitis. Dig Dis Sci 26:532–537.
48. Steinberg WM, Goldstein SS, David ND, Anderson KK, Shammala JM (1985) Predictive value of a low serum trypsinogen. Dig Dis Sci 30:547–551.
49. Durie PR, Forstner GG, Gaskin KJ, Moore DJ, Cleghorn GJ, Wong SS, Corey ML (1986) Age-related alterations of immunoreactive pancreatic cationic trypsinogen in sera from cystic fibrosis patients with and without pancreatic insufficiency. Pediatr Res 20:209–213.
50. Rinderknecht H, Renner IG, Carmack C (1978) Trypsinogen variants in pancreatic juice of healthy volunteers, chronic alcoholics and patients with pancreatitis and cancer of the pancreas. Gut 20:886–891.
51. Borgstrom A, Ohlsson K (1976) Radioimmunological determination and characterization of cathodal trypsin-like immunoreactivity in normal human plasma. Scand J Clin Lab Invest 36:809–814.
52. Hedstrom J, Leinoner J, Sainio V, Senmon U-H (1994) time-resolved immunofluorometric assay of trypsin-2 complexed with alpha-1-antitrypsin in serum. Clin Chem 40: 1761–1765.
53. Koehn HD, Mostbeck A (1981) Age-dependence of immunoreactive trypsin concentrations in serum [Letter]. Clin Chem 27:502.
54. Moffat A, Marks V, Gamble DR (1980) Serum immunoreactive trypsin concentrations in diabetic children. J Clin Pathol 33:871–975.
55. Andriulli A, Masoero G, Fico D, Zayo P, Marchetto M (1986) Evocative test of serum pancreatic enzymes to bombesin in chronic pancreatitis. Am J Gastroenterol 81:562–565.
56. Lankisch PG, Marthey G, Otto J, Koop H, Talawicar M, Willins B (1982) Exocrine pancreatic function in diabetes mellitus. Digestion 25:211–216.
57. Moss DW, Henderson AR (1994) Enzymes. In: Tietz textbook of clinical chemistry, 2nd ed., Burtis CA, Ashwood ER, eds., Philadelphia, PA: W.B. Saunders; pp. 871–876.
58. Lawson N, Chesner I (1994) Tests of exocrine pancreatic function. Ann Clin Biochem 31:305–314.
59. Lesi C, Melzi D'Eril DV, Scotta MS, Zonil, Malagniti P (1988) A new fecal chymotrypsin method for evaluating the exocrine pancreatic function in different pancreatic diseases. Int J Pancreatol 203–208.

60. Durr HK, Otte M, Forrell MM, Bode JC (1978) Fecal chymotrypsin: a study on its diagnostic value by comparison with the secretin-cholecystokinin test. Dig 404–409.
61. Gutierrez LV, Baron JH (1972) A comparison of Boots and GIH secretin as stimuli of pancreatic secretion in human subjects with or without chronic pancreatitis. Gut 13: 721–725.
62. Gullo L, Pezzilli R, Ventrucci M, Barbara L (1990) Caerulein induced plasma amino acid decrease: a simple, sensitive, and specific test of pancreatic function. Gut 31: 926–929.
63. Durr GH-K (1984) The secretin-pancreozymin (caerulin)-test. Methodological problems. In: Pancreatities—concepts and classification, Gyr KE, Singer MX, Sorles H, eds., Amsterdam: Excerpta Medica, pp. 261–266.
64. Otte M (1979) Pankreasfunktionsdiagnostik. Internist 20:331–340.
65. Heij HA, Obertop H, van Blankenstein M, Nix GAJJ, Westbroek DL (1987) Comparison on endoscopic retrograde pancreatography with functional and histological changes in chronic pancreatitis. Acta Radiol 28:289–293.
66. Lankisch PG (1981) Exocrine pancreatic function tests. Gut 23:777–798.
67. Henderson AR, Tietz NW, Rinker MS (1994) Gastric, pancreatic, and intestinal function. In: Tietz textbook of clinical chemistry, 2nd ed., Burtis CA, Ashwood ER, eds., Philadelphia, PA: WB Saunders; pp. 1604–1616.
68. Hoek FJ (1988) The PABA test for evaluation of exocrine pancreatic function: a review of the literature. Neth J Med 32:143–156.
69. Scharpe S, Iliano L (1987) Two indirect tests of exocrine pancreatic function evaluated. Clin Chem 33:5–12.
70. Mitchell CJ, Humphrey CS, Bullen AW, Kelleher J, Losowsky MS (1979) Improved diagnostic accuracy of a modified oral pancreatic function test. Scand J Gastroenterol 14:737–741.
71. Berg JD, Chesner IM, Allen-Narker RA, Buckley BM, Lawson N (1986) Exocrine pancreatic function as determined in a same day test with use of bentiromide and *p*-aminosalicylic acid. Clin Chem 32:1010–1012.
72. Lang C, Gyr K, Tonko I, Conen D, Stadler GA (1984) Value of serum PABA as a pancreatic function test. Gut 408–512.
73. Tanner AR, Robinson DP (1988) Pancreatic function testing: serum PABA measurement is a reliable and accurate measurement of exocrine function. Gut 29:1736–1740.
74. Lankisch PG, Brauneis J, Otto J, Goke B (1986) Pancreolauryl and NBT-PABA tests. Are serum tests more practical alternatives to urine tests in the diagnosis of exocrine pancreatic insufficiency? Gastroenterology 90:350–354.
75. Weizman Z, Forstner G, Gaskin K, Kopelman H, Wong S, Durie P (1985) Bentiromide test for assessing pancreatic dysfunction using analysis of *p*-aminobenzoic acid in plasma and urine. Gastroenterology 89:596–604.
76. Libeer JC, Scharpe SL, Verkerk RM, Deprettere AJ, Schepens PJ (1981) Simultaneous determination of p-aminobenzoic acid, acetyl-*p*-aminobenzoic acid and *p*-aminohippuric acid in serum and urine by capillary gas chromatography with use of a nitrogen-phosphorus detector. Clin Chim Acta 115:119–123.
77. Lawson N, Berg JD, Chesner I (1985) Liquid-chromatographic determination of *p*-aminobenzoic acid in plasma to evaluate exocrine pancreatic function. Clin Chem 31: 1073–1075.
78. Cavallini G, Piubello W, Brocco G, Micciolo R, Chech G, Angelini G, Venini L, Riela A, Dalle Molle L, Vartini I, Scuro LA (1985) Serum PABA and fluorescein in the course of PABA and pancreolauryl test as an index of exocrine pancreatic insufficiency. Dig Dis Sci 30:655–663.
79. Malfertheiner P, Buchler M, Muller A, Ditschuneit H (1987) Fluorescein dilaurate serum test: a rapid, tubeless pancreatic function test. Pancreas 2:53–60.

80. Malfertheiner P, Bucher M, Muller A, Ditschuneit H (1987) Fluorescein dilaurate-serum test nach metoclopramid-und. sekretinstimulation zur pankreasfunktionsprufung. Beitrag zur diagnose der chronischen pankreatis. Z Gastroenterol 25:225–232.
81. Domeschke S, Heptner G, Kolb S, Sailer D, Schneider MU, Domschke W (1986) Decrease in plasma amino acid level after secretin and pancreozymin as an indictor of exocrine pancreatic function. Gastroenterology 90:1031–1038.
82. Gullo L, Pezzili R, Ventrucci M, Barbara L (1990) Caerulein induced plasma amino acid decrease: a simple, sensitive, and specific test of pancreatic function. Gut 31:926–929.
83. Gilinsky NH (1989) Pancreatic function testing. Postgrad Med 86:165–172.
84. Benini L, Senro LA, Menini E (1984) Is the ^{14}C-triolein breath test useful in the assessment of malabsorption in clinical practice? Digestion 29:91–97.
85. Van trappen GR, Rutgeerts PJ, Ghoos YF, Hiele MI (1989) Mixed triglyceride breath test: a non-invasive test of pancreatic lipase activity in the duodenum. Gastroenterology 96:1126–1134.
86. Kato H, Nakao A, Kishimoto W, Nanami T, Harada A, Hayakawa T, Takagi H (1993) ^{13}C-labeled trioctanoin breath test for exocrine pancreatic function-test in patients after pancratoduodenectomy. Am J Gastroenterol 88:64–69.
87. Cole SG, Rossi S, Stern A, Hofmann AF (1987) Cholesterol octanoate breath test. Preliminary studies on a new noninvasive test of human pancreatic exocrine function. Gastroenterology 93:1372–1380.
88. Chen WL, Morishita R, Eguchi T, Kawai T, Sakai M, Tateishi H, Uchino H (1989) Clinical usefulness of dual-label schilling test for pancreatic exocrine function. Gastroenterology 96:1337–1345.
89. Leung JWC, Frost RA, Burgess K, Braganza JM, Slater DM, Cotton PB (1988) Modified dual label Schilling test for pancreatic exocrine function. Clin Chim Acta 174:93–100.
90. Lee MJ, Crook T, Noel C, Levinson, UM (1994) Detergent extraction and enzymatic analysis for fecal long-chain fatty acids, triglycerides and cholesterol. Clin Chem 40:2230–2234.
91. Simko V (1981) Fecal fat microscopy: acceptable predictive value in screening for steatorrhea. Am J Gastroetnerol 75:204–208.
92. Pedersen NT, Halgreen H (1985) Simultaneous assessment of fat maldigestion and fat malabsorption by a double isotope method using fecal radioactivity. Gastroenterology 88:47–54.
93. Koumantakis G, Radcliff FJ (1987) Estimating fat in feces by near-infrared reflectance spectroscopy. Clin Chem 33:502–506.
94. Schneider MV, Demling L, Jones SA, Barker PJ, Domschke S, Heptner G, Domschke W (1987) NMR spectroscopy. A new method for total stool fat quantification in chronic pancreatitis. Dig Dis Sci 32:494–499.
95. Li Y, Chiverton SG, Hunt, RH (1989) Exocrine pancreatic function tests. J Clin Gastroenterol 376–378.
96. Bai JC, Andrush A, Matelo G, Martinez C, Vazquez H, Boerr L, Sambuelli A (1989) Fecal fat concentration in the differential diagnosis of steatorrhea. Am J Gastroenterol 84:27–30.
97. Roberts IM, Poturich C, Wald A (1986) Utility of fecal fat concentrations as screening test in pancreatic insufficiency. Dig Dis Sci 31:1021–1024.
98. Fine KD, Fordtran JS (1992) The effect of diarrhea on fecal fat excretion. Gastroenterology 102:1936–1939.
99. The LB, Stopard M, Anderson S, Grant A, Quantrill D, Wilkinson RH, Jewell DP (1983) Assessment of fat malabsorption. J Clin Pathol 36:1362–1366.
100. Heeley AF, Watson D (1983) Cystic Fibrosis—Its biochemical detection. Clin Chem 29:2011–2018.

101. Sferra TJ, Collins FS (1993) The molecular biology of cystic fibrosis. Annu Rev Med 133–144.
102. Boat TF, Welsh MJ, Baendet AL (1989) Cystic fibrosis. In: The Metabolic Basis of Inherited Disease, 6th ed., Scriver CR, et al. eds., New York: McGraw-Hill, pp. 2649–2680.
103. Welsh MJ (1990) Abnormal regulation of ion channels in cystic fibrosis epithelia. FASEB J 4:2781–2725.
104. Rommens JM, Iannuzzi MC, Karem B, Drumm ML, Melmer G, Dean M, Rozmahel R, Cole JL, Kennedy D, Hidaka N, Zsiga M, Buchwald M, Riordan JR, Tsui L, Collins FS (1989) Identification of the cystic fibrosis gene: chromosome walking and jumping. Science 245:1059–1065.
105. Zielenski J, Rozmahel R, Bozon D, Karem B, Grzelczak Z (1991) Genomic DNA sequence of the cystic fibrosis transmembrane conductance regulator (CFTR) gene. Genomics 10:214–228.
106. Riordan JR, Rommens JM, Kerem B, Alon N, Rozmahel R, Grzelczak Z, Zielenski J, Lok S, Plavsic N, Chou J, Drumm ML, Iannuzzi MC, Collins FS, Rsui L (1989) Identification of the cystic fibrosis gene: cloning and characterization of complementary DNA. Science 245:1066–1073.
107. Trezise AEO, Buchwald M (1991) In vivo cell-specific expression of the cystic fibrosis transmembrane conductance regulator. Nature 353:434–437.
108. Kerem B, Rommens JM, Buchanan JA, Markiewicz D, Cox TK, Chakravarti A, Buchwald M, Tsui L (1989) Identification of the cystic fibrosis gene: genetic analysis. Science 245:1073–1080.
109. The Cystic Fibrosis Genetic Analysis Consortium. (1990) Worldwide survey of the ΔF508 mutation—Report from the Cystic Fibrosis Genetic Analysis Consortium. Am J Hum Genet 47:354–359.
110. Ng ISL, Pace R, Richard MV, Kobayashi K, Kerem B, Tsui L, Beaudet AC (1991) Methods for analysis of multiple cystic fibrosis mutations. Hum Genet 87:613–617.
111. Kristidis P, Bozon D, Corey M, Markiewicz D, Rommens J, Tsui L, Durie P (1992) Genetic determination of exocrine pancreatic function in cystic fibrosis. Am J Hum Genet 50:1178–1184.
112. Strong TV, Smit LS, Turpin SV, Cole JL, Tom Hon C, Markiewicz D, Petty TL, Craig MW, Rosenow EC, Tsui L, Iannuzzi MC, Knowles MR, Collins FS (1991) Cystic fibrosis gene mutation in two sisters with mild disease and normal sweat chloride electrolyte levels. N Engl J Med 325:1630–1634.
113. Anguiano A, Oats RD, Amos JA, Dean M, Gerrard B, Stewart C, Maher TA, White MB, Milunsky A (1992) Congenital bilateral absence of the vas deferens. JAMA 267:1794–1797.
114. Canadian Task Force on the Periodic Health Examination. (1991) Periodic health examination, 1911 update: 4. Screening for cystic fibrosis, Can Med Assoc J 145:629–635.
115. Crossley JR, Smith PA, Edgar BW, Gluckman PD, Elliott RB (1981) Neonatal screening for cystic fibrosis, using immunoreactive trypsin assay in dried blood spots. Clin Chim Acta 113:111–121.
116. Crossley JR, Eliott RB, Smith PA (1979) Dried-blood spot screening for cystic fibrosis in the newborn. Lancet 1:472–474.
117. Hammond KB, Abman SH, Sokel RJ, Accurso FJ (1991) Efficacy of statewide neonatal screening for cystic fibrosis by assay of trypsinogen concentrations. N Engl J Med 325:769–774.
118. Rock MJ, Mischler EH, Farrell PM, Wei L, Bruns WT, Hassemer DJ, Laessig RH (1990) Newborn screening for cystic fibrosis is complicated by the age-related decline in immunoreactive trypsinogen levels. Pediatrics 85:1001–1007.
119. Statement for the National Institutes of Health Workshop on Population Screening for the Cystic Fibrosis gene. (1990) N Engl J Med 323:70–71.

120. Rosenstein BJ, Langbaum TS (1982) Sweat sodium and chloride values. J Pediatr 1001–1002.
121. Webster HL (1983) Laboratory diagnosis of cystic fibrosis. CRS Crit Rev Clin Lab Sci 18:313–338.
122. LeGrys VA, Burnett RW (1994) Current status of sweat testing in North America. Results of the College of American Pathologists need assessment survey. Arch Pathol Lab Med 118:865–867.
123. LeGrys VA, Barlow WK, Bracey A, Gibson LE, Hammond KB, Kraft K, Rosenstein BJ (1993) Sweat Testing: Sample Collection and Quantitative Analysis. NCCLS Document C 34-P.
124. Gibson LE, diSant'Agnese PA, Schwachman H (1985) Procedure for the quantitative iontophoretic sweat test for cystic fibrosis. Cystic Fibrosis Foundation.
125. Hardy JD (1973) Sweat tests in the newborn period. Arch Dis Child 48:316–318.
126. Rosentstein BJ, Langbaum TS (1982) Sweat testing in CF: Not to be taken lightly. J Respir Dis 3:71–76.
127. Kerem E, Corey M, Karem B, Rommens J, Markiewicz D, Levison H, Tsui L, Durie P (1990) The relation between genotype and phenotype in cystic fibrosis-analysis of the most common mutation. N Engl J Med 323:1517–1522.
128. Green MN, Clarke JT, Schwachman H (1958) Studies in CF; protein pattern in meconium ileus. Pediatrics 21:635–637.
129. Hellsing K, Barrljung K, Ceder O, Kollberg H (1982) Meconium screening for cystic fibrosis. An eight-year follow-up study. Acta Paediatr Scand 71:827–832.
130. Roberts IM (1990) Disorders of the pancreas in children. Gastroenterol Clin North Am 19:963–973.
131. Gaskin KJ, Durie RR, Lee L, Hill R, Forstner GG (1984) Colipase and lipase secretion in childhood-onset pancreatic insufficiency: delineation of patients with steatorrhea secondary to relative colipase deficiency. Gastroenterology 86:1–7.
132. Waters DL, Dorney SFA, Gaskin KJ, Gruca MA, O'Halloran M, Wilcken B (1990) Pancreatic function in infants identified as having cystic fibrosis in a neonatal screening program. N Engl J Med 322:303–308.
133. Johansen HK, Nir M, Hoiby N, Koch C, Schwartz M (1991) Severity of cystic fibrosis in patients homozygons and heterozygous for Δ508 mutation. Lancet 337:631–634.
134. Nousia-Arvanitakis S, Arvanitakis C, Desai N, Greenberger NJ (1978) Fecal chymotrypsin compared with PABA test. J Pediatr 734–737.
135. Brown GA, Sule D, Williams J, Puntis JW, Booth IW, McNeish AS (1988) Fecal chymotrypsin: a reliable index of exocrine pancreatic function. Arch Dis Child 63:785–789.
136. Puntis JW, Berg JD, Buckley BM, Booth IW, McNeish AS (1988) Simplified oral pancreatic function test. Arch Dis Child 63:780–784.
137. Hubbard VS, Wolf RO, Lester LA, Egge AC (1984) Diagnostic and therapeutic applications of bentiromide screening test for exocrine pancreatic insufficiency in patients with cystic fibrosis. Comparison with other tests of exocrine pancreatic disease. Dig Dis Sci 29:881–889.
138. Dalzell AM, Heaf DP (1990) Fluorescein dilaurate test of exocrine pancreatic function in cystic fibrosis. Arch Dis Child 65:788–789.
139. Green RM, Austin S, McClena P, Jolliffe S, Weaver LT (1995) Spot urine pancreolauryl test for use in infancy. Arch Dis Child 72:233–234.
140. Green MR, Austin S, Weaver LT (1993) Dual marker one day pancreolauryl test. Arch Dis Child 68:649–652.
141. Cummings JGR, Forsyth JS, Boyd EJS, Frost GJ, Cuschieri A (1986) Diagnosis of exocrine pancreatic insufficiency in cystic fibrosis by use of fluorescein dilaurate test. Arch Dis Child 61:573–575.

142. Forsyth JS (1991) Fluorescein dilaurate test of exocrine pancreatic function in cystic fibrosis [Letter]. Arch Dis Child 66:273.
143. Couper RT, Corey M, Moore DJ, Fisher LJ, Forstner GG, Durie PR (1992) Decline of exocrine pancreatic function in cystic fibrosis patients with pancreatic sufficiency. Pediatr Res 32:179–182.
144. Couper RT, Corey M, Durie PR, Forstner GG, Moore DJ (1995) Longitudinal evaluation of serum trypsinogen measurement in pancreatic-insufficient and pancreatic-sufficient patients with cystic fibrosis. J Pediatr 127:408–413.
145. Heijerman HG, Lamers CB, Bakker W, Dijkman JH (1993) Improvement of fecal fat excretion after addition of omeprazole to pancreas in cystic fibrosis is related to residual exocrine function of the pancreas. Dig Dis Sci 38:1–6.
146. Puntis JWL (1993) Dual marker one day pancreolauryl test [Letter]. Arch Dis Child 69:471.
147. Owyang C, Levitt M (1990) Chronic pancreatitis. In: Textbook of gastroenterology, Yamada T, ed. Philadelphia, PA, J.B. Lippinoctt; pp. 1874–1893.
148. Goebell H, Bode CH, Bastran R (1970) Clinisch asymptomatische funktion storungen des exokuinen pankreas bei chromischen alkoholikern. Dtch Med Wochenschr 95: 808–810.
149. Van Lente F (1993) Free radicals. Anal Chem 374R–377R.
150. Mathew P, Wyllie R, Van Lente F, Caulfield M, Michener W (1991) Antioxidant levels in hereditary pancreatitis [Abstract]. Pediatr Res 29:108A.
151. Delhaye M, Engelholm L, Cremer M (1985) Pancreas divisum: Is it a normal anatomic variant or anomaly. Gastroenterology 89:951–960.
152. Adrian TE, Barnes AJ, Bloom SR (1979) Hypotrypsinemia in diabetes mellitus. Clin Chim Acta 97:213–216.
153. Masoero G, Andriulli A, Bianco A, Benitti V, Marchetto M, De La Pierre M (1982) Diagnostic accuracy of serum cationic trypsinogen estimation for pancreatic diseases. Dig Dis Sci 27:1089–1094.
154. Otte M, Thurmayr R, Thurmayr GR, Forell MM (1976) Diagnostic value of the provocative test with secretin and cholecystokinin/pancreozymin. Scand J Gastroenterol Supp 41 11:88.
155. Owyang C, Scarpello JH, Vinik AI (1982) Correlation between pancreatic enzyme secretion and plasma concentration of human pancreatic polypeptide in health and in chronic pancreatitis. Gastroenterology 83:55–59.
156. Stern AI, Hansky J (1981) Secretin stimulated pancreatic polypeptide: a test for chronic pancreatitis. Aust NZ J Med 11:351–354.
157. Koch MB, Go VL, Dimagno EP (1985) Can plasma human pancreatic polypeptide be used to detect disease of the exocrine pancreas? May Clin Proc 259–265.
158. Malfertheimer P, Ditschuneit H, eds. (1986) Prognostic procedures in pancreatic disease, Berlin, Springer.
159. Lankisch PG, Schreiber A, Otto J (1983) Pancreolauryl test. Evaluation of a tubeless pancreatic function test in comparison with other indirect and direct tests for exocrine pancreatic function. Dig Dis Sci 28:490–493.
160. Lang C, Gyr K, Stadler GA, Gillessen D (1981) Assessment of exocrine pancreatic function by oral administration of *N*-benzoyl-L-tyrosyl-*p*-aminobenzoic acid (Bentiromide): 5 years clinical experience Br J Surg 68:771–775.
161. Boyd EJ, Cumming JG, Cuschieri A, Wood RA, Wormsley KG (1982) Prospective comparison of the fluorescein-dilaurate test with the secretin-cholecystokmin test for pancreatic exocrine function. J Clin Pathol 35:1240–1243.
162. Brayanza JM, Hunt LP, Warwick F (1982) Relationship between pancreatic exocrine function and ductal morphology in chronic pancreatitis. Gastroenterology 1341–1345.

163. Searles H (1986) Etiopathogenesis and definition of chronic pancreatitis. Dig Dis Sci 31: 915–1075.
164. Hayakawa T, Kondo T, Shibata T, Kitagawa M, Nakae Y, Hayakawa S (1994) Trypsin(ogen) content of pancreatic calculi in chronic calcified pancreatitis in man. Dig Dis Sci 39:1345–1350.
165. DiMagno EP, Go VLW, Summerskill WHJ (1973) Relations between pancreatic enzyme outputs and malabsorption in severe pancreatic insufficiency. N Engl J Med 288: 813–817.
166. O'Keefe SJ, Adam J (1984) Assessment of adequacy of pancreatic enzyme replacement with the multiple-phase carbon-14-triolein test. S Afr Med J 66:763–765.
167. Frey CF (1981) Role of subtotal pancreatectomy and pancreticojejunostomy in chronic pancreatitis. J Surg Res 31:361–365.
168. Frey CF, Child CG, Fry W (1976) Pancreatectomy for chronic pancreatitis. Ann Surg 184:403–405.
169. Doty JE, Fink AS, Meyer JH (1989) Alterations in digestive function caused by pancreatic disease. Surg Clin North Am 69:447–465.
170. Dimagno EP, Malagelada JR, Go VLW (1979) The relationships pancreatic ductal obstruction and pancreatic secretion in man. May Clin Proc 54:157–162.
171. Heptner G, Domshcke S, Domschke W (1989) Exocrine pancreatic function after gastrectomy. Specificity of indirect tests. Gastroenterology 97:147–153.
172. Liddle RA (1991) Congenital and hereditary diseases of the pancreas. In: Textbook of gastroenterology, Yamada T, ed. Philadelphia, PA, J.B. Lippincott, pp. 1937–1951.
173. Novis BH, Bank S, Young GO, Marks IN (1975) Chronic pancreatitis and alpha-1-antitrypsin. Lancet 2:748–749.
174. Dossetor JF, Spratt HC, Rolles CJ, Seem CP, Heeley AF. (1989) Immunoreactive trypsin in Schwachman's syndrome. Arch Dis Child 64:395–396.
175. Jones NL, Hofley PM, Durie PR (1994) Pathophysiology of the pancreatic defect in Johanson-Blizzard syndrome: a disorder of acinar development. J Pediatr 125:406–408.
176. Daentl DL, Frias JL, Gilbert EF, Opitz JM (1979) The Johanson-Blizzard syndrome: Case report and autopsy findings. Am J Med Genet 3:129.
177. Muller DP, McCollum JP, Trompeter RS, Harries JT (1975) Proceedings: Studies on the mechanism of fat absorption in congenital isolated lipase deficiency. Gut 16:838.
178. Figarella C, Negri GA, Sarles H (1972) Presence of colipase in congenital pancreatic lipase deficiency. Biochem Biophys Acta 280:205–210.
179. Lowe C, May DC (1951) Selective pancreatic deficiency: absent amylase, diminished trypsin, and normal lipase. Am J Dis Child 82:459.
180. Morris MD, Fisher DA (1967) Trypsinogen deficiency disease. Am J Dis Child 114: 203–205.
181. Tarlow MJ, Hadorn B, Arthurton MW, Lloyd JK (1970) Intestinal enterokinase deficiency. A newly recognized disorder of protein digestion. Arch Dis Child 45:651–656.
182. Lembcke B, Grimm K, Lankisch PG (1987) Raised fecal fat concentration is not a valid indicator of pancreatic steatorrhea. Am J Gastroenterol 82:526–531.

3
Biochemical Indicators of Acute Pancreatitis

Steven C. Kazmierczak

INTRODUCTION

One of the earliest biochemical markers employed for the diagnosis of a particular disease state was reported in 1916 by Stocks *(1)*, who suggested that amylase activity in blood and urine was a sensitive and reliable test for various pancreatic disorders. Since this time, numerous other enzymatic markers of pancreatic disease have been described. Although there is a large body of literature indicating that some of these other tests may provide better diagnostic accuracy of acute pancreatitis when compared with serum amylase, none of these newer tests have replaced amylase. Amylase remains among one of the top 20 most frequently requested clinical assays and is an important component of emergency laboratory services *(2)*. Recent studies, however, have demonstrated that other markers in addition to amylase offer greater clinical specificity for the diagnosis of acute pancreatitis and should replace amylase as the primary test for this disease. As stated by Tietz, "old myths die hard" *(3)*. It will probably take years before the diagnostic utility of these other tests are recognized. This section reviews the diagnostic utility of both the commonly used and more esoteric indicators of acute pancreatitis. The analytes most frequently employed for the diagnosis of acute pancreatitis include amylase and the pancreatic isoenzyme of amylase and lipase. The markers infrequently used, but that may provide good diagnostic and/or prognostic information, include trypsin, phospholipase A (PLA), carboxypeptidase A, and lipase isoforms. Also discussed are some key issues related to the correct interpretation of these tests in certain pathophysiological states such as renal failure. In addition, the utility of some of these studies in the investigation of the etiology of an attack of acute pancreatitis is also reviewed.

AMYLASE

Measurement of serum amylase has long been considered the test of choice in the evaluation of patients with suspected acute pancreatitis. Amylase activities rise within the first 12–24 h following an attack of acute pancreatitis and then decline steadily to normal values over the next 4–7 d. Since amylase is eliminated via renal excretion, patients with impaired renal function may exhibit longer elimination times for the enzyme.

Amylase has widespread acceptance by clinicians for the diagnosis of pancreatic disease. The test can be performed inexpensively and rapidly using instrumentation

From: *Clinical Pathology of Pancreatic Disorders* Edited by: J. A. Lott Humana Press Inc., Totowa, NJ available in most hospital laboratories. Unfortunately, however, the specificity of amylase for the pancreas is poor. Amylase is found in a number of tissues in addition to the pancreas, including the salivary glands, fallopian tubes, and small intestine. Thus, patients presenting with abdominal pain and increased amylase activities in serum may not have pancreatitis. Instead these patients may have hyperamylasemia secondary to intestinal obstruction or ischemia, or disorders affecting the fallopian tubes. It is important to differentiate acute pancreatitis from these other disorders owing to differences in treatment modalities. Patients with the benign condition of macroamylasemia, in which amylase is bound to serum immunoglobulins, may present with greatly increased serum amylase activities, but without other signs or symptoms suggestive of pancreatitis. The incidence of this disorder has been estimated to be 0.5–2.0% of the general population. The combination of immunoglobulin and enzyme results in the formation of a protein complex that is too large to be cleared by the kidneys, and may also prevent or delay elimination via the reticuloendothelial system. Determination of the amylase:creatinine clearance ratio can help in the identification of hyperamylasemia owing to macroamylasemia. However, the amylase:creatinine clearance ratio does not offer any advantage over serum amylase in the diagnosis of acute pancreatitis and should be abandoned for this purpose (4). In addition to the high rate of false-positive test results obtained using serum amylase activity, the finding of acute pancreatitis and normal amylase activities is common (5). Patients with acute pancreatitis owing to ethanol abuse may present with normal or just mild increases in serum amylase activities.

The nonspecificity of amylase for the pancreas can be overcome by analysis of amylase isoenzymes. Amylase seen in many of the disease states causing an increase in serum amylase activities is usually owing to increases in the salivary isoenzymes. The pancreas has the highest concentration of amylase per gram of tissue, and also contains the greatest total amount of amylase relative to any other amylase-containing organ in the body. Amylase is not absorbed by intact gut mucosa. Thus, normal serum concentrations of amylase are derived from leakage of the enzyme into the blood from the pancreatic acinar cells, or via lymphatic drainage from the pancreas or salivary glands. Obstruction of the pancreatic ducts or pancreatic inflammation results in increased cellular enzyme leakage into the blood or the lymphatics. Disorders, which cause an increase in the permeability of the gut mucosa, or cases whereby perforation or rupture of the gastrointestinal tract occurs, may result in the release of large quantities of fluid into the peritoneal or pleural space. This fluid containing large amounts of amylase is eventually drained via the lymphatics into the systemic circulation causing hyperamylasemia (6).

Since the pancreas contains the highest concentration of enzyme per gram of tissue, and is the largest organ containing amylase, acute pancreatitis should result in the greatest increase of enzyme activity in the blood when compared with other disorders associated with increased amylase activity. Many studies have cited the sensitivity and specificity of amylase for acute pancreatitis to be well over 90% when interpreted in conjunction with an appropriate clinical picture (7,8). These values are usually obtained using amylase cutoff values that are four to five times the upper range of the normal reference interval. Thus, when using the Phadebas method for amylase, which has a normal reference interval of 70–300 U/L, many authors consider amylase values of at least 1000–2000 U/L to be diagnostic of acute pancreatitis *(9,10)*. Other studies indicate that amylase is diagnostic of acute pancreatitis when values exceed 2 to "several times" the upper reference interval *(11)*. However, many studies base sensitivities and specificities of amylase for acute pancreatitis on values that exceed the upper range of the normal reference interval only.

Since the diagnostic criteria for acute pancreatitis are loosely defined, a wide range of sensitivities and specificities for amylase have been reported. Another factor influencing these parameters is the use of initial or peak enzyme activities when evaluating the diagnostic performance of these markers. One common approach used in assessing the diagnostic accuracy of amylase and lipase is to evaluate these markers using peak enzyme activities selected retrospectively from serial measurements. However, this type of evaluation of the diagnostic utility is unrealistic; the diagnosis of a life-threatening event, such as acute pancreatitis, requires that medical decisions be based on enzyme findings obtained at admission or early in the course of the disease. The use of peak enzyme data usually leads to falsely increased claims for sensitivity and specificity of the test. Use of peak data may also change the optimal decision threshold of the marker, compared with evaluations based on enzyme data obtained at admission. Use of enzyme data at admission may result in lower reported test sensitivity because of the time delay between the onset of clinical symptoms and appearance of abnormal concentrations in the blood.

A number of studies have challenged the primary diagnostic role of amylase for acute pancreatitis. Many have advocated the use of serum lipase as the primary biochemical test for this disease. In addition, assays for a variety of other pancreatic enzymes, including trypsin, phospholipase A, elastase, and carboxypeptidase, have been developed in order to improve the biochemical diagnosis of acute pancreatitis. However, recent data suggest that when appropriate cutoff intervals are used, the amylase activity obtained at admission may have a diagnostic accuracy for acute pancreatitis equivalent to other available biochemical markers *(8,12,13)*. One recent study evaluated initial, peak, and serial amylase and lipase activities for the diagnosis of acute pancreatitis using a multivariate data approach *(13)*. Analysis of enzyme data by use of a multivariate technique permits a more accurate and unbiased assessment of test utility, because patients can be classified with respect to disease status by use of all available enzyme data. Multivariate approaches, such as those that employ neural networks, classify patients with respect to disease status on the basis of the diagnostic patterns in amylase and lipase that may be subtle and not readily appreciated by human observation. Analysis of both amylase and lipase obtained from over 500 patients has shown that when peak enzyme activities are used for evaluating the diagnostic accuracy of these enzymes, lipase shows significantly better diagnostic utility *(13)*. However, when initial enzyme activities are considered only, no significant difference in diagnostic accuracy between amylase and lipase can be demonstrated. These differences in diagnostic accuracies obtained using either initial or peak enzyme activities may help explain much of the controversy in the literature surrounding the relative merits of amylase vs lipase.

However, evaluation of serial amylase and lipase data by use of neural network analysis reveals significantly better diagnostic utility for lipase than for amylase when serial enzyme data are considered *(13)*. Diagnosis of acute pancreatitis by use of a neural network that used serial lipase data showed greater diagnostic accuracy for acute pancreatitis than either initial, peak, or serial amylase activity. A major limitation of data analysis using neural networks is that rules and representations that the system develops during the process of data evaluation are not readily available to the user. Almost all understanding of the functioning of the neural network comes from observation of the data input into the system (i.e., serial amylase or lipase results) and how the system assigns patients with respect to disease status. In addition, although the neural network may identify patterns in the data that may be useful for the diagnosis of acute pancreatitis, these patterns may not be apparent to the user of the system.

Controversy still exists regarding the diagnostic information gained from the simultaneous measurement of amylase and lipase vs measurement of either enzyme alone. Previous work using a neural network approach showed that serial amylase and lipase measurements did not provide greater diagnostic accuracy for pancreatitis when compared to serial lipase measurements alone *(13)*. However, amylase in conjunction with lipase provided significantly better diagnostic accuracy compared to serial amylase measurements. Another recent study addressing this issue evaluated the initial amylase and lipase results using "AND" and "OR" rules and discriminant function analysis *(12)*. This approach also demonstrated that combinations of both amylase and lipase offer no advantages over using lipase results alone. However, use of a logistic regression discriminant function was found to offer statistically significant superior performance over lipase alone. The successful clinical application of such an approach would necessitate the formulation of a discriminant function rule specific to the particular local population of patients and analytical techniques used for measuring amylase and lipase activity.

Amylase Isoenzymes

The recognition that amylase is produced by multiple tissues, in addition to the pancreas, requires that extreme caution be used in the interpretation of abnormal amylase activities. Whereas an increased serum amylase activity may be a very sensitive indicator of pancreatic injury, the marker suffers from lack of specificity. Hyperamylasemia has been associated with several nonpancreatic disorders that may mimic clinical pancreatitis. These include ruptured ectopic pregnancy, perforated peptic ulcer, appendicitis, choledocholithiasis, and mesenteric artery infarction *(14)*. The vast majority of patients presenting with abdominal pain suggestive of acute pancreatitis and an abnormal value for serum amylase activity will be assigned a diagnosis of acute pancreatitis. However, one study found that only one-third of such patients actually had pancreatitis *(15)*. Patients presenting with abdominal pain associated with alcohol use and who show an abnormally increased serum amylase may be overdiagnosed with acute pancreatitis to an even greater extent. Only 15% of patients of patients falling into the aforementioned category were actually found to have biochemical evidence of acute pancreatitis *(16)*. The use of total amylase only in the evaluation of patients with suspected acute pancreatitis is associated with a high rate of overdiagnosis of the disease. In addition, some patients with acute pancreatitis may present with normal or just mild increases in amylase activity. Although this situation occurs infrequently, it may be seen in patients who present several days after the onset of the disease when amylase activities have declined back into the normal range. In these patients, underdiagnosis of acute pancreatitis is possible.

Attempts to improve the specificity of serum amylase for the diagnosis of acute pancreatitis have led to the development and use of the amylase:creatinine clearance ratio, and the determination of amylase isoenzymes by a variety of methods, including electrophoresis, inhibition of the salivary isoenzyme with use of lectins, and immunoinhibition methods with use of monoclonal antibodies (MAbs) directed against the salivary isoenzyme.

Amylase in serum can usually be separated by electrophoresis into two major fractions termed salivary (S) or pancreatic (P). In turn, each S- and P-type isoenzyme fraction may show three distinct isoform fractions. Three pancreatic isoforms (P_1, P_2, P_3) and three salivary isoforms (S_1, S_2, S_3) may be seen. Except for the P_1 isoform fraction, which is thought to represent a genetic variant, all the other amylase isoforms are produced as a result of posttranslational modification of the P_2 and S_1 forms *(17)*. In patients with acute pancreatitis, the typical findings include a dominant increase in total P-type isoenzyme fraction. This increase can be noted by visual or densitometric review of the electrophoretic gel or by increases in P-type activity measured using quantitative methods.

Detection of the P_3 isoform following electrophoretic separation of amylase has been advocated as a specific marker of acute pancreatitis. This fraction is presumed to occur in patients with acute pancreatitis owing to intrapancreatic proteolytic modification of the other pancreatic isoform fractions. However, the P_3 isoform has been shown to be present in approx 40% of patients with chronic renal insufficiency, limiting its usefulness in this patient population *(18)*. False-positive findings for the P_3 isoform have also been reported in patients with biliary tract disease and in patients with necrosis of the bowel *(19)*. The mechanism by which P_3 is produced in these other disease states is not clear. It has been previously suggested that the P_2 isoform released from the biliary tract or bowel could be modified to produce the P_3 isoform. Although the P_3 isoform may be observed in patients with renal insufficiency or abdominal pain owing to causes other than pancreatitis, the absence of the P_3 isoform virtually excludes a diagnosis of acute pancreatitis.

The determination of the P_3 isoform is further hampered by the fact that its presence on electrophoretic gels is often masked by the S_1 isoform. Insufficient separation of the S_1 and P_3 isoform often does not permit the quantitation of either isoform by densimetric methods. A method used to determine the presence of P_3 accurately has been developed *(20)*. The method developed to measure the P_3 isoform more accurately is the P_3 index. The P_3 index is a measure of the ratio of the P_3 isoform to the S_1 isoform. Normal patients and those with abdominal pathology mimicking pancreatitis, but who do not have the disease typically show a P_3 index >80%.

The P_3 index was developed following early observations that the distance of electrophoretic migration between the main pancreatic isoform, P_2, and the next anodal fraction, P_1, is approx 60% of the distance between the P_2 and S_1 isoform peaks obtained using a standard solution *(20)*. The standard solution is prepared from salivary gland and pancreatic tissue. As a patient with pancreatitis recovers, the distance between the P_2 and P_1 peak increases, and this increase is owing to the gradual disappearance of the P_3 isoform. The P_3 index is calculated as follows:

$$P_3 \text{ index } (\%) = (\text{Distance between } P_2 \text{ and } P_1/\text{Distance between } P_2 \text{ and } S_1) \times 100 \quad (1)$$

Early studies on the diagnostic utility of the P_3 isoform indicated that its determination of this marker may provide better diagnostic accuracy for acute pancreatitis than total amylase or lipase activities *(21)*. However, later studies using greater numbers of patients with a variety of abdominal disorders showed that the P_3 isoform has the same diagnostic accuracy for acute pancreatitis as lipase *(19)*. Use of both the P_3 isoform and lipase in combination does not provide any additional diagnostic information compared with single enzyme determinations.

Similar diagnostic accuracy has also been noted between total pancreatic isoamylase and lipase activities for acute pancreatitis. When appropriate reference cutoffs are applied, lipase and pancreatic amylase demonstrate diagnostic efficiencies of 0.94 and 0.93, respectively *(22)*. The importance of utilizing appropriate reference cutoffs for these indicators of pancreatitis deserve special emphasis. Several investigators describe a "gray zone" that lies between the upper normal reference interval and the cutoff value, which provides the greatest diagnostic efficiency as determined by receiver operator characteristic curve analysis. Recent studies have shown that this "gray zone" is approximately four to five times the upper limit of the normal reference interval *(19,22)*.

In summary, it has been readily shown that total pancreatic amylase activity and the P_3 isoform fraction are equivalent to total lipase activity for the diagnosis of acute pancreatitis. Determination of the P_3 isoform by electrophoretic separation of the various amylase isoforms is both labor-intensive and not amendable to the rapid reporting of test results; these factors severely limit its clinical utility *(23)*. Rapid and accurate measurement of the total pancreatic isoamylase fraction can be readily accomplished with automated immunochemical techniques employing MAbs.

LIPASE

Pancreatic lipase is often considered to be a more sensitive and specific marker for acute pancreatitis compared with total amylase. Until relatively recently, lipase was infrequently requested by clinicians. The test has a long history of being difficult to perform and having poor precision. However, most commercially available assays for lipase now incorporate the important cofactor called colipase. Colipase is present in the blood of patients with pancreatitis, but in concentrations that are highly variable and usually well below what is required to activate pancreatic lipase fully *(24)*. Thus, the addition of colipase has greatly improved the diagnostic utility of lipase on both analytical and clinical grounds. Extremely abnormal lipase values appear to be pathognomonic for pancreatitis. In assays that utilize the colipase cofactor, the increase in lipase is much more pronounced yielding greater diagnostic power of the test.

Early reports on lipase indicated that the enzyme became increased in serum following increases in amylase and returned to within the normal reference interval before amylase. However, recent studies using lipase measured by procedures containing the colipase cofactor suggest that lipase increases sooner, and remains increased longer than amylase *(25)*. The magnitude of increase in lipase above the upper reference limit in patients with acute pancreatitis can vary dramatically depending on what analytical assay is utilized for its measurement. Discrepancies as great as 13 times the upper reference limit cutoff have been observed among the various assays *(26)*. Although results between different assays may correlate, the presence of a strong correlation between different assays does not mean that identical diagnostic accuracies exist between the different methods. For lipase, marked differences in catalytic activity may be observed between the different analytical assays that are available. These differences may have profound effects on the diagnostic accuracy that can be achieved.

Much has been written on the diagnostic utility of lipase vs that of amylase. This topic has been addressed in the Amylase section of this chapter. Recent studies have attempted to utilize the differences in the serum activities of amylase and lipase in order to distinguish among the different causes of pancreatitis, specifically pancreatitis owing to ethanol abuse and pancreatitis owing to biliary obstruction *(27,28)*. The amylase response in patients with acute pancreatitis has been noted, in general, to be lower in ethanol-induced pancreatitis compared to other pathogenesis. It has been suggested that the smaller increase in amylase in patients with ethanol-induced pancreatitis is owing to a chronically diseased pancreas and little amylase reserve in the gland. However, patients with ethanol-induced pancreatitis can produce significant increases in serum lipase activities similar to those observed in patients with pancreatitis owing to other causes *(27)*. This finding does not lend support to the suggestion that a chronic insult to the pancreas owing to repeated ethanol ingestion causes a selective decrease in pancreas amylase activities. Other mechanisms have been proposed to explain the difference in amylase activities seen in alcoholic vs nonalcoholic acute pancreatitis. A difference in the mechanism by which amylase and lipase reach the blood following pancreatic injury might be different in the alcoholic vs the nonalcoholic patient *(27)*. It should be noted however that the clinical utility of the ratio of lipase activity to amylase activity as a means for distinguishing acute pancreatitis owing to ethanol abuse from acute pancreatitis owing to other pathogenesis is still under investigation. Some studies have found this ratio not to be useful in determining the pathogenesis of the disease *(29)*.

The early discrimination of biliary obstruction and acute pancreatitis from pancreatitis owing to other causes, such as ethanol, is essential owing to differences in management of those with biliary pancreatitis. Patients with acute pancreatitis owing to biliary obstruction may be at greater risk for the evolution of pancreatic edema to hemorrhage and necrosis. Persistent ampullary obstruction has been shown to increase the severity of the attack. Thus, a rapid and noninvasive method for differentiating patients with pancreatitis owing to biliary obstruction from other causes has gained considerable interest. In addition to the ratio of lipase to amylase, other markers that have been evaluated for determining the pathogenesis of acute pancreatitis include aspartate and alanine aminotransferase, alkaline phosphatase, γ-glutamyltransferase, and total bilirubin.

Obstruction of the biliary tract causes a rapid increase in pressure within the bile duct with consequent liver cell damage, and release of aspartate and alanine transaminase. Increases in alkaline phosphatase and total bilirubin have also been noted, although significant increases in these tests may not occur if the bile duct is obstructed only transiently. Following passage or removal of the obstruction, a sudden decrease in biliary pressure occurs with rapid normalization of enzyme activities in serum. The rapidity and transient nature of enzyme changes seen in patients with pancreatitis owing to biliary obstruction make it imperative that frequent serial determinations of these analytes be performed. It has been demonstrated previously that aspartate and alanine aminotransferase, as well as amylase may decrease from peak activities that are 10–15 times the upper reference interval to within the normal reference interval within 24 h following removal of a gallstone that has been obstructing the biliary passages *(28)*. The speed by which these enzyme changes occur may explain why some studies fail in their attempts to utilize biochemical markers for the determination of the pathogenesis of acute pancreatitis *(29,30)*.

One recent study that evaluated a series of different biochemical markers for determining the pathogenesis of acute pancreatitis found that alanine aminotransferase was the best test for correctly identifying patients with acute pancreatitis resulting from biliary obstruction from those with pancreatitis owing to other causes *(28)*. In addition to alanine aminotransferase, the only other test that could discriminate biliary from other causes of acute pancreatitis was the ratio of lipase to amylase.

Lipase Isoforms

Measurement of isoenzymes or isoforms of enzymes (e.g., creatinine kinase, lactate dehydrogenase, amylase) can provide diagnostic information that has greater utility than that provided by the total enzyme activity. Pancreatic lipase isoforms have recently been shown also to provide diagnostic information that is much better than that provided by total enzyme activity *(31)*. Pancreatic lipase consists of at least three isoforms that can be separated by electrophoresis. The three lipase isoforms present in pancreatic fluid include L1 and L2, which appear to be pancreatic lipase owing to their reactivity with human antipancreatic lipase antibody. The third isoform, L3, is believed to be cholesterol esterase. The L1 and L2 isoforms are probably posttranslational variants of a single enzyme form. Previous work has shown that human pancreatic juice contains two pancreatic isolipases having isoelectric pHs of 5.80 and 5.85 *(32)*. No immunological differences between the L1 and L2 forms have been shown. It has been speculated that the L2 isoform represents a (pro) colipase complex released from the injured pancreas. Ordinarily, colipase is undetectable in serum because it is presumed to be cleared rapidly from the circulation *(33)*. Detection of an activated form of colipase within this complex may be useful in predicting the presence of peripancreatic fat necrosis or the development of systemic complications related to lipolysis *(34)*. Further work in increasing the current understanding of lipase isoforms and their diagnostic as well as prognostic utility is needed.

The L2 lipase isoform has been shown to have a sensitivity of 100% in patients with acute pancreatitis *(31)*. However, up to 70% of patients with disorders involving the liver or biliary tract have been found to contain the L2 isoform in serum. This finding has been suggested to be the result of extreme sensitivity of the pancreas to inflammation of nearby organs. For the diagnosis of acute pancreatitis, total lipase and the L2 isoform show essentially the same diagnostic sensitivity, although the diagnostic accuracy of L2 appears to be better *(31)*.

TRYPSIN

Trypsin is produced primarily by the pancreas; a very small amount is found in Paneth cells in the intestine *(35)*, and its measurement should provide a specific diagnosis of acute pancreatitis. Once released into the serum, trypsin is immediately complexed by its two main protease inhibitors, α-2-macroglobulin and α-1-protease inhibitor. The majority of the trypsin–α-2-macroglobulin complexes are quickly metabolized by the reticuloendothelial system. Immunoassays developed to quantitate trypsin measure primarily circulating trypsinogen or the α-1-protease inhibitor complexes. Thus, immunoassays fail to differentiate between active enzyme (trypsin) and the parent zymogen (trypsinogen). Specific identification of the α-1-protease inhibitor–trypsin complex in serum may help in the identification of patients with acute, severe pancreatitis who have had release of active protease enzymes into the circulation. Assays that measure both the active and inactive enzyme do not allow this. Thus, the current immunoassays that measure all forms of the enzyme are probably not better at diagnosing acute pancreatitis compared to the standard enzyme assays, such as amylase or lipase.

The recent development of an assay that measures α-2-macroglobulin–trypsin complexes only has been shown to be useful for diagnosing pancreatitis owing to ethanol from pancreatitis resulting from other causes (36). Patients with pancreatitis due to causes other than ethanol were found to have no increase in serum trypsin activity, whereas high concentrations of active trypsin were found in patients with acute alcoholic pancreatitis.

The mechanism by which ethanol-induced pancreatitis causes increased serum trypsin concentrations is not known. Chronic consumption of ethanol can increase the synthesis of trypsinogen, resulting in greater concentrations of the enzyme in pancreatic juice than is found in nondrinkers of ethanol. Another reason may be owing to decreased clearance of the α-2-macroglobulin–trypsin complex by the reticuloendothelial system resulting from ethanol. Further investigation validating these initial studies is warranted.

Another assay designed to measure the amount of trypsinogen that becomes activated in acute pancreatitis utilizes antibodies directed against the C-terminal end of trypsinogen activation peptide. This peptide is produced following activation of trypsinogen to trypsin. The trypsinogen activation peptide is excreted rapidly in the urine. Its measurement in the urine thus provides a useful way for gauging the amount of trypsinogen that has been activated. Peak urinary concentrations of trypsinogen activation peptide occur between 12 and 24 h following the onset of symptoms. Concentrations are much greater in patients with severe disease compared to those with mild disease. Since trypsin can activate proPLA to PLA, it has been suggested that severe acute pancreatitis results from the activation of proPLA by trypsin (37).

PHOSPHOLIPASE A

PLA has been recommended as a useful marker for gauging the severity of acute pancreatitis (38). The enzyme is secreted by the pancreas in an inactive form, and activation by trypsin follows proteolytic cleavage of an activation peptide. Circulating active PLA is thought to attack phospholipids in cells and lung surfactant leading to the development of systemic complications (39). The activity of PLA in serum has therefore been advocated as an indicator of disease severity; greatly increased concentrations are associated with severe hemorrhagic forms of the disease and lesser increases are found in the mild edematous types.

A number of different assays have been developed for the measurement of PLA. Radioimmunological procedures measure concentration of the enzyme, and these values most closely parallel the course of amylase and lipase activity in patients with acute pancreatitis *(40)*. Enzymatic assays have also been developed, and they measure enzyme activity based on the liberation of fatty acids from phospholipid substrates. Catalytic activity of PLA does not necessarily correlate with amylase or lipase activities. This finding has been suggested to indicate that increases in PLA found in patients with necrotizing pancreatitis are not pancreas-derived. Many studies have reported increased PLA activities in association with a wide variety of nonpancreatic disorders including sepsis, malignancy, myocardial infarction, and hematological diseases *(39,41)*.

Recent investigations into the diagnostic and prognostic utility of PLA activity suggest that measurement of catalytic enzyme activity is not always useful in patients with acute pancreatitis *(42)*. Enzyme values were found to be markedly increased in a wide variety of conditions not involving the pancreas. Substantial concentrations of PLA have also been found in leukocytes, and activation of those cells with release of active enzyme into the circulation may explain the increased PLA activities seen in patients with nonpancreatic inflammatory diseases. In addition, association has been demonstrated between an increase in mortality and increased PLA catalytic activity *(41)*. This finding is consistent with the assertion that the significant increases in PLA in serum seen in patients with severe forms of acute pancreatitis are not necessarily derived from the pancreas. Any increase in PLA activity usually occurs late in the course of the disease after the clinical course of the patient has deteriorated considerably.

CARBOXYPEPTIDASE A

Carboxypeptidase A is a pancreatic enzyme that cleaves carboxy-terminal amino acids from proteins. The enzyme shows dramatic increases in the serum following the onset of acute pancreatitis *(43)*. Substantial carboxypeptidase A activity is found in the pancreas with minor amounts (<1% of that found in pancreas) found in intestinal tissue *(43)*. When compared with amylase and lipase, carboxypeptidase A is the most tissue-specific enzyme. Patients with pancreatitis show much greater increases in carboxypeptidase A activity above the upper reference interval compared with amylase and lipase. Mean peak amylase, lipase, and carboxypeptidase A activities in patients with pancreatitis were found to be 9, 23, and 40 times the upper reference limit, respectively. Carboxypeptidase A also increases faster than and remains increased longer than amylase or lipase in patients with pancreatitis.

Techniques developed for measurement of carboxypeptidase A include quantitation of L-phenylalanine released from the substrate by use of affinity chromatography *(44)* and an automated colorimetric method *(45)*. Although the colorimetric method is simple to perform and adaptable to automation, the procedure is subject to severe negative interference by glucose and bilirubin. At bilirubin concentrations of only 30 mg/L, carboxypeptidase A activity is decreased to one-half of its original activity. Glucose concentrations >2000 mg/L show similar negative effects. The effect of these interferents can be eliminated by substitution of an enzymatic, kinetic reaction for the colorimetric indicator reaction *(43)*.

Comparison of the diagnostic utility of carboxypeptidase A with that of amylase and lipase shows that all three enzymes exhibit similar diagnostic accuracies. Although carboxypeptidase A is more specific for the pancreas than amylase or lipase, the presence of renal insufficiency leads to much more frequent increases in the serum activity of this marker when compared with amylase or lipase. The molecular mass of carboxypeptidase A is 35,000 Da, which is less than that of amylase (50,000 Da) and lipase (38,000 Da). Currently, the routine application of carboxypeptidase A measurements for the evaluation of acute pancreatitis is probably not warranted.

ETIOLOGY OF ACUTE PANCREATITIS

Acute pancreatitis can present with a wide spectrum of signs and symptoms ranging from mild discomfort to severe prostration with multiple organ failure. The variability in the presentation of acute pancreatitis and its clinical course has necessitated the establishment of classification schemes in order to provide a basis for the study and treatment of acute pancreatitis and its complications (46).

Throughout the years a number of classification systems have been proposed. Early systems were based primarily on clinical criteria, and classified pancreatitis into acute and chronic forms of the disease. Further expansion of this system gave rise to a third category, chronic relapsing pancreatitis, that was later broadened to cover the wide variety of clinical presentations ranging from painless presentation to the severe fatal form of the disease. Although this classification scheme is easily implemented, it does little to identify the etiologic factors responsible for the development of the disease. In particular, it does not allow an appreciation for the natural course of the disease and the diagnostic and therapeutic aspects that the various etiologies of the disease entail. Identification of the etiology of an attack of acute pancreatitis is essential to prevent recurrences and possible complications. It was only natural that the clinical classification schemes give rise to classification schemes based on etiologic factors. The etiologic factors that have been implicated in the pathogenesis of acute pancreatitis are numerous and varied. A recent review of the subject lists close to 70 conditions that have the potential of initiating acute pancreatitis (47). Unfortunately, given the great number of recognized etiological factors, little is known about the actual mechanisms by which these factors precipitate acute pancreatitis. The etiologic categories can be defined under the general headings of pancreatic duct obstruction, drugs and toxins including ethanol, metabolic causes, trauma, including postsurgical and blunt force, anatomic abnormalities, and idiopathic.

Drugs and Toxins

Reports of drug-induced pancreatitis first appeared in the mid- to late 1950s, when it was noted that cortisone and thiazides could induce acute pancreatitis (48,49). Since then, published reports have identified approx 50 drugs that may be directly responsible for inducing acute pancreatitis (50). The incidence of drug-induced pancreatitis is estimated at <2% (50). A higher incidence has been observed in patients with diseases usually associated with acute pancreatitis. Thus, patients with pre-existing inflammatory bowel disease may experience drug-induced pancreatitis at a rate two to three times greater than that seen in patients without inflammatory bowel disease.

Little information is available concerning the pathogenesis or dose relationship between certain drugs and pancreatitis. For some drugs, a slight relationship has been shown between drug use and the onset of pancreatitis, whereas for others, a very strong association exists. Drugs associated with pancreatitis may be classified into one of three groups: definite association with pancreatitis, possible association, and drugs proposed as causing pancreatitis, but documented evidence for a causal relationship is lacking (51).

Drugs reported to show a definite association with pancreatitis include azathioprine, chlorothiazide, estrogens, furosemide, sulfonamides, tetracycline, and valproate. For all these compounds, pancreatitis develops in some patients taking the drug and disappears following drug withdrawal. In many cases, pancreatitis again develops following reintroduction of the drug. Additional evidence has been obtained from studies of the incidence of pancreatitis in treated and untreated control populations and studies in control and experimental animals given the drug.

Drugs for which an association with pancreatitis is thought to exist include L-asparaginase, corticosteroids, ethacrynic acid, phenformin, and procainamide. For many of these drugs, pancreatitis developed in patients who frequently had serious underlying disease and were on a regimen of multiple drugs. For some compounds, it is often difficult to show a direct relation between a particular drug and pancreatitis owing to these confounding factors.

The majority of drugs fall into the category of "proposed as causing pancreatitis, but lacking in strong documented evidence." Drugs falling into this category include amphetamines, cholestyramine, propoxyphene, histamine, indomethacin, isoniazid, mercaptopurine, opiates, rifampicin, salicylates, cimetidine, and acetaminophen. At present, further documented information regarding the relationship between these drugs and pancreatitis is needed.

Pancreatitis in association with HIV infection with or without the acquired immunodeficiency syndrome (AIDS) has been reported with increasing frequency over the past several years. Acute pancreatitis was once considered to be uncommon in AIDS patients; however, recent studies indicate an increasing incidence of pancreatitis of up to 30% (52). Autopsy studies in patients with AIDS indicate abnormalities in the pancreas in up to 50% (53). Pathologic changes include pancreatic inflammation, fibrosis, and hemorrhage. Opportunistic infection may affect the pancreas in 10% of these individuals.

Biochemical abnormalities in patients with AIDS, such as hyperamylasemia, and hyperlipasemia are frequently found. Up to half of these patients may demonstrate enzyme abnormalities, but otherwise appear asymptomatic; the amylase in these patients is frequently of salivary origin (52). Even though these patients may appear asymptomatic, the finding of increased amylase and lipase activities in the sera of patients taking $2',3'$ dideoxyinosine (ddI) may indicate subclinical or impending pancreatitis (54).

Two drugs, pentamidine and ddI, that are frequently given to patients with AIDS, have been implicated as the causative agents of pancreatitis. Pancreatitis was noted in patients taking ddI during early trials of the drugs with a reported incidence of 1–2.4%. More recent data, however, indicate a much higher incidence ranging from 4–23.5% (55). Patients with AIDS and a prior history of pancreatitis taking high doses of ddI or on long-term therapy with ddI, and who are severely immunocompromised or with poor clinical status appear to be at increased risk of developing pancreatitis. In addition, those receiving both pentamidine and ddI may be at increased risk owing to a cumulative effect of both drugs.

Metabolic Causes of Acute Pancreatitis

Hypercalcemia

Abnormalities in calcium homeostasis, particularly a prolonged or excessive increase in calcium, have been associated with cell damage in many tissues, including the pancreas. Alterations in the concentration of cytosolic-free or ionized calcium can induce a diverse array of cellular responses, including changes in the exocrine, endocrine, neurocrine, and paracrine secretions, as well as alterations in cell growth, cell differentiation, and cell death *(56)*. Other effects of prolonged increases in calcium include the activation of calcium-dependent proteases, phospholipases, and endonucleases, the depletion of high-energy phosphate stores, such as adenosine triphosphate (ATP) owing to the collapse of mitochondrial membrane potentials, and cytoskeletal disruption *(57)*. These effects may account for abnormalities in the acinar cells of the pancreas that occur early in the course of acute pancreatitis.

Studies on the pathophysiology of acute pancreatitis indicate that the crucial early events occur within the acinar cells. Initiating events that result in an abnormal sustained increase of acinar cytosolic calcium may precipitate pancreatitis *(56)*. Initiating factors, such as ethanol abuse, hyperlipidemia, and ductal hypertension, may induce pancreatitis through the common mechanism of raising acinar calcium concentrations.

Ethanol may have direct and indirect effects on acinar cell calcium homeostasis. Direct effects include a decrease in pancreatic muscarinic receptors that may lead to an increase in cholinergic tone and increased susceptibility to excessive cholinergic stimulation of acinar cells *(58)*. Indirect effects of ethanol causing abnormalities in acinar cell calcium concentrations may involve acetaldehyde, the primary metabolite of ethanol. Increased concentrations of acetaldehyde may give rise to the production of oxygen-derived free radicals *(59)*, which may cause peroxidation of membrane lipids with resultant disruption in intracellular calcium homeostasis.

Hyperlipidemia may induce sustained increases in acinar cell calcium concentrations precipitating pancreatitis. Low-density and high-density lipoprotein fractions have been shown to increase calcium concentrations in a variety of cell types.

Obstruction of the pancreatic duct by a gallstone, neoplastic mass, or parasite is a known cause of acute pancreatitis. Some studies suggest that calcium may also play a key role in the induction of pancreatitis in these patients. Ductal hypertension results in increased pressure within the acinar lumen and may impair passage of zymogenes from acinar cells as well as impede acinar cell calcium extrusion. In addition, disruption of the acinar cell plasma membrane may interfere further with calcium homeostasis. Direct support for the role of increased acinar cell calcium concentrations in the pathogenesis of acute pancreatitis in patients with ductal abnormalities comes from the finding that verapamil, a calcium channel blocker, has been shown to ameliorate the course of the disease *(60)*.

Finally, a number of drugs and toxins associated with the development of acute pancreatitis may exert their effects through the increase in acinar cell cytosolic calcium concentrations. For example, organophosphorus insecticides and certain anesthetics can cause an increase in acetylcholine released from autonomic nerve synapses. This accumulation of acetylcholine can lead to stimulation of acinar cells and prolonged increases in acinar cell calcium concentrations. Thiazides may induce pancreatitis owing to their effects at increasing calcium uptake by cells.

Hypertriglyceridemia

Hypertriglyceridemia is a well-recognized cause of pancreatitis; however, the clinical syndrome is not well characterized and the clinical course is ill-defined. Ethanol is thought to play a role in hyperlipidemia. However, it is not certain whether hyperlipidemia results from, or precedes, pancreatitis. Hypertriglyceridemia may result because of a genetic defect in the uptake and metabolism of chylomicrons by cells, or it may be secondary owing to ethanol abuse, diabetes, hypothyroidism, nephrotic syndrome, or use of certain drugs, such as thiazides, estrogen, glucocorticoids, retinoids, and cimetidine.

The frequency of hyperlipidemia in patients with pancreatitis has been reported as ranging from 3–38% *(61)*. There does not appear to be any difference in the course of illness or complications seen in patients with pancreatitis attributed to hyperlipidemia compared with pancreatitis owing to other pathogenesis *(62)*. Acute pancreatitis secondary to hypertriglyceridemia is most often encountered in poorly controlled, obese diabetics. Alcoholics with hypertriglyceridemia are the second most common type of patients presenting with this disorder, whereas nondiabetic, nonalcoholic, nonobese patients with drug- or diet-induced hypertriglyceridemia represent the remaining 15–20% of patients with pancreatitis associated with hypertriglyceridemia *(62)*.

Triglyceride concentrations of <5000 mg/L are rarely, if ever, encountered in patients with hyperlipidemic pancreatitis. Generally, admission triglyceride concentrations in these patients exceed 10,000 mg/L *(62)*. Hyperlipidemic pancreatitis can occur in any age group and has been documented in children with hypertriglyceridemia owing to inborn defects in the lipoprotein lipase system *(63)*.

The mechanism by which hypertriglyceridemia causes pancreatitis is thought to be chemical irritation of pancreatic acinar cells or capillary endothelium by cytotoxic free fatty acids and lysolecithin released by the action of pancreatic lipase or lipoprotein lipase *(64)*. Studies in animals have shown that the addition of free fatty acids to the perfusate of a canine isolated pancreas preparation produced edema and hemorrhage. Some investigators have also found that the pancreas preferentially utilizes lipids as metabolic substrate *(62)*. This preference for fatty acids may explain why the pancreas is rich in lipolytic enzymes and why hyperlipidemia may predispose the pancreas to injury.

Postoperative Pancreatitis

Postoperative pancreatitis has been described as a consequence of gastric surgery, biliary tract surgery, renal and liver transplantation, and cardiovascular surgery *(65,66)*. Postoperative pancreatitis also occurs following surgery not involving the abdomen. Patients suffering postoperative pancreatitis usually experience more frequent complications and higher mortality than patients experiencing pancreatitis owing to other pathogenesis. Complications of postoperative pancreatitis, such as pseudocyst, are more common. The higher mortality rate may be the result of the diagnosis being missed more frequently in this patient population as well as other concomitant disease processes being present. Postoperative pancreatitis may be difficult to recognize, particularly following procedures involving the abdomen, because incisional pain may mask pancreatic abdominal pain, the use of analgesics may blunt the abdominal pain, and because ileus is a common finding in patients undergoing abdominal surgery. The incidence of postoperative pancreatitis has been difficult to establish. In patients who are studied at autopsy, it is often difficult to establish whether the patient died of acute pancreatitis or whether acute pancreatitis was a consequence of the terminating event *(65)*.

Factors claimed to be responsible for causing postoperative pancreatitis are numerous, although the exact mechanisms are uncertain. Direct pancreatic injury as a consequence of abdominal surgery has long been the obvious candidate. However, pancreatitis occurring as a result of extra-abdominal surgery suggests that some other mechanism(s) must also be responsible. Pancreatic ischemia has been frequently suggested as a cause of postoperative pancreatitis, especially in patients placed on cardiopulmonary bypass. In these individuals, pancreatic injury may be mediated by oxygen-derived free radicals *(67)*. Production of these free radicals may be caused by the conversion of the enzyme xanthine dehydrogenase to xanthine oxidase. Previous studies have shown that inhibition of xanthine oxidase can provide some degree of protection to the ischemic pancreas *(67)*. In addition to ischemia as a cause for activation of xanthine oxidase, endogenous pancreatic enzymes, such as chymotrypsin, are potent catalysts of the proteolytic conversion of xanthine dehydrogenase to the oxidase form. Thus, the pancreas may be especially susceptible to injury from free radicals owing to its ability to convert xanthine dehydrogenase to xanthine oxidase via proteolytic cleavage.

Other mechanisms suggested as initiating postoperative pancreatitis include the use of perioperative medications, especially calcium replacement therapy *(68)*. Also, the production of microthrombi with resultant pancreatic ischemia, especially in patients undergoing cardiac valve replacement therapy, has been suggested as another mechanism of postoperative pancreatitis *(66)*. Other postulated factors include obstruction of the pancreatic duct and infections. In patients undergoing organ transplantation, the use of immunosuppressive, drugs such as azathioprine and corticosteroids, may be responsible for initiating pancreatitis.

Pancreatitis following endoscopic retrograde cholangiopancreatography (ERCP) is a serious problem that often requires prolonged hospitalization and surgical intervention. In addition to acute pancreatitis, other complications of ERCP include infection of a pre-existing pseudocyst, sepsis related to cholangitis, and injury from the instrument itself. The incidence of pancreatitis following ERCP has been reported as 1–5%, although the incidence of hyperamylasemia has been reported to be as high as 70% *(69,70)*. There is conflicting evidence concerning the severity of post-ERCP pancreatitis. Most reports suggest that pancreatitis following this procedure is relatively mild with few complications and infrequent mortality. However, in one series, 50% of patients who developed pancreatitis following ERCP required prolonged hospitalization, aggressive nutritional support, or surgical therapy *(69)*. Mortality in these same patients was 13%. Several factors have been implicated in the pathogenesis of post-ERCP pancreatitis. The type and ionic strength of contrast material used, the volume of contrast material injected, and repeated injections of the pancreatic duct have all been cited as factors. Successful treatment of ERCP-induced pancreatitis requires early recognition and institution of appropriate therapy. Further investigations into the exact mechanisms by which ERCP induces pancreatitis are needed so that complications can be prevented.

Ethanol

The association between ethanol consumption and acute pancreatitis is well documented, and has been known for over 100 yr. Alcohol usually accounts for the greatest number of episodes of pancreatitis in males, whereas females tend to have pancreatitis more often from biliary obstruction. Ethanol-induced pancreatitis can develop following binge drinking; however, it usually develops in patients following chronic ingestion of large quantities of alcohol over a prolonged period, usually at least 7–10 yr *(71)*.

Many theories for the pathogenesis of alcohol-induced pancreatitis have been proposed. Mechanisms include alcohol-induced stenosis of the sphincter of Oddi resulting in pancreatic hypersecretion, biliary pancreatic reflux, duodenal-pancreatic reflux, and alcohol-induced reduction of pancreatic blood flow *(71)*. Another mechanism recently proposed suggests that toxic metabolites of ethanol are involved in the generation of free radial species, which are responsible for pancreatic injury. Both the superoxide radical and hydroxyl radical appear to be important early mediators of this injury.

The primary metabolite of ethanol oxidation is acetaldehyde. Acetaldehyde is an excellent substrate for the enzyme xanthine oxidase. Xanthine oxidase is present in normal tissue primarily as the dehydrogenase form, termed xanthine dehydrogenase. Xanthine dehydrogenase must be converted to the oxidase form prior to metabolism of acetaldehyde. This conversion can be readily achieved in the pancreas by the action of proteolytic enzymes released from the inflamed pancreas. A period of pancreatic ischemia is also required before acetaldehyde induces the injury seen in pancreatitis. The ischemia is necessary for the conversion of xanthine dehydrogenase to xanthine oxidase *(72)*. Free radicals are generated when acetaldehyde is oxidized by xanthine oxidase. The administration of compounds, such as superoxidase dismutase and catalase, scavengers of free radicals, and allopurinol, an inhibitor of xanthine oxidase, have been found to minimize this injury. These findings lend further support for the role of toxic oxygen metabolites in the pathogenesis of ethanol-induced pancreatitis.

Another mechanism whereby alcohol may induce pancreatitis is through a reduction in pancreatic blood flow. Pancreatitis has been observed in association with low blood flow rates. Studies of the effect of alcohol on pancreatic perfusion have also demonstrated that high doses of ethanol can reduce pancreatic blood flow without altering systemic circulatory parameters *(73)*. Alcohol administration is associated with decreased pancreatic hemoglobin oxygen saturation, despite stable hemoglobin content and systemic cardiorespiratory parameters. These findings may be owing to a state of pancreatic ischemia produced by a reduction in capillary blood flow *(73)*. The pancreas, in particular, may be more susceptible to ethanol-induced perfusion disturbances compared to other organs. Hemoglobin oxygen saturation has been noted not to be affected in kidney or stomach following ethanol administration.

Other mechanisms have also been suggested by which ethanol may cause pancreatic hypoxia. A reduction in capillary blood flow following ethanol administration may result in edema of the acinar cells with consequent compression of the capillaries *(74)*.

Another mechanism of ethanol-induced pancreatitis may be via aggregation of erythrocytes. Aggregation of erythrocytes has been demonstrated in the bulbar conjunctiva following acute ethanol intoxication *(75)*.

Anatomic Abnormalities

Anatomic abnormalities of the pancreas have been reported to cause acute pancreatitis. The most common anatomic variant of the pancreas is pancreas divisum. This condition results from a failure of the dorsal and ventral pancreatic ducts to fuse during embryological development. Pancreas divisum has been implicated as the source of 10–20% of cases of previously unexplained pancreatitis. However, the debate still continues regarding whether this condition is a cause of acute pancreatitis. Pancreas divisum affects 5–7% of the general population. Some investigators suggest that the development of pancreatitis in patients with pancreas divisum is common *(76)*. The mechanism by which pancreas divisum causes pancreatitis is owing to stenosis.

The dorsal portion of the pancreas drains through the minor papilla, whereas the ventral portion drains through the major papilla. Since the bulk of pancreatic secretions drain via the minor papilla, functional obstruction is created, because the minor papilla is too small for the volume of secretions presented to it. In patients with this condition, surgical enlargement of the accessory ampulla may help to mitigate or prevent further episodes of pancreatitis. It has been suggested that aggressive examination of patients with unexplained or idiopathic pancreatitis may uncover a large percentage of those with pancreas divisum as a cause of the pancreatitis that can be corrected surgically *(77)*.

Other anatomical abnormalities that may result in pancreatitis include dysfunction of the sphincter of Oddi or ampullary stenosis. The incidence of this problem is unknown. However, these conditions may be responsible for some cases of unexplained pancreatitis.

Infection

A variety of infectious agents have been associated with the development of acute pancreatitis. Viral, bacterial, and parasite causes have been documented. Viral infections associated with the development of acute pancreatitis include mumps, rubella, Coxsackie B, Epstein-Barr virus, cytomegalovirus, hepatitis A, B, non-A and non-B.

Opportunistic infections affecting the pancreas in individuals who are immunocompromised because of infection with HIV create a substantially increased risk for the development of pancreatitis. It is thought that up to two-thirds of cases of pancreatitis in patients with HIV are owing to infection. Agents implicated in causing pancreatitis in these patients include cytomegalovirus, cryptococcus, *Toxoplasma gondii*, Cryptosporidium, *Mycobacterium tuberculosis*, and *Mycobacterium avium* complex *(78)*. The remaining one-third of cases of pancreatitis associated with HIV infection are thought to be induced by some of the drugs that these patients take.

Infestation and obstruction of the biliary system by parasites can also cause pancreatitis. The most common agent is *Ascaris*.

Biliary Obstruction

The exact frequency of pancreatitis owing to biliary obstruction is unknown. Some reports indicate that the incidence may be high as 60–80%. The true incidence of biliary pancreatitis is most likely a reflection of the type of patient population served by a particular institution. Hospitals that administer to a predominantly male patient population, especially if of a lower socioeconomic status (e.g., Veteran's Administration Hospitals), will probably see a fairly low incidence of biliary pancreatitis; the majority of patients in this group have alcohol-associated pancreatitis. Gallstone pancreatitis is seen more frequently in females.

The association between acute pancreatitis and gallstones is owing to impaction and transient obstruction of the ampulla of Vater by a migrating gallstone *(79)*. However, acute pancreatitis develops in only 4–8% of patients with cholelithiasis *(80)*. Factors that may predispose some patients with gallstones to pancreatitis include the number and size of gallstones in the gallbladder, and the anatomy and motor function of the biliary tract.

The early detection of biliary obstruction in patients with acute pancreatitis is essential because of differences in management of these patients vs patients with acute pancreatitis owing to other pathogenesis. Patients with acute pancreatitis resulting from biliary obstruction may be at greater risk for the evolution of pancreatic edema to hemorrhage and necrosis, because persistent ampullary obstruction has been shown to increase the severity of the attack *(81)*. Although most cases of biliary pancreatitis are self-limiting, severe acute pancreatitis is seen in 20% of these patients, and is associated with increased morbidity and mortality. Although the debate regarding the optimal timing (early vs delayed) of stone removal and the best approach (surgical vs endoscopic) has yet to be settled, patients with acute pancreatitis owing to biliary obstruction often benefit from biliary decompression *(82)*.

Ultrasonography is the test of choice for the detection of cholelithiasis; however, it gives only indirect evidence in support of a biliary pathogenesis of acute pancreatitis. A spectrum of ultrasound findings can be seen in patients with gallstone disease. These findings range from the presence of sludge in the gallbladder, the presence of "sludge balls" composed of mucus and crystals, microcalculi, and stones *(83)*. It has been speculated that up to 75% of patients with pancreatitis for which no cause can be found is owing to the presence of biliary sludge or microcalculi that are not readily discerned on ultrasound examination. However, examination of duodenal fluid for crystals or microcalculi will often show these entities to be present. Several conditions can predispose individuals to supersaturation of bile with resultant formation of crystals and stones. These include prolonged fasting, pregnancy, and individuals on a diet low in calories for purposes of weight loss.

Attempts to discriminate biliary from nonbiliary origins of acute pancreatitis by use of radiologic contrast studies have proven unreliable, especially in the early stages of the disease when accurate diagnosis is essential. Biochemical markers, including aspartate aminotransferase, alanine aminotransferase, alkaline phosphatase, γ-glutamyltransferase, and total bilirubin, have also been evaluated in an effort to discriminate biliary from nonbiliary pancreatitis. Some studies have found these markers helpful in discriminating biliary from nonbiliary pancreatitis, whereas others have found them of limited diagnostic utility *(27–29)*.

The ampullary obstruction causes a rapid increase in bile duct pressure with consequent liver cell damage, and release of aspartate aminotransferase and alanine aminotransferase. Increases in alkaline phosphatase and bilirubin have also been observed in patients with biliary pancreatitis. However, significant increases in these may not occur if the bile duct is obstructed only transiently. Passage or removal of gallstones that have been obstructing the biliary tract results in a sudden decrease in biliary pressure and normalization of enzyme activities. The rapidity and transient nature of enzyme changes in patients with pancreatitis owing to biliary obstruction make it essential that frequent serial determinations be performed.

ASSESSMENT OF THE SEVERITY OF ACUTE PANCREATITIS

Assessment of the severity of acute pancreatitis plays an important role in the treatment plan. Severe cases of acute pancreatitis can often be cured by medical treatment if the disease is restricted to interstitial inflammation. However, if pancreatic necrosis develops, the patient has a high risk of local infection and generalized sepsis that can lead to multiple system organ failure. In patients who develop pancreatic necrosis, prompt surgical removal of necrotic tissue can significantly improve patient outcome. Patients with pancreatic necrosis who have surgery delayed past the onset of systemic complications have significantly higher postoperative mortality compared to those patients who are quickly identified as requiring surgery. Thus, it is important that patients with evolving pancreatic necrosis be quickly identified so that appropriate treatment may be given.

Approximately 85–90% of attacks of acute pancreatitis are self-limiting and pass without significant morbidity within 3–7 d. The remaining 10–15% of attacks are more severe and are associated with a 50% mortality *(84)*. The ability to predict disease severity accurately and to monitor the course of an attack is advantageous for a number of reasons including:

1. To ensure that intensive therapy is targeted at patients with severe attacks and to evaluate the efficacy of such therapy;
2. To allow for the early detection of complications;
3. To satisfy requirement for entry of patients into therapeutic trials; and
4. To facilitate the comparison of disease severity of patients that present to different institutions *(85)*.

The system used for the prediction of disease severity should be sufficiently sensitive so that intensive therapy is not withheld inappropriately.

The most severe episodes of acute pancreatitis and those associated with the highest mortality are the first and second attacks of acute pancreatitis. However, an exception to this rule is pancreatitis associated with hyperlipidemia. In these cases, any episode may be severe with a fatal outcome *(86)*. Pancreatitis that occurs as a result of ethanol abuse is associated with lower mortality when compared with pancreatitis owing to other causes.

Many schemes have been developed for use as predictors of disease severity. The types of predictors may be based on one or more combination of the following: clinician's assessment, multiple prognostic criteria, results of the peritoneal tap, computerized scanning, and use of biochemical test results *(87)*. In addition, the definition of severity itself may differ. For example, some studies define severe disease as the presence of hemorrhagic or necrotizing pancreatitis, whereas others define disease severity in terms of complications, mortality, or spending more than a predetermined number of days (e.g., 7) in an intensive care unit.

Prediction of severity based on clinical assessment is often inaccurate, especially when performed early in the course of the disease. Initial clinical assessment can predict approx 40% of those who will develop severe disease. However, when performed within 24 h following admission, clinical assessment can predict up to 75% of patients likely to develop severe disease *(88)*. Thus, some mechanism for identifying patients early in the course of the disease would be of great benefit. A clinical assessment in terms of sensitivity and specificity has shown that the clinician's assessment has poor sensitivity, but excellent specificity for predicting disease severity *(87)*.

The use of multiple prognostic criteria for establishing disease severity has gained wide acceptance since being established by Ranson in 1974 *(89)*. This classification scheme was based on the findings of 11 clinical and biochemical factors. Five of these factors were determined on admission, and the other six were determined during the ensuing 48 h. Mortality was found to be <1% if two or fewer risk factors were present, 40% if five or six risk factors were found, and essentially 100% if seven or more signs were present. This scoring system has been found to classify approx 90% of patients accurately with respect to disease severity. The original list proposed by Ranson has since been modified by others. The Glasgow score first proposed in 1978 utilized nine of the original criteria proposed by Ranson, although with some modifications to the cutoff values *(90)*. A re-evaluation of the Glasgow score in 1984 revealed that the diagnostic accuracy of the scoring system could be improved if aspartate aminotransferase (AST) was removed as one of the predictive factors.

In addition to the scoring systems developed by Ranson and the Glasgow score, other severity scores have been developed. The original Acute Physiology and Chronic Health Enquiry score (APACHE) is based on 34 physiologic variables, the sum of which yields a score *(91)*. The underlying utility of the APACHE score is that the severity of acute disease can be assessed by quantifying the degree of abnormality of multiple physiologic variables. The APACHE II classification system is a revised version of the original APACHE scheme; however, only 14 clinical and biological parameters are used, instead of the original 34. An advantage of the APACHE II score over the Ranson or Glasgow scores is that the former can be evaluated immediately on admission and throughout the whole hospital stay; this allows for a more rapid prognostic classification of the patient.

A variety of other scoring systems have also been developed. The Simplified Acute Physiology Score (SAPS) is derived from the APACHE score. Evaluation studies comparing these different systems have demonstrated that the APACHE II score is superior to the other prognostic classification schemes *(85)*. Reasons given for its superior performance include the use of all the major risk factors that influence outcome from disease and the semiquantitative use of varying weights assigned to increasingly abnormal values instead of a qualitative "yes" or "no" answer. The use of a semiquantitative weighting scheme provides for a greater range of values between mild and severe attacks. Unfortunately, however, none of the scoring systems is particularly good at predicting late complications; in addition, the prediction of a pancreatic pseudocyst is poor *(92)*.

A simplified approach for classification of patients with respect to disease severity is the use of single prognostic indicators. Whereas the APACHE and Ranson scores rely on a multitude of biochemical and clinical indicators, the use of a single, relatively inexpensive, rapid, and reliable blood or urine test to replace the cumbersome multiple criteria scores would be advantageous (93).

A variety of enzyme and other protein markers have been proposed for gauging severity in acute pancreatitis. Although increases in amylase and lipase are the hallmarks of pancreatitis, increases in a multitude of other enzymes are observed, some of which have been proposed as prognostic indicators. It is unfortunate that although amylase and lipase are universally used for the diagnosis of pancreatitis, the magnitude of increase in either enzyme has no prognostic value. One study of 417 patients with acute pancreatitis found that the mortality rate was greater in patients with amylase activities < 1000 U/L compared to those with amylase activities much >1000 U/L (94). However, the P_3 isoamylase fraction has been found to be of prognostic significance (95). In one study, approx 90% of patients with an unfavorable outcome had an increase in the P_3 isoamylase at the time of discharge (96). Thus, careful follow-up of patients with increased P_3 isoamylase at the time of discharge may be appropriate.

Neutrophil Elastase

Data suggest that excessive activation and release of endogenous humoral mediators from polymorphonuclear neutrophils, monocytes, and macrophages may be responsible for the severity of complications in acute pancreatitis. The activation of neutrophils and monocytes at sites of inflammation results in the release of biologically active products. The products include proteolytic enzymes, such as elastase, reactive oxygen species, and cytokines, such as interleukin (IL)-1, IL-6, IL-8, and tumor necrosis factor. Elastase is a serine protease that can degrade elastin, collagen, clotting factors, immunoglobulins, protease inhibitors, and transport proteins, such as ferritin. Normally, individuals are well protected against the effect of proteolytic enzymes, because 60% of plasma proteins function as protease inhibitors (97). The effects of elastase include increased pulmonary vascular resistance, decreased cardiac output, pulmonary leukostasis, and disseminated intravascular coagulation (98). Elastase concentrations in plasma have been shown to correlate directly with severity of acute respiratory distress syndrome, sepsis, and multiple organ failure (99,100).

Numerous studies have demonstrated good prognostic accuracy for patients with acute pancreatitis using neutrophil elastase (101–103). The time-course of this test reveals that maximal concentrations are attained 24–48 h following disease onset, and increased concentrations are associated with worsening prognosis. Although test procedures are available commercially, measurement of elastase is not performed routinely in most clinical laboratories. In addition, leukocytes contain high concentrations of the enzyme. The latter requires the careful and prompt separation of plasma from the specimen following blood collection.

Acute-Phase Proteins

The acute phase of pancreatitis is characterized by certain predictable changes in the production of pancreatic proteins and other markers of inflammation and injury. Whereas the expression and production of many pancreatic enzymes and other proteins decrease following the onset of acute pancreatitis, the production of certain stimuli, including cytokines and tumor necrosis factor, is enhanced. These agents are produced from the damaged tissue and from activated mononuclear cells. Cytokines elicit the biological effects that are characteristic of the acute phase response.

The proteins that are characteristic of the acute-phase response are divided into one of two classes based on their pattern of regulation by cytokines *(104)*. Synthesis of class 1 acute-phase proteins, including C-reactive protein (CRP), haptoglobin, and α-1-acid glycoprotein, is induced by IL-1 or a combination of IL-1 and IL-6. The class 2 acute-phase proteins, such as α-2-macroglobulins, α-1-antichymotrypsin, pancreatitis-associated protein (PAP), and fibrinogen, are regulated primarily by IL-6 and glucocorticoids *(105)*.

C-Reactive Protein

Increased concentrations of CRP in patients with acute pancreatitis are owing to activation of the monocyte-macrophage system *(106)*. Concentrations >150 mg/L have been shown to be highly suggestive of severe acute pancreatitis *(107)*. Maximal CRP concentrations generally are reached 2–4 d following the onset of disease. The prolonged time-course of CRP is thus of limited clinical utility. At 48 h postonset, CRP was no better at predicting severity than a multiple criteria scoring system *(107)*. The use of CRP as a prognostic indicator also suffers from the nonspecificity of this test for pancreatic disease. Individuals with any other type of acute inflammatory process may show increased CRP concentrations. However, even the limitations of CRP should not preclude its use; the analyte is readily available in most laboratories, is easy to perform, and is relatively inexpensive.

Trypsinogen Activation Peptide (TAP)

A new marker of disease severity that has not been extensively evaluated is urinary concentrations of TAP. The use of TAP to predict severity is based on the concept that mild pancreatitis occurs in patients without activation of trypsinogen to trypsin. If the amount of activated trypsin exceeds the availability of antiproteases to inhibit trypsin activity, then release of active trypsin into the systemic circulation occurs with its adverse effects. Thus, the amount of active trypsin with concomitant production of TAP is directly related to disease severity.

TAP is a five amino acid compound that is released from trypsin following activation. Although free trypsin is normally rapidly complexed to antiprotease inhibitors, TAP is not. Since TAP has a low molecular weight and is unbound in serum, it is rapidly excreted into urine following its formation. One study that evaluated urinary TAP, serum CRP, and the Glasgow criteria for discriminating mild from severe acute pancreatitis found TAP the best indicator of disease severity on admission and at 24 h following admission *(108)*.

Pancreatitis-Associated Protein (PAP)

Another relatively new marker of disease severity is PAP. This protein is barely detectable in normal pancreatic tissue; however, following the onset of acute pancreatic damage, the enzyme is synthesized in the acinar cells of the pancreas. The increased synthesis of PAP by the acinar cells following pancreatic injury is unique; the synthesis of pancreatic enzymes is normally repressed during the acute phase of an attack *(109)*. This finding may partially explain why serum pancreatic enzyme activities quickly decline following their initial rise and why severe attacks of acute pancreatitis are often associated with lower enzyme activities when compared with mild attacks *(110)*.

PAP is a secretory protein and leaks into the bloodstream following its synthesis. PAP may offer some advantages when compared to other protein markers, such as TAP and CRP. PAP is expressed in response to pancreatic damage, whereas TAP is produced from trypsinogen whose synthesis is repressed during acute pancreatitis. PAP might also offer better specificity for pancreatic damage when compared to CRP, because the latter is not synthesized by the pancreas.

In addition to acute pancreatitis as a cause of increased serum PAP concentrations, long-term chronic use of ethanol has been found to lead to approx 10-fold increases in serum PAP *(111)*. The highest concentrations have been observed 2 d following cessation of ethanol use. These patients did not develop other signs of symptoms suggestive of acute pancreatitis, and the results further support the suggestion that heavy long-term consumption of ethanol induces subclinical pancreatic damage, but not clinical pancreatitis.

Concentrations of PAP obtained following admission have been found not to correlate with the severity of pancreatitis. Apparently, the induction of PAP gene expression starts several hours following the onset of an attack, after which PAP concentrations may increase more than 100 times baseline values within a few days *(112)*. Thus, PAP is most likely a useful test in the follow-up of patients with acute pancreatitis. Monitoring of PAP during the acute phase of an attack may provide information on the development and severity of the disease. An initial rise followed by a persistent decrease in PAP concentrations appears to predict recovery; consistently increased concentrations are associated with poor outcome. Unfortunately, no procedures for measuring PAP are available commercially.

Complement

Activation of complement with release of anaphylatoxins has been demonstrated in patients with acute pancreatitis *(113)*. Activation of the complement system can occur owing to proteases, such as trypsin, or from tissue injury as a result of hypoperfusion, thermal injury, or mechanical trauma. In addition, the complement system can be activated in patients with acute pancreatitis who have intravascular coagulation and fibrinolysis *(114)*.

Anaphylatoxins including $C3_a$ and $C5_a$ are formed from C3 and C5 following the activation of complement. $C3_a$ and $C5_a$ mediate an increase in vascular permeability, induce contractions of smooth muscle, cause release of histamine from mast cells and basophils, and may even impair cardiac function *(97)*. The active anaphylatoxins ($C3_a$ and $C5_a$) are inactivated by an anaphylatoxin-inactivator enzyme. However, even when inactivated, $C5_a$ still retains the ability to stimulate neutrophils.

Activation of the complement system also results in the formation of a terminal–complement complex, and the presence of this complex in plasma indicates that complete activation of complement has occurred. Patients with moderate to severe pancreatitis have higher concentrations of activated and inactivated anaphylatoxin $C3_a$ as well as the terminal complement complex when compared to patients with mild pancreatitis.

Interleukin-6

Experimental studies have shown that IL-6, which is released primarily by activated mononuclear phagocytes, is the principal mediator of the acute-phase protein response of which CRP is an important component *(115)*. Serum concentrations of IL-6 begin to rise during the first 24 h following the onset of an attack of acute pancreatitis and peak between 24 and 36 h. Peak concentrations of CRP occur between 36 and 48 h following the onset of symptoms. Thus, measurement of IL-6 concentrations may allow earlier prediction of disease severity owing to its earlier rise when compared with CRP. One study of 24 patients found that serum IL-6 concentrations obtained on admission could distinguish between mild and severe attacks of acute pancreatitis *(116)*. IL-6 measured at admission provided a diagnostic accuracy of 75% compared with an admission diagnostic accuracy for CRP of 54%. When peak IL-6 and CRP concentrations were used to gauge disease severity, both markers provided a diagnostic accuracy of 83%.

Measurement of IL-6 may be performed using a bioassay procedure or by use of immunoassay-based methods that are available commercially. The major drawback of the bioassay procedure is its turn around time of 5 d; the immunoassay procedures can provide results within 6 h *(116)*.

Tumor Necrosis Factor

Tumor necrosis factor (TNF) is another multifunctional cytokine that is involved in the acute-phase response to trauma, bacterial infection, and inflammation *(117)*. TNF is a potent inducer of secretion of IL-6 from leukocytes and therefore appears in the circulation earlier than IL-6. Once released into the circulation, TNF induces the activation of the enzyme PLA_2 and mediates the release of toxic oxygen-derived metabolites, causing necrotic cell lysis that finally results in hemorrhagic necrosis *(118)*. Increased concentrations have been observed in a variety of conditions, including sepsis, and in patients with multiorgan failure.

The role of TNF in the evaluation of the severity of acute pancreatitis is still not completely defined. One study found that increased TNF concentrations in serum during the first 24 h of an attack were helpful in predicting complicated and fatal pancreatitis *(119)*. However, later studies have not corroborated these findings *(117)*. Possible explanations for these differences may be owing to the rapid time-course in which TNF rises and falls in serum. In those patients with septic shock where TNF concentrations may reach extraordinary values, the increase occurs for a few hours only *(120)*. Since circulating TNF has a half-life of only 5–25 min, those studies that evaluated TNF as a marker of disease severity, and collected only one sample or collected one sample every few days could have easily missed the rapid rise and fall of TNF *(117,120)*. It appears that appropriate use of TNF as a marker of disease severity requires frequent serial sampling. The utility of TNF as a marker of disease severity has not yet been adequately addressed, and further studies are needed to define its role.

Ribonuclease

Increased activity of ribonuclease in serum has been reported in a variety of conditions, including acute necrotizing pancreatis, pancreatic cancer, and other neoplastic diseases *(121)*. Ribonuclease is useful for the discrimination of patients with acute interstitial pancreatitis from those with acute necrotizing pancreatitis; the latter have increased ribonuclease activities *(121)*. An earlier study found that only one of 25 patients with normal ribonuclease activities developed evidence of pancreatic necrosis, whereas 11 of 13 patients with increased ribonuclease developed a pancreatic abscess or necrosis *(122)*.

The utility of ribonuclease for the identification of patients with severe acute pancreatitis is limited by several factors. Most notable is the effect of impaired renal function on serum ribonuclease. Increasing serum ribonuclease values correlate directly with increasing serum creatinine concentrations. Ribonucleases are low-mol-wt proteins that are eliminated predominantly by the kidneys. Thus, ribonuclease may be a useful marker for severe cases of pancreatitis in the absence of renal insufficiency. Unfortunately, renal insufficiency is a common finding in patients with acute necrotizing pancreatitis. Another factor that hampers evaluation of the clinical utility of this test is the fact that several different isoenzymes of ribonuclease are present in serum, each possessing its pH optimum and substrate specificity. Thus, it is often difficult to compare results obtained by different investigators owing to differences in the methods used to measure ribonuclease activity. A third factor that can interfere with ribonuclease measurements is the effects of hemolysis. Erythrocytes have been found to contain inhibitors of ribonuclease activity and can therefore lead to falsely decreased measurements of ribonuclease activity.

Antiproteases

Following the onset of an attack of acute pancreatitis, high concentrations of pancreatic secretory enzymes are released into the circulation. The finding that protease activity is usually absent following the onset of acute pancreatitis is because active proteases are scavenged by protease inhibitors present in the circulation. Evidence that active proteases are released into the circulation is provided by the finding that antiproteases, such as α-2-macroglobulin, are decreased in patients with acute pancreatitis. It is one of two primary protease inhibitors that preferentially bind activated proteolytic enzymes, including trypsin, chymotrypsin, and elastase. In patients with acute pancreatitis, α-2-macroglobulin concentrations decrease in proportion to the severity of the attack *(123)*. Binding of proteases by α-2-macroglobulin results in the formation of a complex that is cleared from the circulation by the reticuloendothelial system. The protease–antiprotease complex has a half-life of approx 10 min compared with several hours for the uncomplexed form.

The trypsin binding capacity of α-2-macroglobulin has been reported to decrease to 70–80% of normal following an attack of acute pancreatitis *(124)*. The lowest concentrations usually occur 3–9 d following the onset of an attack.

Another important protease inhibitor present in serum is α-1-antiprotease. In human serum, 90% of trypsin inhibitory capacity is attributable to α-1-antiprotease with α-2-macroglobulin accounting for much of the remainder. α-1-antiprotease is an acute-phase reactant. Concentrations of this protein begin to rise soon after the onset of symptoms of an attack of acute pancreatitis and peak between 3 and 7 d. The most severe attacks of acute pancreatitis are often associated with the greatest increase in α-1-antiprotease *(125)*.

Not all studies have been able to demonstrate good diagnostic utility of antiproteases for discriminating mild from severe attacks of acute pancreatitis *(107,126)*. Reported positive and negative predictive values for α-2-macroglobulin and α-1-anti-trypsin measured during the first 48 h of an attack were 82 and 67%, and 59% and 50%, respectively *(127)*. Another study found that LD had a diagnostic accuracy of 82% compared with diagnostic accuracies of just 71 and 69% for α-2-macroglobulins and α-1-antitrypsin, respectively *(126)*.

Phospholipase A (PLA)

Measurement of PLA has been advocated as a test for the severity of acute pancreatitis; greatly increased activities of PLA are associated with severe hemorrhagic forms of the disease, and lesser increases are found in the mild edematous type *(128,129)*. PLA that reaches the circulation is converted from its proenzyme form to active PLA by trypsin. No inhibitors are present in serum to mediate the action of active PLA, and it is thought to play an important role in the cause of pulmonary insufficiency often associated with acute pancreatitis. The enzyme has been found to destroy lecithin found in pulmonary surfactant as well as in cell membranes.

Although many studies have found an association between PLA activity and severity of disease *(128–130)*, one has not *(131)*. Increased PLA activities are found in a wide variety of conditions not involving the pancreas, including liver disease, renal failure, trauma, surgery, and cardiac disease *(131)*. Thus, although PLA may contribute to the organ necrosis and mortality of patients with acute pancreatitis, increased PLA is not specific for dysfunction of any one organ system or for any clinical syndrome. Substantial quantities of PLA have been found in leukocytes *(132)*. Release of PLA into the circulation following the activation of these cells may explain the increased PLA activities seen in patients with nonpancreatic inflammatory disorders.

Measurement of PLA in serum may be performed by the quantitation of active enzyme present or by measurement of immunoreactive PLA concentrations. Controversy still exists regarding what method, enzymatic vs immunologic, should be used for measurement of PLA *(133)*. One study showed that enzymatic, but not immunologic PLA measurements provided good positive and negative predictive value of 71 and 82%, respectively, for detecting pancreatic necrosis *(134)*. However, other studies have indicated that immunoreactive PLA is a more sensitive marker than enzymatic PLA for detecting severe cases of acute pancreatitis *(135)*.

Body Mass Index

One easily obtained parameter that may provide prognostic information is the body mass index. One study has shown that patients with a body mass index of >30 kg/m^2, as derived from the patient's height and weight, had poorer outcomes following acute pancreatitis more frequently than patients who were not significantly overweight *(136)*.

Methemalbumin

The recognition of a brown pigment in the serum of patients with hemorrhagic pancreatitis was noted by Edmondson in 1952 *(137)*. The pigment was later characterized as methemalbumin, and its use as a marker of hemorrhagic pancreatitis was further characterized *(138)*. Methemalbumin is produced via the oxidation of heme that is initially produced from the breakdown of retroperitoneal hemoglobin into heme by pancreatic enzymes. Heme is oxidized to hematin, which is absorbed into the systemic circulation were it combines with albumin to form methemalbumin. Methemalbumin concentrations increase within the first 24 h following the onset of an attack and remain increased for several days.

Studies that have used methemalbumin as an indicator of disease severity have produced variable results *(139,140)*. When used as a predictor of death and complications, methemalbumin has been found to be relatively insensitive *(140)*; however, if methemalbumin is used as a predictor of mortality only, then test sensitivity increases substantially with the predictive value of an abnormal test result often exceeding 90% *(87)*. Thus, methemalbumin measurements appear to be most useful as an indicator of the severest types of acute pancreatitis. When used in this way, methemalbumin is more useful than the criteria of Ranson for predicting fatal attacks of acute pancreatitis *(139)*.

Peritoneal Tap

Similar to methemalbumin in its ability to predict the severest cases of acute pancreatitis is the peritoneal tap. The peritoneal tap may also be used to differentiate an acute surgical abdomen from acute pancreatitis. Aspiration of dark, nonodorous, prune juice-colored fluid is characteristic of severe necrotizing pancreatitis, whereas fluid obtained from the patient with a perforated viscus is usually foul-smelling and contains bacteria *(141)*. A study of 79 patients using peritoneal lavage found that the severest attacks of acute pancreatitis could be expected when one of the following was present:

1. Aspiration of more than 10 mL of fluid irrespective of color;
2. Free fluid of dark color; and
3. A straw- or darker colored lavage return fluid *(140)*.

The presence of pancreatic enzymes in lavage fluid has also been investigated as a means for predicting disease severity. Using a scoring system based on the relative activities of amylase and lipase in peritoneal fluid to their respective serum activities, Robert et al. *(142)* found that the presence of both amylase and lipase in peritoneal fluid having activities greater than those seen in serum could identify patients most likely to have a fatal outcome. The mortality rate for the patients studied was just 5% when none or only one enzyme was higher in peritoneal fluid than in serum. However, when both amylase and lipase were present in greater activities in peritoneal fluid compared with their serum activities, the mortality rate was 29%. The major disadvantage of the peritoneal tap is the invasive nature of the procedure. Complications, such as viscus puncture, are unusual with a reported incidence of <1% *(141)*.

COMPLICATIONS OF ACUTE PANCREATITIS

The pancreas is capable of releasing a great quantity of potent vasoactive peptides, hormones, and enzymes following an insult, such as acute pancreatitis. The wide array of biochemical mediators can induce a variety of derangements both locally and systemic. The various prognostic criteria that are employed to gauge disease severity are early indicators of potential metabolic derangements. Although hypocalcemia, hyperglycemia, and hypertriglyceridemia are usually considered to be the common metabolic complications, acute pancreatitis may also cause a diverse array of derangements that can, in the severest cases, result in multiple organ system failure and death.

Local Complications

Hemorrhage

A variety of mechanisms can result in hemorrhage in patients with acute pancreatitis. Gastrointestinal hemorrhage occurring in association with pancreatic inflammation has been reported with an incidence ranging from approx 1–40%. The cause of hemorrhage may be the result of several mechanisms, including coexistent peptic ulcer disease, stress gastritis, pre-existent esophageal varices, or erosion of a major blood vessel secondary to a pancreatic pseudocyst, necrosis, or abscess. Elastase and other pancreatic enzymes that are released by recurrent or persistent pancreatic inflammation can weaken and erode the wall of the peripancreatic vasculature leading to hemorrhage.

Hemorrhage into the gastrointestinal tract may also be caused by a pancreatic pseudocyst; hemorrhage into a pseudocyst is a relatively frequent and catastrophic event. This mechanism also involves erosion and weakening of peripancreatic vasculature following enzymatic attack. A blood vessel in close proximity to the wall of a pseudocyst may rupture into the pseudocyst. If a communication exists between the pseudocyst and the pancreatic duct, then blood and fluid present in the pseudocyst will be discharged into the duodenum.

Pseudocyst

Pancreatic pseudocysts consist of a fibrous capsule containing necrotic tissue, blood, and secretions. The fluid within the pseudocyst is often rich in proteolytic enzymes. Pseudocysts are commonly associated with chronic pancreatitis, and they may develop in up to 50% of patients with severe, acute inflammation *(143)*. Clinical symptoms of a pancreatic pseudocysts are similar to those accompanying acute pancreatitis, and include abdominal pain, fever, vomiting, and occasionally mild jaundice.

Pseudocysts may form in a variety of locations. They can be found within the pancreas, posterior to the pancreas, in the pararenal spaces, or in the mediastinum. The walls of the pseudocyst are composed of whatever tissue structures first limit its spread. Encapsulation of the pseudocyst occurs owing to evoked inflammatory reactions with the eventual formation of a fibrous wall. This maturation process generally takes from 4–6 wk for the capsule to thicken sufficiently to hold sutures *(143)*. Further growth of a pseudocyst may occur owing to osmotic influx of fluid in response to tissue necrosis within the pseudocyst *(144)*.

Diagnosis of a pancreatic pseudocyst is by use of imaging studies. Approximately 40% of patients with a pseudocyst will have a palpable mass. In 27% of patients, pseudocysts will undergo spontaneous resolution within 3 wk *(145)*; spontaneous resolution after 3 wk is an uncommon occurrence. Pseudocysts are classified as chronic if they remain for longer than 6 wk.

Pseudocysts can cause a variety of potentially lethal complications. Those located at the head of pancreas may cause duodenal obstruction or compress the common bile duct, resulting in obstructive jaundice. Splenic vein thrombosis may result in splenic infarction or cause hypersplenism owing to congestive splenomegaly. Similarly, thrombosis of the portal vein may cause extrahepatic portal hypertension and esophageal varices. Another important complication of pseudocysts is infection, resulting in an abscess.

Pancreatic Abscess

Pancreatic abscesses occur as a complication in 4% of patients admitted with acute pancreatitis. The incidence of abscess formation increases with the severity of the attack *(144)*. The direct relationship between disease severity and abscess formation probably reflects the amount of tissue necrosis. In patients with a fatal attack of acute pancreatitis, abscesses are found in 50–70% of cases *(146)*.

Because the term "pancreatic abscess" has often been loosely used to describe a variety of infected processes in the region of the pancreas, the term "infected pancreatic necrosis" has been suggested to represent diffuse, infected pancreatic and peripancreatic necrosis, and fluid collections that occur as a complication of acute pancreatitis *(147)*.

Pancreatic abscess can occur as a result of pancreatitis from any etiology. It is more commonly seen in acute rather than chronic pancreatitis, unlike pseudocysts that are more frequently found in patients with chronic pancreatitis.

The diagnosis of pancreatic abscess by use of biochemical indices is not reliable, because standard laboratory studies are generally nonspecific *(148)*. An increase in leukocytes is usually noted, whereas albumin and total calcium concentrations are generally decreased. Serum amylase is increased in fewer than 50% of patients at the time of diagnosis of a pancreatic abscess. In addition, results of liver function studies, including aspartate aminotransferase, alkaline phosphatase, and bilirubin, are within normal limits in the majority of patients with pancreatic abscess. Other laboratory parameters that have been proposed for the evaluation of pancreatic abscess include ribonuclease *(148)*, CRP, α-1-antitrypsin, and α-2-macroglobulin *(149)*. However, none of these tests have good diagnostic accuracy for the detection of pancreatic abscess. At present, computed tomography is the best diagnostic tool for abscess detection; abscess-specific changes are seen in approx 75% of patients *(148)*.

Phlegmon

A pancreatic phlegmon is produced as a result of secondary infection of the pancreas and retroperitoneal tissue in patients with necrotizing pancreatitis. The incidence of phlegmon has been reported to be as high as 18% and may be higher in patients with severe attacks of acute pancreatitis *(144)*. Patients with phlegmon may present with fever, increased amylase and lipase, abdominal pain or tenderness, and leukocytosis. Detection of phlegmon by ultrasound or computed tomography scan is achievable in 30–60% of patients. An abdominal mass is palpable in approx 15% of cases.

BIOCHEMICAL DISTURBANCES ASSOCIATED WITH ACUTE PANCREATITIS

The ability of the pancreas to produce a variety of potent vasoactive peptides, hormones, and enzymes often leads to complications involving other organ systems.

Some of these complications involving the lungs, heart, liver, and kidneys are often not associated with any detectable structural changes occurring in these organ systems. Evidence suggests that biochemical disturbances that occur in patients with acute pancreatitis are primarily responsible for initiating major organ failure.

Hypocalcemia

Hypocalcemia is a frequent finding in patients with acute pancreatitis, reportedly occurring in 30–60% of patients with the disease *(150)*. A strong correlation has been established between patient prognosis and the magnitude of hypocalcemia *(151)*. The exact mechanism for hypocalcemia in acute pancreatitis is still unresolved. Several mechanisms working alone or in conjunction with one another may be responsible.

The sequestration of calcium by saponification of calcium salts in areas of fat necrosis has long been a popular theory for the pathogenesis of hypocalcemia. However, calcium sequestration in areas of fat necrosis has been shown to be insufficient to explain the hypocalcemia seen in these patients. Infusion of calcium into patients with acute pancreatitis and who are hypocalcemic is of little benefit *(152)*. In addition, the amount of calcium sequestered during the process of saponification typically amounts to <2 g, an amount insufficient to cause hypocalcemia owing to the abundant skeletal stores of readily mobilized calcium. Thus, sequestration of calcium in areas of fat necrosis is not considered to be an adequate mechanism accounting for the hypocalcemia seen in patients with acute pancreatitis.

The rapid development of hypoalbuminemia in patients with acute pancreatitis has been suggested to play a predominant role in hypocalcemia. The exact pathogenesis of hypoalbuminia is not certain; possible causes include diminished hepatic synthesis, increased catabolism, urinary loss, or redistribution of albumin within various body compartments. Approximately half of the total amount of calcium in blood is bound to serum proteins with albumin accounting for 80% of the protein-bound calcium. Thus, when the hypocalcemia is corrected by taking into account the serum albumin concentrations, the incidence of "true" hypocalcemia is relatively low. Imrie et al. *(153)* reported that although 68% of their study patients were initially designated as hypocalcemic, the incidence of true hypocalcemia, obtained by correcting serum calcium concentrations for albumin, was only 12%. Measurement of ionized calcium rather than total calcium in serum has been advocated as the best method for assessing calcium status in patients with pancreatitis. However, other investigators have demonstrated decreases in ionized calcium in humans with acute pancreatitis *(154)*, as well as in animals *(155)*, suggesting that hypoalbuminia alone cannot account for hypocalcemia in all patients with acute pancreatitis.

Hypomagnesemia has been implicated in the hypocalcemia of acute pancreatitis owing to the inhibition of both parathyroid hormone (PTH) secretion and its action on calcium mobilization by osteoclasts. The relationship between magnesium concentrations and its role in the hypocalcemia of acute pancreatitis is controversial. Hypomagnesemia is not a consistent finding in patients with acute pancreatitis and magnesium replacement therapy in those patients who are deficient is not always beneficial *(153)*.

The role of hormone imbalances in the pathogenesis of hypocalcemia in acute pancreatitis is controversial. Increased secretion of glucagon may result in hypocalcemia by directly inhibiting bone resorption or by releasing calcitonin *(156)*. However, not all investigators have found a relationship between these hormones and hypocalcemia *(152)*.

Derangements in the calcium–PTH axis are also often cited as the cause of hypocalcemia in acute pancreatitis. PTH concentrations in patients with acute pancreatitis have been reported as being decreased *(156)*, normal *(157)*, and even increased *(158)*. Decreased PTH concentrations in patients with acute pancreatitis and hypocalcemia have often been attributed to a relative deficiency of PTH owing to failure of the parathyroid glands to maintain secretion of the hormone *(159)*.

An alternative explanation for the decrease in PTH concentrations following acute pancreatitis may be owing to inactivation of PTH by proteolytic enzymes released from the injured pancreas. Brodrick et al. *(160)* reported that the biological activity of bovine PTH, as measured using a chicken kidney plasma membrane adenyl cyclase assay system, is readily degraded by sera from patients with acute pancreatitis. These results suggest that degradation of PTH, as well as other relevant peptides governing calcium homeostasis (e.g., calcitonin), may play an important role in the hypocalcemia of patients with acute pancreatitis.

Hyperlipidemia

Hyperlipidemia in association with acute pancreatitis has been reported in some series to be as high as 50% *(161)*. The hyperlipidemia observed in these patients is usually characterized by abnormally increased triglyceride concentrations of >12,000 mg/L and normal cholesterol concentrations. In some patients, cholesterol concentrations may even be decreased as a consequence of stress.

Some studies have shown a direct relationship between the degree of hypertriglyceridemia and disease severity *(161,162)*. In one study, all patients with triglyceride concentrations greater than approx 18,000 mg/L (20 mmol/L) developed necrotizing pancreatitis *(161)*. In addition, a direct association between hypercholesterolemia and pancreatic necrosis has also been observed. Patients with acute pancreatitis and hyperlipidemia also have a higher likelihood of developing acute respiratory distress syndrome. Embolization of agglutinated lipid particles in lung and other organs, including the kidney, heart, and brain, is another serious concern in these patients.

The issue of whether hypertriglyceridemia is a pre-existing metabolic disorder in these patients, or if it occurs as a consequence of acute pancreatitis is unresolved. Some studies suggest that patients who develop acute pancreatitis have an abnormality in the metabolism of chylomicrons *(163)*. This abnormality causes the pancreatic interstitium to have increased triglyceride concentrations. Lipase present in pancreatic juice results in the production of cytotoxic free fatty acids, which are able to initiate the autodigestive process in the pancreas. In addition, increased serum concentrations of chylomicrons and chylomicron remnants may cause damage to the pancreatic capillaries owing to release of cholesterol crystals during lipolysis that can induce ischemic lesions.

Patients with hyperlipidemia that occurs secondarily to disease states, such as hypothyroidism, diabetes mellitus, pregnancy, and chronic renal failure, are also at increased risk for developing acute pancreatitis. However, the pathogenesis of hyperlipidemia in many patients with acute pancreatitis is not readily explained. The abnormally increased triglycerides in these patients is thought to be secondary to necrosis of peripancreatic fat *(161)*. Other studies suggest that inhibition of postheparin lipoprotein lipase and acute deficiency of glucagon may lead to hyperlipidemia in acute pancreatitis *(164)*.

Hyperglycemia

Increased glucose concentrations in serum (>2000 mg/L) have been used as an indicator of poor prognosis. Up to half of patients with acute pancreatitis will develop mild transient hyperglycemia. Another 30% of patients will demonstrate glycosuria, and from 2–10% may develop frank diabetes *(164)*. In addition to hyperglycemia, hypoglycemia has been also noted to occur in <5% of patients *(164)*.

A variety of mechanisms may be responsible for the hyperglycemia in acute pancreatitis. Glucose metabolism is altered in these patients by an increased ratio of glucagon to insulin, resulting in a relative resistance to insulin *(165)*. These patients may also have impaired function of the β-cells and decreased insulin secretion that can further contribute to poor glucose utilization and hyperglycemia. Other hormone imbalances that may contribute to hyperglycemia include increased concentrations of growth hormone, cortisol, and catecholamines.

Individuals with acute pancreatitis exhibit a number of metabolic similarities when compared with patients who are septic. These similarities include an increased expenditure of energy mediated through a hypermetabolic state with increased oxidation of amino acids, increased ureagenesis, and increased gluconeogenesis. These patients also exhibit a net decrease in protein synthesis often leading to malnutrition. Patients with severe, acute pancreatitis often exhibit a hypermetabolic state. The rate of endogenous glucose production has been found to be significantly higher in these patients. However, despite the increase in endogenous glucose production, there is a significant decrease in the percentage of glucose uptake by cells. This imbalance between glucose production and metabolism can also lead to hyperglycemia.

The hypermetabolic state observed in patients with severe, acute pancreatitis is characterized by a fall in systemic vascular resistance and a rise in cardiac output leading to a marked increase in visceral and muscle blood flow and consumption of oxygen. The increase in oxygen consumption and corresponding increased caloric need are met through a variety of mechanisms. The utilization of branched-chain amino acids (isoleucine, leucine, and valine) as substrates for gluconeogenesis and peripheral oxidation is handled through increased catabolism of body protein stores and increased ureagenesis. In addition to increased concentrations of branched-chain amino acids, increased concentrations of aromatic amino acids have also been observed. The excess of amino acids within the circulation can result in the accumulation of aromatic amino acids within the central nervous system and production of false neurotransmitters, such as octopamine and phenylethanolamine.

The extremely high catabolic rates in patients with pancreatitis may result in nitrogen losses as great as 40 g/24 h. Administration of glucose to those patients can serve to inhibit urea production and reduce protein catabolism.

Disseminated Intravascular Coagulation (DIC)

Patients with acute pancreatitis may exhibit coagulation disturbances ranging from scattered intravascular thrombolysis to fatal DIC. Clinically significant DIC is characterized by production of microthrombi and consumption of clotting factors and complement, and is seen occasionally in patients with severe acute pancreatitis. However, subclinical coagulation disorders occur more frequently in these patients; they often exhibit a hypercoagulable state with increased concentrations of fibrinogen and factor VIII. Fibrinogen concentrations peak by d 6 or 7 following onset of the disease. In patients with severe, acute pancreatitis, the occurrence of DIC with associated defibrination, thrombocytopenia, decreased factor VII, and prolongation of the thrombin time has been described frequently *(150)*.

Studies in animals have shown that the concentration of platelets and fibrinogen falls immediately following the onset of acute pancreatitis *(166)*. This initial drop is followed by a subsequent rebound, and in fact, the increased concentrations of fibrinogen and platelets found in patients several days after the onset of acute pancreatitis may represent a rebound from the initial low values occurring shortly after disease onset.

The mechanism for the coagulation disorders seen in patients with acute pancreatitis is not clear. The release of active trypsin into the circulation has been suggested as a cause *(167)*. Induction of DIC in dogs has been accomplished following iv infusion of trypsin *(168)*. Infusion of other pancreatic enzymes, including amylase or lipase, has been found not to induce coagulation disturbances. Other mechanisms postulated to cause this condition include imbalances in the ratio of proteases to antiproteases, an increase in the reactivity of the reticuloendothelial system, and loss of fibrinogen from the circulation owing to vascular injury *(169)*.

The treatment of patients with acute pancreatitis who develop DIC is difficult. To suppress the activation of proteolytic enzymes, the use of enzyme inhibitors, such as aprotinin, has been studied. Unfortunately, the use of aprotinin in patients with acute pancreatitis has been met with limited success *(170)*. The use of nafamostat mesilate may be beneficial to these patients. This synthetic protease inhibitor is able to penetrate the acinar cells of the pancreas readily owing to the low molecular weight of the drug and its strongly amphophilic properties. Studies have shown that nafamostat mesilate is effective for the treatment of both acute pancreatitis and disseminated intravascular coagulation *(171)*.

Systemic Complications of Acute Pancreatitis

During the first week following the onset of acute pancreatitis, severe cases are often complicated by multisystem organ failure. The organ systems most commonly affected include the renal, pulmonary, and cardiovascular systems. Cardiovascular collapse owing to bleeding or myocardial infarction is also possible. A variety of late complications may occur, typically after the second week of illness, such as pseudocyst and abscess formation. A variety of unusual complications, including gastrointestinal hemorrhage, gastric varices, and pancreatic encephalopathy associated with confusion, delusions, and coma, may also occur. Purtscher's angiopathic retinopathy owing to retinal arteriolar obstruction may result in sudden blindness. Pancreatic inflammation may result in obstruction, necrosis, or fistulization of the adjacent colon, whereas the spread of peripancreatic inflammation may result in splenic rupture or hematoma formation *(172)*.

The likelihood of organ failure is closely related to the type of pancreatitis. In patients with edematous pancreatitis, systemic complications develop in fewer than

10%. However, patients with sterile necrotizing pancreatitis develop systemic complications in up to 60% of cases, whereas those with infected pancreatic necrosis almost always exhibit systemic complications *(173)*.

Pulmonary Complications

Clinical evidence of lung injury has been described in up to 70% of patients with acute pancreatitis. Severe lung injury, manifested as acute respiratory distress syndrome or acute respiratory failure, has been reported in approx 15% of patients *(174)*. The exact mechanism for respiratory complications is uncertain. A wide variety of endogenous substances and cellular elements released from necrotic cells have been postulated. Experimental evidence suggests that activated pancreatic proteases, free fatty acids, activated PLA, activated neutrophils, activated complement, and kinins may play an important role *(175)*.

Pulmonary injury found in patients with acute pancreatitis is difficult to distinguish clinically and pathologically from the acute respiratory distress syndrome *(174)*. These pulmonary complications can vary in severity from mild to life-threatening, and may be grouped into various stages depending on the severity of the lesion *(150,164)*.

The first stage that affects the majority of patients with acute pancreatitis is hypoxemia. Approximately two-thirds of patients will develop tachypnea, mild respiratory acidosis, and hypoxemia during the first 48 h following admission *(176)*. In these patients, physical examination is normal, and abnormalities in chest radiographs are infrequently seen. Approximately one-half of patients demonstrate arterial oxygen tensions of 71 mmHg or below. Severe hypoxia, defined as arterial PO_2 of <60 mmHg, was found in one study in up to 45% of patients *(177)*. This same study also found that those patients with arterial oxygen tensions of less than approx 50 mmHg had a mortality rate of more than 30%. A right to left intrapulmonary shunting of up to 30% of cardiac output as a result of ventilation and perfusion mismatch is thought to be the major cause of hypoxia *(178)*.

Patients who are experiencing their first attack of acute pancreatitis are more likely to develop hypoxia compared to those individuals with a history of previous attacks; the reason for this is unknown. No correlation has been established between the hypoxemia found in these patients and patient age, severity of the attack, pancreatic enzyme activities, serum calcium concentrations, amount of fluid or blood products administered, or estimated fluid sequestration *(150,164)*.

Patients with hypoxemia who show both clinical and radiographic abnormalities of respiratory function may be categorized as reaching stage II. The most common radiographic abnormalities include pulmonary infiltrates or atelectasis, pleural effusions, and pulmonary edema. Patients who reach this stage experience considerably higher morbidity and mortality compared with those in stage I.

Pleural effusions are usually small; however, massive effusions have been described in patients with pancreatitis attributed to ethanol abuse *(179)*. Biochemically, the effusions are characterized by increased amylase activities of up to 30 times greater than corresponding serum activities, protein concentrations >30 g/L, and a fluid:serum LD ratio >0.6 *(172)*. Most pleural effusions are absorbed spontaneously following resolution of pancreatic inflammation.

Patients who exhibit severe dyspnea and extreme hypoxemia that is refractive to increased inspired oxygen concentrations are classified as having stage III respiratory complications. The most serious respiratory complications is the adult respiratory distress syndrome. Not only does acute pancreatitis cause acute respiratory distress syndrome, but the syndrome can exacerbate existing pancreatic injury *(180)*. Thus, a cycle of pancreatic and respiratory injury is created, which if unchecked, can quickly lead to multiple organ system failure. The association of adult respiratory distress syndrome is present in up to 20% of patients with acute pancreatitis with a mortality rate of approx 50%. Adult respiratory distress syndrome typically occurs between 48 h and 1 wk following the onset of acute pancreatitis. Autopsy findings show that the morphological changes seen in the lungs cannot be differentiated from those seen in patients with adult respiratory distress syndrome owing to other pathogenesis, including shock, sepsis, and severe trauma. The incidence of adult respiratory distress syndrome is highest in patients with hemorrhagic pancreatitis, although patients with interstitial edematous pancreatitis are also at risk.

A variety of mechanisms have been postulated in the pathogenesis of respiratory failure in patients with acute pancreatitis. The most frequently cited mechanism involves the release of large quantities of proteases from the inflamed pancreas; they enter the circulation following pancreatic injury and include trypsin, chymotrypsin, and elastase. The release of proteases can cause the breakdown of cellular constituents, pulmonary surfactant, and elastic tissue. In addition, activated proteases can cause the activation of the coagulation and complement cascades.

Another enzyme that has been implicated in the pulmonary damage seen in these patients is PLA. PLA is a lecithinase that cleaves one fatty acid from lecithin, the principal component of pulmonary surfactant, to form lysolecithin and free fatty acids. In addition to the effect of PLA in destroying pulmonary surfactant, the enzyme may also cause breakdown of the phospholipid layer of cell membranes resulting in cell lysis. The action of arachidonic acid formed by the action of PLA on the cell membrane phospholipids may result in the generation of thromboxane A_2, causing increased leukocyte adherence and leukocyte-dependent vascular injury to the lung. Also, the liberated free fatty acid may contribute to further injury. Owing to the potential adverse effects of PLA present in the circulation, this enzyme is considered to play a major role in the pathogenesis of pulmonary injury.

Another mechanism that may play a role in pulmonary injury involves activation of the complement cascade. Some complement fragments, especially C5a, are leukotactic and may cause entrapment of leukocytes within the lung. Activated neutrophils within the lung can produce pulmonary damage owing to release of lysosomal enzymes, generation of oxygen free radicals, or release of arachidonic acid metabolites.

The presence of fibrin and platelet microthrombi in the pulmonary vessels observed at autopsy of patients dying from acute pancreatitis suggests that pulmonary intravascular coagulation and platelet aggregation had occurred. Fibrinogen and platelet concentrations have been observed to be decreased in patients with pancreatitis. Activation of the coagulation cascade may occur as a result of release of trypsin into the circulation. Studies in animals suggest that iv administration of either lipase or PLA substances, both of which that are also present in patients with acute pancreatitis, does not produce thrombosis *(166)*.

A variety of other factors in addition to release of trypsin may contribute to the formation of microthrombi in patients with acute pancreatitis. These factors include acidosis, circulatory shock, and the inhibition of fibrinolysis secondary to the inhibition of plasminogen activation.

Many studies have indicated a role for the generation of free fatty acids following lipolysis in the pulmonary damage seen in acute pancreatitis *(181)*. A high incidence of hypertriglyceridemia has been noted in patients with respiratory failure, suggesting that increased serum triglyceride concentrations may play an etiologic role in the development of pulmonary insufficiency.

Hypertriglyceridemia is often seen in individuals without pulmonary injury, suggesting that hypertriglyceridemia by itself is not responsible for pulmonary insufficiency. Experimental studies suggest that lipoprotein lipase that is present in high concentrations within the pulmonary capillaries may become activated. The activated lipoprotein lipase can cleave fatty acids from triglycerides, causing the release of large quantities of free fatty acids within the lungs. The unbound fatty acids can induce injury to the alveolar membrane, leading to an increase in pulmonary extravascular water, interstitial and intra-alveolar edema, and intrapulmonary shunting *(181)*.

One final mechanism that may play a minor role in pulmonary injury is activation of the kallikrein-kinin system, leading to the production of bradykinin from kininogen. Acute pancreatitis results in the liberation of kallikrein and trypsin from the pancreas; they are probably responsible for the generation of bradykinin from its precursors. The ability of bradykinin to increase lung vascular permeability in patients with acute pancreatitis is small and does not play an important role in the lung injury seen in these patients.

Cardiovascular Complications

Cardiovascular disturbances found in patients with acute pancreatitis include electrocardiographic abnormalities, hemodynamic disturbances, and pericardial effusion. The changes in cardiac function in patients with acute pancreatitis have not been found to be associated with structural abnormalities within the myocardium, suggesting that myocardial depression in acute pancreatitis is of metabolic origin. A variety of biochemical mediators that have profound effects on the cardiovascular system have been described in these patients. Increases in vascular permeability owing to formation of bradykinin and increases in prostaglandins with a decrease in systemic vascular resistance have been described *(182,183)*. The existence of a myocardial depressant factor released from the acinar cells in patients with acute pancreatitis has also been suggested *(184)*.

Electrocardiographic changes in acute pancreatitis are relatively common. Arrythmia, conduction abnormalities, and changes in the T wave and QT period are frequently seen *(185)*. ST elevation is a rare occurrence in these patients. Several hypotheses have been proposed to explain these changes. Electrolyte abnormalities, such as hypokalemia, hypocalcemia, and hyponatremia, are common in acute pancreatitis, and can modify the repolarization phase on the electrocardiogram. Electrocardiographic changes may also be induced by hemodynamic disturbances, such as profound hypotension causing myocardial ischemia, and conduction disturbances. These changes have been especially noted in patients with pre-existing cardiac abnormalities and cardiomyopathy secondary to ethanol abuse *(186)*.

Hypovolemia occurs early in the course of an attack of acute pancreatitis and is associated with poor prognosis *(187)*. With aggressive volume replacement therapy, hypovolemia is now an infrequent complication of acute pancreatitis. Hypovolemia develops owing to loss of fluid into the peripancreatic spaces and systemic tissues. Fluid loss is owing primarily to an increase in the permeability and a decreased resistance in the peripheral circulation. These effects may be induced by the release of vasoactive peptides, such as bradykinin. In addition, the development of hypoalbuminemia, nausea with vomiting, and sequestration of fluid within the bowel may further contribute to volume loss.

Gastrointestinal disorders presenting with epigastric pain are an important part of the differential diagnosis of acute myocardial infarction. The mistaken diagnosis of acute myocardial infarction in a patient with acute pancreatitis can result in serious consequences owing to withholding of appropriate therapy or initiation of inappropriate measures, such as thrombolytic therapy; the latter given to a patient with acute pancreatitis can exacerbate the underlying disease process *(188)*.

Renal Complications

Acute renal failure is an infrequent, although serious, complication of acute pancreatitis. Mortality in patients who reach this state still remains approx 80%. The extent of tubular necrosis has been shown to be related to the degree of pancreatic inflammation, and is most severe in patients with pancreatitis caused by biliary obstruction or following postoperative complications *(189)*.

Renal failure was believed to be caused by hypovolemia and hypotension alone. However, other factors also play an important role. Some studies suggest that a hypercoagulable state, possibly enzyme-induced, may be an important factor in the pathogenesis of renal insufficiency. Histologic findings of prominent deposits of IgG, fibrin, and fibrinogen in the glomerular capillaries lend support to this hypothesis.

Another mechanism that may also play a role in renal failure involves the release of platelet-activating factor from the ischemic pancreas inducing the release of platelet-activating factor that owing to its potent vasoactive properties, causes a marked decrease in renal blood flow and glomerular filtration rate through either constriction of vascular smooth muscle cells or mesangial cell contraction.

Subcutaneous Fat Necrosis

Subcutaneous fat necrosis in association with acute pancreatitis is a rare complication. Fat necrosis is not localized to any one specific area, and may be found on the buttocks, thighs, upper arms, and trunk. Fat necrosis can accompany pancreatitis in association with malignancy, trauma, and biliary obstruction; however, it appears to occur more frequently in men with pancreatitis attributed to alcohol abuse.

Joint lesions involving the metatarsal, interphalangeal, wrist, knee, and ankle joints are often associated with subcutaneous fat necrosis *(190)*. The joint lesions are clinically identical to gout. However, serum uric acid concentrations may not be increased.

The significance of these lesions is that in some patients with acute pancreatitis, they are the patient's only complaint on presentation *(191)*. The pathogenesis of subcutaneous fat necrosis is poorly understood. It has been postulated that these lesions occur secondarily to the release of active pancreatic enzymes into the circulation or lymphatic drainage. Lipase has been implicated in reports of strongly positive intracellular staining of adipocytes with an MAb specific for pancreatic lipase *(192)*. A more likely explanation for the development of these lesions is that subcutaneous fat necrosis and joint lesions develop in those patients who are deficient in protease inhibitors, such as α-1-antitrypsin and α-2-macroglobulin. Thus, in these patients, circulating active proteolytic and/or lipolytic enzymes would be able to exert their effects in systemic sites. This mechanism would help explain why this syndrome is so rare, in contrast to the relative frequency of pancreatitis. It would also explain why these lesions occur in some patients who are otherwise asymptomatic for pancreatic disease.

Pancreatitis and Multiple System Organ Failure

Multiple system organ failure associated with acute pancreatitis is very similar to that seen in patients with trauma, burns, or other catastrophic illness. Advances in supportive care have increased the number of patients who survive the acute phase of the disease. However, in a minority of patients, acute pancreatitis progresses to multiple system organ failure with poor prognosis. The prevalence of multiple system organ failure in acute pancreatitis is approximately 20% *(187)*, and the mortality rate is proportional to the number of organs involved. In patients with four organ systems failing, mortality is virtually 100%. One study found that the mean number of organ system failures in survivors was 1.4 vs 3.2 in patients who did not survive *(193)*.

The development of organ failure has been shown to be influenced by factors, such as the patient's age, local complications, pre-existing diseases, and systemic infection. Of these factors, systemic infection has been shown to be an important initiating factor for the development of multiple organ system failure *(187,194)*. The predominance of enteric Gram-negative bacteria in both local and systemic infections in patients with acute pancreatis suggests that translocation of intestinal flora from the gastrointestinal tract may be primarily responsible in the pathogenesis of infection and multiple organ system failure *(187,195)*. Studies in animals have shown that reducing the amount of intestinal flora can significantly improve survival in acute pancreatitis. Unfortunately, data for humans with acute pancreatitis confirming these results is lacking.

Pancreatitis-Associated Retinopathy

Retinal lesions in association with acute pancreatitis are a rare complication, being first documented and described in 1975 *(196)*. The retinal lesions are similar to these described by Purtscher in 1910 *(197)* in patients with head trauma in whom sudden loss of vision occurred within hours following injury. The severity of visual impairment can vary widely ranging from complete recovery to permanent impairment. No specific therapy is known.

The mechanism of trauma-induced retinopathy is thought to be owing to retinal ischemia produced by arterial occlusive disease. The exact cause of ischemic retinal injury in patients with acute pancreatitis has not been identified. Initially, obstruction of retinal arteries by fat emboli was the purported mechanism. Evidence for this included the finding of fat emboli in some patients with retinopathy owing to causes other than pancreatitis, and because arterial fat emboli have been found in other organ systems in patients with acute pancreatitis.

Recent studies suggest that other mechanisms are responsible for the retinopathy of acute pancreatitis. One hypothesis involves the generation of activated complement factor 5 by proteolytic enzymes released from the inflamed pancreas *(198)*. The active factor 5 can induce the aggregation of granulocytes leading to microvascular occlusion by microemboli. However, this mechanism alone cannot account for all cases of pancreatitis-associated retinopathy.

A fairly strong relationship has been found between retinopathy in acute pancreatitis and excessive ethanol consumption. However, the association between the two is not well understood. It has been suggested that a nutritional deficit, toxin exposure, or some other risk factor associated with alcohol ingestion or alcoholism may be responsible *(198)*.

The development of retinopathy has been found by some to have prognostic significance *(199)*. Retinopathy was four times more frequent in patients with multiple system organ failure than in those without any organ system failure. In addition, the frequency of retinopathy in nonsurvivors was twice that seen in survivors. Thus, the retinopathy of pancreatitis may have prognostic significance; its onset indicates a poor prognosis and the likelihood of development of multiple organ system failure.

SUMMARY

Biochemical Indicators

Measurement of amylase activity in serum has remained the primary biochemical test for the evaluation of patients with suspected acute pancreatitis for over 80 yr. Even with its acknowledged shortcomings, including nonspecificity for the pancreas and increases in patients with renal insufficiency, amylase remains one of the top 20 most commonly requested laboratory tests. Attempts to improve the nonspecificity of amylase have led to methods for the measurement of amylase isoenzymes. Increases in the amount of P type amylase on the presence of the P3 isoform have been advocated as more specific markers of pancreatic damage. However, use of amylase isoenzymes on the P3 isoform have been found to provide similar diagnostic accuracy to that of lipase alone.

Lipase is often considered to be the most useful marker of acute pancreatitis available today. Previous problems with the analysis of lipase have been largely overcome by the use of colipase which is an important cofactor for the enzyme. Measurement of lipase in conjunction with amylase may be useful in the evaluation of the pathogenesis of acute pancreatitis. Calculation of the ratio of lipase to amylase has been found by some to allow differentiation of pancreatitis owing to ethanol abuse from other causes; the ratio of lipase to amylase being much higher in ethanol-induced pancreatitis.

Lipase has recently been shown to be composed of two isoforms, L1 and L2, which are probably posttransitional variants of a single enzyme form. Preliminary studies have shown the diagnostic accuracy provided by measurement of the L2 isoform to be better than that provided by total lipase activity.

In addition to amylase and lipase, several other biochemical markers of acute pancreatitis have been evaluated for their effectiveness in detecting pancreatic injury.

Assays have been developed for trypsin, phospholipase A, and carboxypeptidase A. Although these markers may provide greater diagnostic accuracy for acute pancreatitis than amylase or lipase, and may even allow for the severity of an attack to be determined, none of these markers have been implemented to any great extent.

Etiology of Acute Pancreatitis

A great number of etiologic factors have been recognized with the potential of initiating acute pancreatitis. Drug-induced pancreatitis has been attributed to more than 50 drugs. Therapy with ddI has most recently been implicated as a causative agent of acute pancreatitis. This compound is frequently used in patients with AIDS. Acute pancreatitis associated with patients taking ddI has been reported with an incidence of 4–23.5%.

Metabolic disturbances implicated in causing acute pancreatitis include hypercalcemia and hypertriglyceridemia. Prolonged or excessive increases in calcium concentrations has been associated with cell damage in many tissues, including the pancreas. A variety of factors have been found that lead to increases in acinar cell calcium concentrations. These initiating factors include ethanol abuse, hyperlipidemia, ductal hypertension, and certain drugs and toxins.

Hypertriglyceridemia is well-recognized as a cause of acute pancreatitis. Hypertriglyceridemia may be genetic in origin or it may be secondary to various causes including ethanol abuse, diabetes, hypothyroidism, nephrotic syndrome, or certain drugs. Mechanisms of hypertriglyceride-induced pancreatitis include chemical irritation caused by the release of cytotoxic free fatty acids or increases in acinar cell calcium concentrations as discussed previously.

Postoperative pancreatitis has been described in patients undergoing abdominal surgery as well as following surgery not involving the abdomen. Factors thought responsible for postoperative pancreatitis include direct pancreatic injury in patients undergoing abdominal surgery; pancreatic ischemia, especially in patients placed on cardiopulmonary bypass; use of perioperative medications such as calcium replacement therapy; the production of microthrombi with resultant pancreatic ischemia, pancreatic duct obstruction; and infarction. Pancreatitis associated with ERCP has been reported to occur in up to 5% of individuals undergoing this procedure. The incidence of hyperamylasemia in patients undergoing this procedure has been reported to be as high as 70%.

The association between ethanol abuse and acute pancreatitis has been known for well over a century. Ethanol induced pancreatitis usually develops following chronic ingestion of alcohol for at least 7–10 yr. Several theories have been proposed to explain the pathogenesis of ethanol-induced pancreatitis. These mechanisms include alcohol-induced stenosis of the sphincter of Oddi, the production of free radical compounds following the metabolism of ethanol, and a reduction in pancreatic blood flow mediated by ethanol.

Anatomic abnormalities have also been reported to cause acute pancreatitis. Pancreas divisum is the most common anatomic variant of the pancreas and has been implicated by some as the source of 10–20% of cases of pancreatitis for which no other causes can be found. Other anatomic abnormalities that may predispose an individual to pancreatitis include dysfunction of the Sphincter of Oddi and ampullary stenosis.

Pancreatitis owing to biliary obstruction has been reported as the most common cause of pancreatitis in women, with ethanol being the most common cause in men. The most common cause of biliary obstruction is caused by gallstones. However, obstruction can be also be the result of tumors or parasites.

Assessment of Severity of Acute Pancreatitis

Assessment of the severity of acute pancreatitis plays an important role in the treatment plan. Severity assessment helps ensure that intensive therapy is targeted at patients with the severest attacks and allows the early detection of complications. Many schemes have been developed for use in gauging disease severity. Those include clinical assessment, multiple prognostic criteria, peritoneal tap, computerized scanning, and use of biochemical test results.

Severity assessment based on clinical assessment is often inaccurate, especially when performed early in the course of the disease. The use of multiple prognostic criteria has gained greater acceptance. Classification of disease severity by use of multiple prognostic criteria include that of Ranson, the Glasgow score, the APACHE and APACHE II scores, and the simplified acute physiology score. Studies have demonstrated that the APACHE II score is superior to these other classification schemes.

A more simplified approach for classifying patients with respect to disease severity relies on the use of single prognostic indicators. A variety of enzymes and other protein markers have been suggested for this purpose. These markers include neutrophil elastase, C-reactive protein, trypsinogen activation peptide, pancreatitis-associated protein, complement, interleukin-6, tumor necrosis factor, ribonuclease, antiproteases including α-2-macroglobulins and α-1-antitrypsin, phospholipase A_2, and methemalbumin. Other single prognostic indicators include the peritoneal tap and determination of the body mass index.

Complications of Acute Pancreatitis

Acute pancreatitis can result in the release of a wide array of biochemical substances that can induce a variety of derangements, both local and systemic. Local complications include hemorrhage, pseudocyst, pancreatic abscess and phlegmon.

Biochemical disturbances that can occur as a result of acute pancreatitis may be primarily responsible for initiating major organ failure in severe attacks. These disturbances include hypocalcemia, hypomagnesemia, hyperlipidemia, and hyperglycemia. Coagulation disturbances range from scattered intravascular thrombolysis to fatal disseminated coagulation.

Severe cases of acute pancreatitis are often complicated by multisystem organ failure. Organ systems most commonly affected include the renal, pulmonary, and cardiovascular systems. Pulmonary injury has been described in up to 70% of patients with acute pancreatitis. A variety of mechanisms may be responsible for the pathogenesis of respiratory failure. The most frequently cited mechanism involves the release of large quantities of proteases from the inflamed pancreas. Activation of the complement cascade may result in recruitment of neutrophils within the lung and damage due to release of lysosomal enzymes. Another mechanism for pulmonary injury may involve activation of lipoprotein lipase within the pulmonary capillaries with cleavage of fatty acids from the increased concentrations of triglycerides seen in these patients.

Cardiovascular disturbances seen in patients with acute pancreatitis include electrocardiographic abnormalities, hemodynamic disturbances, and pericardial effusion. Electrocardiographic changes have attributed to electrolyte abnormalities and hemodynamic disturbances.

Renal complications are an infrequent although serious complication of acute pancreatitis. Factors suggested to play a role include a hypercoagulable state and the release of platelet-activating factor which causes a marked decrease in renal blood flow. Other complications associated with severe cases of acute pancreatitis include subcutaneous fat necrosis, joint lesions involving the metatarsal, interphalangeal, wrist, knee, and ankle, and pancreatitis-associated retinopathy.

REFERENCES

1. Stocks P (1916) The quantitative determination of amylase in blood, serum, and urine as an aid to diagnosis. Q J Med 9:216–232.
2. Schmidt E, Schmidt FW (1990) Advances in the enzyme diagnosis of pancreatic diseases. Clin Biochem 23:383–394.
3. Tietz N (1988) Amylase measurements in serum-old myths die hard. Clin Chem Clin Biochem 26:251–253 (editorial).
4. Gross JB, Levitt MD (1979) Post-operative evaluation of amylase/creatinine clearance ratio in patients without pancreatitis. Gastroenterology 77:497–498.
5. Claiven PA, Robert J, Meyer P, Borst F, Hauser H, Herrman F, et al. (1989) Acute pancreatitis and normoamylasemia, not an uncommon combination. Ann Surg 210: 614–620.
6. Eckfeldt JH, Levitt MD (1989) Diagnostic enzymes for pancreatic disease. Clin Lab Med 9:731–743.
7. Steinberg W, Goldstein SS, Davis ND, Shamma J, Anderson K (1985) Diagnostic assays in acute pancreatitis. A study of sensitivity and specificity. Ann Intern Med 102:576–580.
8. Winslet M, Hall C, London NJM, Neoptolemos JP (1992) Relation of diagnostic serum amylase levels to aetiology and severity of acute pancreatitis. Gut 982–986.
9. Mayer AD, McMahon MJ, Confield AP, Cooper MJ, Williamson RCN, Dickson AP, et al. (1985) Controlled clinical trial of peritoneal lavage for the treatment of severe acute pancreatitis. N Engl J Med 312:399–404.
10. MRC Multicentre Trial (1977) Death from acute pancreatitis. Lancet ii:632–635.
11. Clave P, Guillaumes S, Blanco I, Nabau N, Merce J, Farre A, et al. (1995) Amylase, lipase, pancreatic isoamylase, and phospholipase A in diagnosis of acute pancreatitis. Clin Chem 41:1129–1134.
12. Corsetti JP, Cox C, Schulz TJ, Arvan DA (1993) Combined serum amylase and lipase determinations for diagnosis of suspected acute pancreatitis. Clin Chem 39:2495–2499.
13. Kazmierczak SC, Catrou PG, VanLente F (1993) Diagnostic accuracy of pancreatic enzymes evaluated by use of multivariate data analysis. Clin Chem 39:1960–1965.
14. Jensen DM, Royse VL, Bonello JN, Schaffner J (1987) Use of amylase isoenzymes in laboratory evaluation of hyperamylasemia. Dig Dis Sci 32:561–568.
15. Weaver DW, Bouwman DL, Walt AJ, Clink D, Resto A, Stephany J (1982) A correlation between clinical pancreatitis and isoenzyme patterns of amylase. Surgery 92:576–580.
16. Bloch RS, Weaver DW, Bowman DL (1983) Acute alcohol intoxication: Significance of the amylase level. Ann Emerg Med 12:294–296.
17. Mifflin TE, Hortin G, Bruns DE (1986) Electrophoretic assays of amylase isoenzymes and isoforms. Clin Lab Med 6:583–599.
18. Legaz ME, Kenny MA (1976) Electrophoretic amylase fractionation as an aid in diagnosis of pancreatic disease. Clin Chem 22:57–62.

19. Panteghini M, Pagani F (1989) Diagnostic value of measuring pancreatic lipase and the P_3 isoform of the pancreatic amylase isoenzyme is serum of hospitalized hyperamylasemic patients. Clin Chem 35:417–421.
20. Frost SJ (1978) A simple quantitative index of the P_3 amylase isoenzyme in the diagnosis of acute pancreatitis. Clin Chim Acta 87:23–28.
21. Leclerc P, Forest JC (1983) Variations in amylase isoenzymes and lipase during acute pancreatitis, and in other disorders causing pancreatitis. Clin Chem 29:1020–1023
22. VanLente F, Kazmierczak SC (1989) Immunologically derived pancreatic amylase, pancreatic lipase, and total amylase compared as predictors of pancreatic inflammation. Clin Chem 35:1542.
23. Kazmierczak SC, Van Lente F, McHugh AM, Katzin WE (1988) Macryoamylasemia with a markedly increased amylase clearance ratio in a patient with renal cell carcinoma. Clin Chem 34:435–438
24. Borgstroem B (1977) The action of bile salts and other detergents on pancreatic lipase and the interaction with colipase. Biochim Biophys Acta 488:381–391.
25. Gwozdz GP, Steinberg WM, Werner M, Henry JP, Pauley C (1990) Comparative evaluation of the diagnosis of acute pancreatitis based on serum and urine enzyme assays. Clin Chim Acta 187:243–254.
26. Lessinger JM, Ferard G (1994) Plasma pancreatic lipase activity: From analytical specificity to clinical efficiency for the diagnosis of acute pancreatitis. Eur J Clin Chem Clin Biochem 32:377–381.
27. Tenner SM, Steinberg W (1992) The admission serum lipase: amylase ratio differentiates alcoholic from nonalcoholic acute pancreatitis. Am J Gastroenterol 87:755–758.
28. Kazmierczak SC, Catrou PG, Van Lente F (1995) Enzymatic markers of gallstone induced pancreatitis identified by ROC curve analysis, discriminant analysis, logistic regression, likelihood ratios, and information theory. Clin Chem 41:523–531.
29. Jaakkola M, Sillanaukee , Lof K, Koivula T, Nordback I (1994) Blood tests for detection of alcoholic cause of acute pancreatitis. Lancet ii:1328–1329.
30. Dammann HG, Dopner M, Wichert PV, Harders H, Hornborstel H (1980) Gallstones and acute pancreatitis (letter). Lancet i:308.
31. Lott JA, Lu CJ (1991) Lipase isoforms and amylase isoenzymes: assays and application in the diagnosis of acute pancreatitis. Clin Chem 37:361–368.
32. DeCaro A, Figarella C, Amie J (1977) Human pancreatic lipase: a glycoprotein. Biochim Biophys Acta 490:411–419.
33. Junge W, Leybold K (1982) Detection of colipase in serum and urine of pancreatitis patients. Clin Chim Acta 123:293–302.
34. Rosenblum JL (1991) Serum lipase activity is increased in disease states other than acute pancreatitis: amylase revisited. Clin Chem 37:315–316.
35. Bohe M, Borgstrom A, Lindestom C, Ohlsson K (1986) Pancreatic endoproteases and pancreatic secretory trypsin inhibitor immunoreactivity in human Paneth cells. J Clin Pathol 39:786–793.
36. LeMoine O, Devaster JM, Deviere J, Thiry P, Cremer M, Ooms HA (1994) Trypsin activity: a new marker of acute alcoholic pancreatitis. Dig Dis Sci 39:2634–2638.
37. Heath DI, Cruickshank A, Gudgeon AM, Jehanli A, Shenkin A, Imrie CW (1995) The relationship between pancreatic enzyme release and activation and the acute-phase protein response in patients with acute pancreatitis. Pancreas 10:347–353.
38. Schmidt D, Hoffman GE (1987) Activity of phospholipase A compared in serum of patients with pancreatic and nonpancreatic diseases. Clin Chem 33:594–595.
39. Nevalainen TJ (1988) Phospholipase A2 in acute pancreatitis. Scand J Gastroenterol 23: 897–904.
40. Eskola JV, Nevalainen TJ, Kortesvo P (1988) Immunoreactive pancreatic phospholipase A_2 in serum from patients with acute pancreatitis. Clin Chem 34:1052–1054.

41. Hoffman GE, Hiefinger R, Steinbrueckner B (1989) Serum phospholipase A in hospitalized patients. Clin Chim Acta 183:59–64.
42. Kazmierczak SC, Van Lente F, Hodges ED (1991) Diagnostic and prognostic utility of phospholipase A activity in patients with acute pancreatitis: comparison with amylase and lipase. Clin Chem 37:356–360.
43. Kazmierczak SC, Van Lente F (1989) Measuring carboxypeptidase A with a centrifugal analyzer: analytical and clinical considerations. Clin Chem 35:251–255.
44. Peterson LM, Homquist B, Bethune JL (1982) A unique activity assay for carboxypeptidase A in human serum. Anal Biochem 125:420–426.
45. Saruta H, Ashihara Y, Sugiyama M, Roth M, Miyagawa E, Kido Y, et al. (1986) Colorimetric determination of carboxypeptidase A activity in serum. Clin Chem 32:748–751.
46. Bradley EL (1993) A clinically based classification system for acute pancreatitis. Arch Surg 128:586–590.
47. Steinberg W, Tenner S (1994) Acute pancreatitis. New Engl J Med 330:1198–1210.
48. Zion MM, Goldberg B, Suzman MM (1955) Corticotrophin and cortisone in the treatment of scleroderma. Q J Med 24:215–227.
49. Johnston DH, Cornish AL (1959) Acute pancreatitis in patients receiving chlorothiazide. JAMA 170:1054–1056.
50. Lankisch PG, Drogen M, Gottesleben F (1995) Drug induced acute pancreatitis: incidence and severity. Gut 37:565–567.
51. Mallory A, Kern F (1980) Drug-induced pancreatitis: a critical review. Gastroenterology 78:813–820.
52. Murthy UK, DeGregorio F, Oates RP, Blair DC (1992) Hyperamylasemia in patients with the Acquired Immunodeficiency Syndrome. Am J Gastroenterol 87:332–336.
53. Zazzo JF, Pichon F, Regnier B (1987) HIV and the pancreas. Lancet i:1212–1213 (letter).
54. Pelucio MT, Rothenhaus T, Smith M, Ward DJ (1995) Fatal pancreatitis as a complication of therapy of HIV infection. J Emerg Med 13:633–637.
55. Maxson CJ, Greenfield SM, Turner JL (1992) Acute pancreatitis as a common complication of 2'3'-dideoxyinosine therapy in the acquired immunodeficiency syndrome. Am J Gastroenterol 87:708–713.
56. Ward JB, Petersen OH, Jenkens SA, Sutton R (1995) Is an elevated concentration of acinar cytosolic free ionized calcium the trigger for acute pancreatitis. Lancet 346:1016–1019.
57. Nicotera P, Bellomo G, Orrehius S (1992) Calcium-mediated mechanisms in chemically induced cell death. Annu Rev Pharmacol Toxicol 32:449–470.
58. Gronroos JM, Kaila T, Kietaranta AJ (1994) Alcohol, pancreatic muscarinic receptors and acute pancreatitis. Exp Toxicol Pathol 45:503–505.
59. Wisner J, Green D, Ferrell L, Renner I (1988) Evidence for a role of oxygen derived free radicals in the pathogenesis of cerulein induced acute pancreatitis in rats. Gut 29:1516–523.
60. Leahy A, Darzi A, Grace P (1992) Verapamil is beneficial in a model of acute pancreatitis after endoscopic retrograde cholangiopancreatography. Br J Surg 79:1241.
61. Taskes PP (1990) Hyperlipidemic pancreatitis. Gastroenterol Clin North Am (4):783–791.
62. Fortson MR, Freedman SN, Webster PD (1995) Clinical assessment of hyperlipidemic pancreatitis. Am J Gastroenterol 90:2134–2139.
63. Chait A, Brunzell JD (1991) Chylomicronemia syndrome. Adv Intern Med 37:249–273.
64. Calderon P, Furnelle J, Christopher J (1979) In vivo lipid metabolism in the rat pancreas. Biochem Biophys Acta 574:379–422.
65. Lankisch PG, Schirren CA, Kunze E (1991) Undetected fatal acute pancreatitis: why is the disease so frequently overlooked. Am J Gastroenterol 86:322–336.
66. Kazmierczak SC, VanLente F (1988) Incidence and source of hyperamylasemia following cardiac surgery. Clin Chem 34:916–919.

67. Sanfrey H, Bulkley GB, Cameron JL (1985) The pathogenesis of acute pancreatitis. The source and role of oxygen-derived free radicals in three different experimental models. Ann Surg 201:633–639.
68. Fernandez del Castillo C, Harringer W, Warshaw AL, Vlahakes GJ, Koski G, Zaslavsky AM, et al. (1991) Risk factors for pancreatic cellular injury after cardiopulmonary bypass. New Engl J Med 325:382–387.
69. Stanten R, Frey CF (1990) Pancreatitis after endoscopic retrograde cholangiopancreatography. Arch Surg 1245:1032–1035.
70. La Ferla G, Gordon S, Archibald M, Murray WR (1986) Hyperamylasemia and acute pancreatitis following endoscopic retrograde cholangiopancreatography. Pancreas 1: 160–163.
71. Singh M, Simsek H (1990) Ethanol and the pancreas. Gastroenterology 98:1051–1062.
72. Nordback IH, Olson JL, Chacko VP, Cameron JL (1995) Detailed characterization of experimental acute alcoholic pancreatitis. Surgery 117:41–49.
73. Foitzik T, Fernandez-del Castillo C, Rattner DW, Klar E, Warshaw AL (1995) Alcohol selectively impairs oxygenation of the pancreas. Arch Surg 130:357–361.
74. Dib JA, Cooper-Vastola SA, Meirelles RF Jr, Bagchi S, Caboclo JL, Holm C (1993) Acute effects of ethanol and ethanol plus furosemide on pancreatic capillary blood flow in rats. Am J Surg 166:18–23.
75. Bloch EH, McQuarrie IG (1988) Early observations of the circulation made by in vivo microscopy during acute ethanol intoxication. Alcohol Clin Exp Res 12:298–300.
76. Richter JM, Schapiro RH, Mulley AG, Warshaw AL (1981) Association of pancreas divisum and pancreatitis and its treatment by sphincteroplasty of the accessory ampulla. Gastroenterology 81:1104–1110.
77. Feeler ER (1984) Endoscopic retrograde cholangiopancreatography in the diagnosis of unexplained pancreatitis. Arch Intern Med 144:1797–1799.
78. Steinberg W, Tenner S (1994) Acute pancreatitis. N Engl J Med 330:1198–1210.
79. Parti MG, Pellegrini CA (1990) Gallstone pancreatitis. Surg Clin North Am 70:1277–1295.
80. Moreau JA, Zinsmeister AR, Melton LJ, DiMagno EP (1988) Gallstone pancreatitis and the effect of cholecystectomy: a population based cohort study. Mayo Clin Proc 63: 466–473.
81. Fan ST, Lai ECS, Mok FPT, Lo CM, Zheng SS, Wong J (1993) Early treatment of acute biliary pancreatitis by endoscopic papillotomy. N Engl J Med 328;226–232.
82. Neoptolemos JP (1991) Acute biliary pancreatitis. Ital J Gastroenterol 23:570–573.
83. Calleja GA, Barkin JS (1993) Acute pancreatitis. Med Clin North Am 77:1037–1056.
84. Leese T, Shaw D (1988) Comparison of three Glasgow multifactorial prognostic scoring systems in acute pancreatitis. Br J Surg 75:460–462.
85. Larvin M, McMahon MJ (1989) APACHE II score for assessment and monitoring of acute pancreatitis. Lancet ii:20120–5.
86. Jacobs ML, Daggett WM, Civette JM, Vasu MA, Lawson DW, Warshaw AL, et al. (1976) Acute pancreatitis: analysis of factors influencing survival. Ann Surg 185:43–51.
87. Steinberg WE (1990) Predictors of severity of acute pancreatitis. Gastroenterol Clin North Am 4:849–861.
88. McMahon MJ, Playforth MJ, Pickford IR (1980) A comparative study of methods for the prediction of severity of attacks of acute pancreatitis. Br J Surg 67:22–25.
89. Ranson JH, Rifkind KM, Roses DF, Fink SD, Eng K, Spencer FC (1974) Prognostic signs and the role of operative management in acute pancreatitis. Surg Gynecol Obstet. 139:69–81.
90. Imrie CW, Benjamin IS, Ferguson JC, McKay AJ, Mackenzie I, O'Neill J (1978) A single-centre double-blind trial of Trasylol therapy in primary acute pancreatitis. Br J Surg 65:337–341.

91. Knaus WA, Zimmerman JE, Wagner DP, Draper EA, Lawrence DE (1981) APACHE-acute physiology and chronic health evaluation: a physiologically based classification system. Crit Care Med 9:591–597.
92. Imrie CW (1995) Prognosis of acute pancreatitis. Ann Ital Chir 66:187–189.
93. Chui DW, Grendell JH (1993) Acute pancreatitis. Curr Opin Gastroenterol 760–766.
94. Winslet M, Hall C, London NJM, Neoptolemos JP (1992) Relation of diagnostic serum amylase levels to aetology and severity of acute pancreatitis. Gut 33:982–986
95. Collins REC, Frost SJ, Spittlehouse KE (1982) The P_3 isoenzyme of serum amylase in the management of patients with acute pancreatitis. Br J Surg 69:373–375.
96. Navarro S, Aused R, Casals E, Elena M, Garcia-Puges AM, Adrian MJ, et al. (1987) Value of the P_3 isoamylase fraction as an indicator of the long-term prognosis in acute pancreatitis. Br J Surg 174:405–407.
97. Goris RJA (1990) Mediators of multiple organ failure. Intern Care Med 16:S192–S196.
98. Solomkin JS, Cotta LA, Satoh PS, Hurst JM, Nelson RD (1985) Complement activation and clearance in acute illness and injury: evidence for C5a as a cell directed mediator of ARDS in man. Surgery 97:668–678.
99. Dusswald KH, Jochum M, Schram W, Fritz H (1985) Released granulocyte elastase: an indicator of pathobiochemical alterations in septicemia after abdominal surgery. Surgery. 98:892–899.
100. Zheutlin LM, Thonar EJ-MA, Jacobs ER, Hanley ME, Balk RA, Bone RC (1986) Plasma elastase in the ARDS. J Crit Care 1:39–44.
101. Gross V, Scholmerich J, Leser HG, Salm R, Lausen M, Ruckaver K, et al. (1990) Granulocyte elastase in assessment of severity of acute pancreatitis. Dig Dis Sci 35:97–105.
102. Uhl W, Büchler M, Malfertheiner P, Martini M, Beger HG (1991) PMN-elastase in comparison with CRP, antiproteases, and LDH as indicators of necrosis in human acute pancreatitis. Pancreas 3:253–259.
103. Domígues-Muñoz JE, Carballo F, Garcia MJ, de Diego JM, Ráago L, Simón MA, et al. (1991) Clinical usefulness of polymorphonuclear elastase in predicting the severity of acute pancreatitis: results of a multicentre study. Br J Surg 78:1230–1234.
104. Baumann H, Prowse KR, Marinkovic S, Won KA, Jahreis GP (1989) Stimulation of hepatic acute phase response by cytokines and glucocorticoid. Ann NY Acad Sci 557: 280–295.
105. Dusetti NJ, Britz EM, Mallo GV, Dagorn J-C, Iovanna JL (1995) Pancreatitis-associated protein I (PAP I), an acute phase protein induced by cytokines. J Biol Chem 270: 22471–22421.
106. Viedma JA, Pérez-Mateo M, Agulló J, Dominguez JE, Carballo F (1994) Inflammatory response in the early prediction of severity in human acute pancreatitis. Gut 35:822–827.
107. Wilson C, Heads A, Shenkin A, Imrie CW (1989) C-reactive protein, antiproteases and complement factors as objective markers of severity in acute pancreatitis. Br J Surg 76: 177–181.
108. Gudgeon AM, Heath DI, Hurley P, Jehanli A, Patel G, Wilson C, et al. (1990) Trypsinogen activation peptides in the early prediction of severity of acute pancreatitis. Lancet i:4–8.
109. Iovanna JL, Keim V, Michel R, Dagorn J-C (1991) Pancreatic gene expression is altered during acute experimental pancreatitis in the rat. Am J Physiol 261:G485–489.
110. Iovanna JL, Keim V, Nordback I, Montalto G, Camarena J, Letoublon C, et al. (1994) Serum levels of pancreatitis-associated protein as indicators of the course of acute pancreatitis. Gastroenterology 106:728–734.
111. Nordback I, Jaakkola M, Iovanna JL, Dagorn J-C (1995) Increased serum pancreatitis associated protein (PAP) concentration after long term alcohol consumption: further evidence for regular subclinical pancreatic damage after heavy drinking? Gut 36: 117–120.

112. Iovanna JL, Orelle B, Keim V, Dagorn J-C (1991) Messenger RNA sequence and expression of rat pancreatitis-associated protein, a lectin-related protein overexpressed during acute experimental pancreatitis. J Biol Chem 266:24,664–24,669.
113. Heideman M, Hugli TE (1984) Anaphylatoxin generation in multisystem organ failure. J Trauma 24:1038–1043.
114. Horn JK, Ranson JHC, Goldstein IM, Weissler J, Coratolo D, Taylor R, et. al. (1980) Evidence of complement metabolism in experimental acute pancreatitis. Am J Pathol 101:205–215.
115. Moshage HJ, Roelofs HMJ, Van Pelt JF, Hazenberg BPC, Van Leeuwen MA, Limburg PC, et al. (1988) The effect of interleukin-1, interleukin-6 and its interrelationship on the synthesis of serum and amyloid A and C-reactive protein in primary cultures of adult human hepatocytes. Biochem Biophys Res Commun 115:112–117.
116. Heath DI, Cruickshank A, Gudgeon M, Jehanli A, Shenkin A, Imrie CW (1993) Role of interleukin-6 in mediating the acute phase response and potential as an early means of severity assessment in acute pancreatitis. Gut 34:41–45.
117. Paajanen H, Laato M, Jaakkola M, Pulkki K, Niinikoski J, Nordback I (1995) Serum tumor necrosis factor compared with C-reactive protein in the early assessment of severity of acute pancreatitis. Br J Surg 82:271–273.
118. Fiers W (1991) Tumor necrosis factor. Characterization at the molecular, cellular and in vivo level. FEBS Lett 285:199–212.
119. Exley AR, Leese T, Holliday MP, Swann RA, Cohen J (1992) Endotoxemia and serum tumor necrosis factor as prognostic markers in severe acute pancreatitis. Gut 33: 1126–1128.
120. Damas P, Ledoux D, Nys M, Vrindts Y, DeGroote D, Franchimont P, et al. (1992) Cytokine serum levels during severe sepsis in human IL-6 as a marker of severity. Ann Surg 215:356–362.
121. Kemmer TP, Malfertheiner P, Büchler M, Kemmer ML, Ditschuneit H (1991) Serum ribonuclease activity in the diagnosis of pancreatic disease. Int J Pancreatol 8:23–33.
122. Warshaw AL, Kang-Hyun L (1979) Serum ribonuclease elevation and pancreatic necrosis in acute pancreatitis. Surgery 86:227–234.
123. Banks RE, Evans SW, Alexander D, Van Leuven F, Whicher JT, McMahon MJ (1991) Alpha$_2$ macroglobulin state in acute pancreatitis. Raised values of α$_2$ macroglobulin-protease complexes in severe and mild attacks. Gut 32:430–434.
124. Lasson A, Ohlsson K (1984) Protease inhibitors in acute human pancreatitis. Correlation between biochemical changes and clinical course. Scand J Gastroenterol 19:779–786.
125. McMahon MJ, Bowen M, Mayer AD, Cooper EH (1984) Relation of alpha 2-macroglobulin and other antiproteases to the clinical features of acute pancreatitis. Am J Surg 147:164–170.
126. Uhl W, Büchler M, Malfertheiner P, Martini M, Berger HG (1991) PMN-elastase in comparison with CRP, antiproteases, and LDH as indicators of necrosis in human acute pancreatitis. Pancreas 16:253–259.
127. Leese T, Shaw D, Holliday M (1988) Prognostic markers in acute pancreatitis: can pancreatic necrosis be predicted? Ann R Coll Surg Engl 70:227–232.
128. Schmidt D, Hoffman GE (1987) Activity of phospholipase A compared in serum of patients with pancreatic and non-pancreatic disease. Clin Chem 33:594–595.
129. Nevalainen TJ (1989) The role of phospholipase A$_2$ in acute pancreatitis. Klin Wochenschr 67:180–182.
130. Bird NC, Goodman AJ, Johnson AG (1989) Serum phospholipase A$_2$ activity in acute pancreatitis: an early guide to severity. Br J Surg 76:731–732.
131. Kazmierczak SC, Van Lente F, Hodges ED (1991) Diagnostic and prognostic utility of phospholipase A activity in patients with acute pancreatitis: comparison with amylase and lipase. Clin Chem 37:356–360.

132. Flesch I, Schonhardt T, Ferber E (1989) Phospholipases and acyltransferases in macrophages. Klin Wochenschr 67:119–122.
133. Kazmierczak SC, Van Lente F, Hodges ED (1994) Utility of serum phospholipase A measurement. Clin Chem 37:1799–1801.
134. Büchler M, Malfertheiner P, Schadlich H, Nevalainen TJ, Friess H, Beger HG (1989) Role of phospholipase A_2 in human acute pancreatitis. Gastroenterology 97:1521–1526.
135. Escola JV, Nevalainen TJ, Kortesno P (1988) Immunoreactive pancreatic phospholipase A_2 and catalytically active phospholipase A2 in serum from patients with acute pancreatitis. Clin Chem 34:1052–1054.
136. Fennell IC, Bornmann PC, Weakley SP, Terblanche J, Marks I (1993) Obesity, an important prognostic factor in acute pancreatitis. Br J Surg 80:484–486.
137. Edmondson HA, Berne CJ, Homann RE (1952) Calcium, potassium, magnesium and amylase disturbances in acute pancreatitis. Am J Med 12:34–38.
138. Northam BE, Rowe DS, Winstone NE (1963) Methemalbumin in the differential diagnosis of acute hemorrhagic and edematous pancreatitis. Lancet i:348–351.
139. Lankish PG, Schirren CA, Otto J (1989) Methemalbumin in acute pancreatitis: An evaluation of its prognostic potential and comparison with multiple prognostic parameters. Am J Gastroenterol 84:1391–1395.
140. McMahon MJ, Playforth MJ, Pickford IR (1980) A comparative study of methods for prediction of severity of attack of acute pancreatitis. Br J Surg 637:22–25.
141. Corfield AP, Cooper MJ, Williamson RC, Mayer AD, McMahon MJ, Dickinson AP, et al. (1985) Prediction of severity in acute pancreatitis: prospective comparison of three prognostic indices. Lancet ii:403–407.
142. Robert JH, Meyer P, Rohner A (1986) Can serum and peritoneal amylase and lipase determinations help in the early prognosis of acute pancreatitis. Ann Surg 203:163–168.
143. Potts JR (1988) Acute pancreatitis. Surg Clin North Am 68:281–299.
144. Warshaw AL (1974) Inflammatory masses following acute pancreatitis: phlegmon, pseudocyst, and abscess. Surg Clin North Am 54:621–636.
145. Bradley EL, III, Gonzalez AC, Clements JL, Jr (1976) Acute pancreatitis pseudocysts: incidence and implications. Ann Surg 184:734–737.
146. Becker JM, Pemberton JH, DiMagno EP, Ilstrup DM, McIlrath DC, Dozios R (1984) Prognostic factors in pancreatic abscess. Surgery 96:455–461.
147. Bradley EL, III (1987) An alternative approach to infected pancreatic necrosis. Infect Surg Feb.:85–95.
148. Warshaw AL, Jin G (1985) Improved survival in 45 patients with pancreatic abscess. Ann Surg 202:408–417.
149. Buchler M, Malfertheiner P, Uhl W (1985) Serum parameters to detect pancreatic necrosis. Dig Dis Sci 30:966 (abstract).
150. Pitchumoni CS, Agarwal N, Jain NK (1988) Systemic complications of acute pancreatitis. Am J Gastroenterol 83:597–606.
151. Ranson JH, Rifkind KM, Roses DF, Fink SD, Eng K, Localio SA (1974) Objective early identification of severe acute pancreatitis. Am J Gastroenterol 61:443–451.
152. Weir CG, Lesser PB, Drop LJ, Fischer JE, Warshaw AL (1975) Hypocalcemia of acute pancreatitis. Ann Intern Med 83:185–189.
153. Imrie CW, Allam BF, Ferguson JC (1976) Hypocalcemia of acute pancreatitis: the effect of hypoalbuminemia. Curr Med Res Opinion 4:101–116.
154. Hauser CJ, Kamrath RO, Sparks J, Shoemaker WC (1983) Calcium homeostasis in patients with acute pancreatitis. Surgery 94:830–835.
155. Izquierdo R, Bermes E, Sandberg L, Saxe A, Oslapas R, Prinz RA (1985) Serum calcium metabolism in acute experimental pancreatitis. Surgery 98:1031–1037.
156. Imrie CW, Beastall GH, McKay AJ, Campbell FC, Gordon D, O'Neill J (1983) Calcitonin and parathyroid hormone (PTH) levels in clinical acute pancreatitis. Gut 24:A597 (abstract).

157. Robertson GM, Moore EW, Switz DM, Sizemore GW, Estep HL (1976) Inadequate parathyroid response in acute pancreatitis. N Engl J Med 294:512–516.
158. McKay C, Beastall GH, Imrie CW, Baxter JN (1994) Circulating intact parathyroid hormone levels in acute pancreatitis. Br J Surg 81:357–360.
159. Condon JR, Ives D, Knight MJ, Day J (1975) The aetiology of hypocalcemia in acute pancreatitis. Br J Surg 62:115–118.
160. Brodrick JW, Largman C, Ray SB, Geokas MC (1981) Proteolysis of parathyroid hormone in vitro by sera from acute pancreatitis patients. Proc Soc Exp Biol Med 167: 588–596.
161. Muñoz JE, Malfertheiner P, Ditschuneit HH, Blanco-Chavez J, Uhl W, Büchler M, et al. (1991) Hyperlipidemia in acute pancreatitis: relationship with etiology, onset and severity of the disease. Int J Pancreatol 10:261–267.
162. Dickson AP, O'Neill J, Imrie CW (1984) Hyperlipidaemia, alcohol abuse and acute pancreatitis. Br J Surg 71:685–688.
163. Rollan A, Guzman S, Pimental F, Nervi F (1990) Catabolism of chylomicron remnants in patients with previous acute pancreatitis. Gastroenterology 98:1649–1654.
164. Agarwal N, Pitchumoni CS (1993) Acute pancreatitis: a multisystem disease. The Gastroenterologist 1:115–128.
165. Havala T, Shronts E, Cerra F (1989) Nutritional support in acute pancreatitis. Gastroenterol Clin North Amer 18:525–542.
166. Kwaan HC, Anderson MC, Gramatica L (1971) A study of pancreatic enzymes as a factor enzymes as a factor in the pathogenesis of disseminated intravascular coagulation during acute pancreatitis. Surgery 69:663–672.
167. Ranson JHC, Lackner H, Berman IR, Sohinella R (1972) The relationship of coagulation factors to clinical complications of acute pancreatitis. Surgery 81:502–511.
168. Kwaan HC, Anderson MC, Gramatica L (1971) A study of pancreatic enzymes as a factor in the pathogenesis of disseminated intravascular coagulation during acute pancreatitis. Surgery 69:663–672.
169. Wardle EN (1973) Fibrinogen and albumin catabolism in experimental pancreatitis in the rat. J Surg Res 15:122–131.
170. Anonymous (1980) Morbidity of acute pancreatitis; the effect of aprotinin and glucagon. Gut 21:334–339.
171. Murakawa M, Okamura T, Shibuya T, Harada M, Otsuka T, Niho Y (1992) Use of synthetic protease inhibitor for the treatment of L-asparaginase-induced acute pancreatitis complicated by disseminated intravascular coagulation. Ann Hematol 64:249–252.
172. Basran GS, Ramasubramanian R, Verma R (1987) Intrathoracic complications of acute pancreatitis. Br J Dis Chest 81:326–331.
173. Uhl W, Buchler M, Beger HG (1993) A clinicopathological classification of acute pancreatitis. In: Standards in pancreatic surgery, Berger HG, Buchler M, Malfertheiner P, eds. Berlin-Heidelberg, Springer Verlag, pp. 34–43.
174. Guice KS, Oldham KT, Johnson KJ, Kunkel RG, Morganroth ML, Ward PA (1988) Pancreatitis-induced acute lung injury: an ARDS model. Ann Surg 208:71–77.
175. Malik AB (1983) Pulmonary edema after pancreatitis: role of humoral factors. Circ Shock 10:71–80.
176. Ranson JH, Turner JW, Roses DF, Rifkind KM, Spencer FC (1974) Respiratory complications in acute pancreatitis. Ann Surg 179:557–566.
177. Imrie CW, Ferguson JC, Murphy D, Blumgart LH (1977) Arterial hypoxia in acute pancreatitis. Br J Surg 64:185–188.
178. Murphy D, Pack AI, Imrie CW (1980) The mechanism of arterial hypoxia occurring in acute pancreatitis. Q J Med 49:151–163.
179. Semba D, Wada Y, Ishihara Y, Kaji T, Kuroda A, Marioka Y (1990) Massive pancreatic pleural effusion: pathogenesis of pancreatic duct disruption. Gastroenterology 99:528–532.

180. Nicod L, Leuenberger PH, Seydoux C, Rey F, Van Melle G, Perret C (1985) Evidence for pancreas injury in adult respiratory distress syndrome. Am Rev Respir Dis 131: 696–699.
181. Kimura T, Toung JK, Margolis S, Bell WR, Cameron JL (1980) Respiratory failure in acute pancreatitis: The role of free fatty acids. Surgery 87:509–513.
182. Malik AB (1983) Pulmonary edema after acute pancreatitis: role of humoral factors. Circ Shock 10:71–80.
183. Cobo JC, Abraham E, Bland RD, Shoemaker WC (1984) Sequential hemodynamic and oxygen transport abnormalities in patients with pancreatitis. Surgery 95:324–330.
184. Altimari AF, Prinz RA, Leutz DW, Sandberg L, Kober PM, Raymond RM, et al. (1986) Myocardial depression during acute pancreatitis: fact or fiction? Surgery 100:724–731.
185. Faintuch J, Abrahao MM, Glacaglia LR (1989) Electrocardiographic changes in pancreatitis. Argentina Bras Cardiol 52:259–260.
186. Mautner RK, Seigel LA, Giles TD, Kayzer J (1982) Electrocardiographic changes in acute pancreatitis. South Med J 75:317–320.
187. Tran DD, Cuesta MA, Schneider AJ, Wesdorp RIC (1993) Prevalence and prediction of multiple organ system failure and mortality in acute pancreatitis. J Crit Care 8:145–153.
188. Cafri C, Basok A, Katz A, Abuful A, Gilutz H, Battler A (1995) Thrombolytic therapy in acute pancreatitis presenting as acute myocardial infarction. Int J Cardiol 49:279–281.
189. Frey CE (1965) Pathogenesis of nitrogen retention in pancreatitis. Am J Surg 109:747–755.
190. Bennett RG, Petrozzi JW (1975) Nodular subcutaneous fat necrosis: manifestations of silent pancreatitis. Arch Dermatol 11:896–898.
191. Higgins E, Ive FA (1990) Subcutaneous fat necrosis in pancreatic disease. Br J Surg 77: 532–533.
192. Dhawan SS, Acosta FJA, Poppiti RJ, Barkin JS (1990) Subcutaneous fat necrosis associated with pancreatitis: histochemical and electron microscopic findings. Am J Gastroenterol 85:1025–1028.
193. Malangoni MA, Richardson JD, Shalleross JC, Seiler JG, Polk HC Jr (1986) Factors contributing to fatal outcome after treatment of pancreatic abscess. Ann Surg 203:605–613.
194. Tran DD, Groeneveld ABJ, van der Meulen J, Nauta JJ, Strack van Schijndel RJ, Thijs LG (1990) Age, chronic disease, sepsis, organ system failure and mortality in a medical intensive care unit. Crit Care Med 18:474–479.
195. Runkel NSF, Moody FG, Smith GS, et al. (1991) The role of the gut in the development of sepsis in acute pancreatitis. J Surg Res 1:18–23.
196. Inkeles DM, Walsh JB (1975) Retinal fat emboli as a sequela to acute pancreatitis. Am J Ophthalmol 80:935–938.
197. Purtscher O (1910) Noch unbekannte befunde nach schadeltrauma. Ber Dtsch Ophthalmol Ges 36:294–307.
198. Semlacher EA, Chan-Yan C (1993) Acute pancreatitis presenting with visual disturbances. Am J Gastroenterol 88:756–759.
199. Hollo G, Tarjanyi M, Varga M, Flautner L (1993) Retinopathy of pancreatitis indicates multiple-organ failure and poor prognosis in severe acute pancreatitis. Acta Ophthalmol 72:114–117.

4
Neoplastic Disorders of the Pancreas

Peter Muscarella II, William Fisher, Jerome A. Johnson, and W. Scott Melvin

INTRODUCTION

Primary neoplasms of the pancreas present with a wide variety of clinical syndromes and represent various tumors. The majority have extremely high mortalities, although prognosis is dependent on histopathological type. Early and accurate diagnosis improves survival, but is difficult. Pancreatic neoplasms may be classified as tumors of the exocrine pancreas, tumors of the endocrine pancreas, and atypical neoplasms, such as lymphomas, mesotheliomas, and sarcomas. Benign masses of the pancreas are common, especially when associated with pancreatitis, and the differentiation can be quite difficult. Traditionally, the diagnosis is based on histologic confirmation, but it is obviously advantageous to diagnose these lesions correctly prospectively or preoperatively. This chapter will focus on the relevant laboratory tests that are appropriate in the evaluation of individuals with the most common classes of pancreatic tumors.

The overwhelming majority of pancreatic cancers are of exocrine origin. Laboratory testing may be helpful in diagnosing these lesions. Conventional laboratory tests, tumor-specific antigens, and oncofetal or hormonal antigens have all been evaluated extensively in pancreatic adenocarcinoma, although no single test has been shown to be absolutely diagnostic for exocrine pancreatic malignancies. There is evidence that combining tests may be helpful. Endocrine tumors of the pancreas are rare and account for about 2% of pancreatic neoplasms. Their prognosis, however, is much better than that of ductal adenocarcinoma, and it is important that they be properly identified. The majority of pancreatic endocrine tumors are hormonally active, allowing an opportunity to diagnose, classify, and follow these lesions. Unlike exocrine pancreatic tumors, clinical laboratory testing is a vital element in the workup of these tumors and has been well described for the majority of islet cell tumors. In fact, the understanding of pancreatic endocrine tumors has become a paradigm for the study of other hormonally active neoplasms. The underlying mechanisms and roles of these tests merit attention. Atypical neoplasms, as defined here, are exceedingly rare, and abnormal laboratory studies have not been shown to be associated with their presence. Exploratory laparotomy is indicated for diagnosis and possible treatment in suspected cases. Consequently, these lesions will not be included in this discussion.

TUMORS OF THE EXOCRINE PANCREAS

Laboratory Diagnosis

Approximately 98% of pancreatic neoplasms are of exocrine origin *(1)* and, of these, the vast majority are ductal adenocarcinomas. Although various tumor markers have been extensively studied, the results of laboratory tests in the diagnosis and management of exocrine pancreatic neoplasms do not have a firm role at this point in time. Instead, diagnosis has relied mainly on imaging techniques, such as ultrasound, computerized tomography (CT) scan, angiography, and endoscopic retrograde cholangiopancreatology (ERCP), as well as surgical or percutaneous biopsy. In evaluating the role of laboratory tests and their relationship to pancreatic neoplasms, it is essential that the objectives of these studies be clearly defined. These objectives may include:

1. Potential for screening high-risk asymptomatic populations for the disease;
2. The ability to detect the presence (preferably at an early stage) of the disease in suspected cases;
3. Proven validity as prognostic indicators; and
4. The ability to detect recurrence or progression of tumor spread after treatment has been initiated.

Perhaps the most significant role tumor markers may play in the future is as a screening tool in asymptomatic populations at risk for pancreatic cancer. Warshaw and Swanson *(2)* predicted that this, in fact, may be impossible. Even if a near perfect test was developed that was inexpensive, simple to perform, noninvasive, and demonstrated 99% sensitivity and 99% specificity in detecting pancreatic cancer, it would still generate 99 false positives (FP) for every true positive (TP), given a low prevalence (0.01%) of pancreatic cancer in the general population. It must then be decided what to do with this information. Simply following all of these patients until a lesion is discovered by standard localization techniques would eliminate any advantage gained by early detection on outcome in terms of earlier treatment. Their conclusion was that any screening tool would need to be coupled with a corresponding localization technique before any benefit would be gained. Despite the seemingly bleak possibility of developing an adequate marker for the diagnosis of pancreatic cancer, it should be noted that significant advances have been made for other solid cancers in the past decade. These include serum carcinoembryonic antigen (CEA) for colon cancer, α-fetoprotein (AFP) for hepatocellular carcinoma, serum CA125 for ovarian cancer, serum prostate-specific antigen for prostate cancer, and serum calcitonin for medullary carcinoma of the thyroid *(3)*. Indeed, there has been a enormous amount of research in this area over recent years, and it remains to be seen whether or not an adequate screening test for pancreatic cancer will be developed. At the current time, screening for pancreatic cancer is not justified, except in individuals in whom there is a high suspicion for pancreatic cancer or in those with pancreatic masses demonstrated on imaging studies.

Laboratory studies for the detection of pancreatic adenocarcinoma can be divided into two groups: conventional serum laboratory studies and tumor markers. Tumor markers may then be subclassified as tumor-related antigens, serum enzyme activity measurements, and oncofetal or hormone products. The role of conventional laboratory studies and tumor markers in the diagnosis and management of ductal pancreatic cancers will be discussed below; these studies are listed in Table 1. In

Table 1
**Laboratory Serum Measurements Useful
in the Diagnosis of Exocrine Pancreatic Cancers**

Conventional tests	Tumor-related antigens
Alkaline phosphatase	CEA
Direct and indirect bilirubin	CA 19-9
ALT/AST	CA-50
Amylase/lipase	CA-195
Glucose	Span-1
Serum enzyme activities	DU-PAN-2
Elastase 1	CAR-3
Ribonuclease	CA-242
GT II	CA-494
Hormonal or oncofetal antigens	CAM-43
β-2-microglobulin	TATI
AFP	TPA
βHCG	TPSA
POA	PCAA
	LAI

addition, multivariate analyses, which utilize a battery of tumor markers, will be addressed.

When evaluating the adequacy of a test in detecting a disease state, as well as differentiating its presence from those of other benign and malignant disease entities, various terms are often used. These will be defined here for purposes of clarity. Sensitivity is the ability to detect a disease state in its presence (TP/[TP + FN]) and specificity is the ability to exclude a disease state in its absence (TN/[TN + FP]). The positive predictive value is the proportion of positive test results that correctly identifies a disease state (TP/[TP + FP]), whereas the negative predictive value is the proportion of negative tests that correctly identifies the absence of a disease state (TN/[TN + FN]). Finally, diagnostic accuracy is defined as the average of sensitivity and specificity.

Conventional Laboratory Studies

Numerous serum laboratory values may be abnormal in pancreatic adenocarcinoma. However, these are highly nonspecific, and do not discriminate pancreatic cancer from benign pancreatic disease and other GI malignancies. Nevertheless, these studies still play a major role in the diagnosis of pancreatic cancer by raising suspicion for the presence of malignancy.

Liver function tests, such as alkaline phosphatase, bilirubin, and the serum transaminases, may be elevated. Again, these are highly nonspecific, and may be elevated in other benign and malignant processes involving the liver or its biliary drainage. In cases of pancreatic cancer, elevation of these values is often a reflection of biliary obstruction by tumor or metastatic liver involvement. Serum activities of the pancreatic enzymes, amylase, and lipase, may be elevated, indicating active areas of inflammation in the pancreas. Local inflammatory responses are common in pancreatic cancer, and these nonspecific tests are of little use in differentiating pancreatic cancer from pancreatitis. The clinical uses of other pancreatic enzymes will be described below. Finally, serum glucose concentrations are a significant, although nonspecific, indicator of pancreatic cancer. An elevated glucose concentration may reflect islet-cell destruction by a tumor or the influence of other tumor-related hormonal factors. There is clearly a relationship between diabetes and pancreatic cancer. New-onset diabetes, in the absence of other known risk factors, should raise clinical warning flags for the presence of a pancreatic tumor.

Tumor Markers

Tumor-Related Antigens

Tumor-related antigens can be defined as a group of antigens, usually identified by a monoclonal antibody (MAb), for which elevated serum concentrations may be associated with the presence of a malignant tumor. With the advent of hybridoma technology, large numbers of tumor-related antigens have been identified in the past decade. A subset of these have proven to be clinically useful in the diagnosis and management of various cancers, including those of the colon, prostate, ovary, and pancreas. As far as pancreatic cancer is concerned, the literature concerning tumor-related antigens has become vast. MAbs against sialylated carbohydrate determinants present on mucinous antigens (specifically the MUC1 core polypeptide) *(4)*, in particular, have been extensively studied. These include CA19-9, DU-PAN-2, and Span-1.

Despite numerous studies involving their use, tumor-related antigens have not replaced imaging modalities in diagnosing pancreatic cancer owing to inadequate sensitivities and specificities of existing analytes and/or assays for these analytes. Data obtained from patients with "early" pancreatic cancer demonstrate even lower sensitivities in detecting these conceivably curable tumors. Current data support the use of serum concentrations of tumor-related antigens in the prognosis and follow-up of known cases of pancreatic cancer as well as in augmenting other diagnostic modalities and for confirming clinical suspicion of pancreatic cancer. In addition, antigen concentrations in pure pancreatic juice obtained by cannulation of the pancreatic duct may play a role in the diagnosis of early tumors.

CARCINOEMBRYONIC ANTIGEN

The role of serum CEA concentration in the management of colon cancer has been clearly defined *(5)*. At the present time, CEA is not used in diagnosing colon cancer. Instead, preoperative and postoperative concentrations are used to determine prognosis as well as the likelihood of occult metastatic disease. Serial serum CEA concentrations are obtained following surgical resection, since elevated values are early indicators of recurrent or metastatic disease and indications for reoperation.

Elevated serum concentrations of CEA have been found in association with pancreatic cancer; prior to the assay for CA19-9, CEA was the only available tumor marker for use in diagnosing pancreatic cancer. The major drawbacks of CEA in diagnosing pancreatic cancer were problems with inadequate sensitivities and specificities, especially in differentiating pancreatic cancer from other GI cancers. Using a normal value of <5 ng/mL, sensitivities of 36–80% and specificities of 58–95% have been reported *(6)*. Numerous other studies have compared the sensitivity and specificity of serum CEA and CA19-9 for detecting pancreatic cancer *(7)*. In most of these studies, healthy controls as well as controls with benign pancreatic disease, benign nonpancreatic GI disease, nonpancreatic GI malignancy, and benign systemic disease were included. CA19-9 is clearly superior in diagnosing pancreatic cancer, with an overall sensitivity of 82% and specificity of 83%, as opposed to 56% and 75% for CEA. In addition, CA19-9 is better able to differentiate pancreatic cancer from pancreatitis. At the present time, CA19-9 is preferred over CEA in diagnosing suspected cases of pancreatic cancer. The measurement of CEA is not indicated in the routine workup of these patients.

CEA concentrations may still play a role in prognosis and follow-up for patients with resectable pancreatic cancer. In a study of 87 patients with resectable pancreatic cancer, Yasue et al. demonstrated that preoperative CEA was a good prognostic indicator *(8)*. Using multivariate analysis, they found that patients with preoperative CEA values <2.5 ng/mL have significantly improved survivals over those with CEA >2.5 ng/mL. Patients with higher CA19-9 concentrations had shorter survival times. However, this difference was not statistically significant. Postoperatively, CEA and CA19-9 concentrations were both shown to be statistically significant predictors of survival. There are reports of conflicting data, but this study indicates that preoperative CEA values may be superior to CA19-9 in determining the prognosis for patients undergoing pancreatic resection.

The measurement of CEA concentrations in pure pancreatic juice obtained at the time of ERCP has been used to diagnose adenocarcinoma of the pancreas. In this procedure, the main pancreatic duct is cannulated, and pure pancreatic juice is aspirated after pancreatic stimulation by iv bolus injection of secretin (1 U/kg). Retrospective analysis of serial pancreatic juice CEA concentrations in a patient thought to have chronic pancreatitis demonstrated a doubling prior to the later diagnosis of pancreatic cancer *(9)*. At the time of increase, there was no radiological evidence of tumor. In studies of early pancreatic cancer (<2 cm, primary tumor size), CEA in pancreatic juice demonstrated 71.4% sensitivity and 93.3% specificity in differentiating pancreatic cancer from chronic pancreatitis *(10)*. In the same study, pancreatic juice CEA concentrations were shown to be superior to both CA19-9 and pancreatic oncofetal antigen (POA) concentrations in detecting pancreatic cancer. By contrast, serum tumor markers were of no value. When combined with cytologic analysis of the same fluid, pancreatic juice CEA values improved the diagnostic accuracy of cytology alone from 84.4–93.8%. Despite these encouraging data, obtaining pure pancreatic juice remains an invasive, costly, and technically challenging procedure. The administration of secretin with concomitant instrumentation of the pancreatic duct may provoke significant pancreatitis. Because of this, the collection of pure pancreatic juice at ERCP is extremely limited and not currently recommended.

CA19-9

CA19-9 is by far the most extensively studied tumor-related antigen used in the diagnosis and management of pancreatic cancer. Assays for CA19-9 were originally developed with a MAb raised against the colon cancer tumor cell line SW1116 *(11)*. CA19-9 was initially shown to be expressed in ~60% of human colorectal carcinomas *(12)*. CA19-9 has subsequently proven to have more clinical utilization in relation to pancreatic cancer and cancers of the hepatobiliary system than to colorectal cancers. The antigenic determinant of the MAb to CA19-9, MAb 1116 ns 19–9, has been characterized as sialosyl-fucosyl-lacto-tetraose *(13)*. This corresponds to a sialylated Lewis[a] blood group antigen or sialyllacto-*N*-fucopentaose II *(14)*. The Lewis gene encodes for a fucosyltransferase enzyme, which fucosylates sialylated Lewis[c] antigen (sialyllact-*N*-tetraose). Five to 7% of the Western population lacks the gene and is unable to produce the sialyllated Lewis[a] antigen corresponding to CA19-9 *(15)*. Lewis[a] (–) individuals with pancreatic cancer should hypothetically not have detectable CA19-9 in their serum. Several reports have proven this to be untrue *(16)*.

The CA19-9 epitope has been identified in association with membrane glycolipids and glycoproteins, or mucins, secreted by various exocrine tissues, including the pancreas *(17)*. It is believed that the neoplastic transformation of pancreatic cells leads to increased expression of sialylated Lewis[a] antigens. Secretion of these antigens into the extracellular space and pancreatic ductal obstruction conceptually leads to increased serum concentrations in patients with pancreatic cancer.

Radioimmunoassay is the usual method for the assay of serum CA19-9 and is widely available. Numerous normal range values have been proposed in the literature for various purposes, but <37 U/mL is considered to be the normal value.

The majority of data concerning the utility of serum CA19-9 concentrations have been obtained from patients with known pancreatic cancer. In an early study done by Safi et al. *(18)*, concentrations >37 U/mL were present in 92% of patients with pancreatic cancer, and those >120 U/mL were present in 77% of patients. CA19-9 values were shown to be adequate in differentiating pancreatic cancer from benign disease, but were commonly elevated in nonpancreatic GI malignancies. For example, 19% of colorectal cancers and 37% of gastric cancers had CA19-9 concentrations above 37 U/mL. These numbers were reduced to 10 and 21%, respectively, when a cutoff of 120 U/mL was used. The authors' conclusion was that CA19-9 values >120 U/mL are an indication for invasive diagnostic procedures of the pancreas. It should be noted that 65% of patients with cholangiocarcinomas and papillary bile duct carcinomas had CA19-9 values >120 U/mL. Finally, CA19-9 concentrations positively correlated with tumor stage. Elevated concentrations of CA19-9 were found in only 66% of stage I tumors, whereas 96% of patients with stage III tumors had elevated values.

Although CA19-9 concentrations are nonspecifically elevated in other GI cancers, they are suitable for differentiating benign pancreatic disease, such as pancreatitis, from pancreatic cancer. This is significant because patients with pancreatitis may harbor malignancies, and pancreatic cancer may present as pancreatitis. In one case-control study, CA19-9 values were able to distinguish pancreatic cancer from pancreatitis in 93% of cases, using an upper normal of 37 U/mL *(19)*. They were also able to distinguish pancreatic cancer from nonpancreatic digestive diseases in 73% of cases. Other studies have shown CA19-9 elevations in 27% of patients with chronic pancreatitis and 28% of patients with acute pancreatitis *(20)*.

Malesci et al. studied the diagnostic value of CA19-9 prospectively in patients presenting with symptoms consistent with pancreatic cancer *(21)*. Using a cutoff value of 40 U/mL, elevated CA19-9 concentrations demonstrated 83% sensitivity and 61% specificity in detecting pancreatic cancer. Jaundice is known to cause nonspecific elevation of CA19-9 values *(22)*, and by eliminating patients who presented with jaundice and raising the cutoff to 120 U/ml, the authors were able to demonstrate an increase in the positive predictive value (PPV) from 0.85–1.0. Diagnostic CA19-9 values improved the PPV of conventional imaging from 0.82–0.93 and the negative predictive value (NPV) from 0.94–1.0. CA19-9 determinations, however, were unable to eliminate the use of imaging. One patient with negative imaging and an elevated CA19-9 value proved not to have pancreatic cancer at laparotomy. The positive correlation between CA19-9 and tumor stage was confirmed, with elevated CA19-9 in 66% of stage I tumors and 85% of stage III tumors. The authors concluded that CA19-9 could play a limited role in diagnosing pancreatic cancer. Its use should be limited to the anicteric population because of FPs in jaundiced patients. In addition, CA19-9 could not eliminate the necessity for conventional imaging, although it was suggested that negative CA19-9 values combined with negative imaging could eliminate the need for further invasive procedures, including laparotomy and laparoscopy. Ritts et al. confirmed these results. This group evaluated 2467 patients who presented with characteristic abdominal pain or weight loss >10% of baseline total body weight (23). Receiver operating characteristic calculations were used to elect cutoff values of 100 U/mL. Using this cutoff, the PPV for elevated CA19-9 concentrations was 87% in jaundiced patients. The PPV was 97% and the NPV was 87% in nonjaundiced patients. When used in combination with a definitive imaging study, PPVs and NPVs were both raised to 100%. The authors concluded that the cutoff value could probably be decreased with improvements in the quality of modern imaging.

The above data demonstrate the utility of CA19-9 in symptomatic patients with advanced disease, but do not indicate any possible role in detecting disease in asymptomatic populations. Because of the increased chance for curative surgical resection in patients whose tumors are diagnosed early, asymptomatic patients would benefit most from an early screening tool. As far as small tumors are concerned, CA19-9 concentrations are elevated in 60.7% of tumors <2 cm in diameter and 73% of those <4 cm in diameter (24). Because of this, the available data does not support a role for CA19-9 as a screening tool in asymptomatic patients. In one prospective study, Satake et al. used abdominal ultrasound, CA19-9 and elastase 1 to screen 12,830 patients for pancreatic tumors (25). Only four (0.03%) pancreatic cancers were identified. Of these, one patient underwent curative surgery. This regimen was not effective in identifying early cancers. The regimen was considered cost effective, however, in symptomatic patients. Of 8706 symptomatic patients, 141 cases of pancreatic cancer were identified, of which 47 patients underwent potentially curative resection. In addition, 62 other GI cancers were identified.

The positive correlation between CA19-9 values and tumor stages indicates that CA19-9 values may be good predictors of tumor resectability. Patients with preoperative CA19-9 concentrations >1000 U/ml rarely are found to have resectable disease, although one of nine patients with a CA19-9 >1000 U/mL in the series done by Glenn et al. did prove to have a resectable tumor (26). In a retrospective analysis of 53 patients undergoing laparotomy for pancreatic cancer, only 1 patient with a CA19 concentration >300 U/mL was found to have resectable disease (27) and this tumor was highly invasive, indicating that CA19-9 values >300 U/mL may be a contraindication for laparotomy even in the absence of radiographic evidence of unresectability, a recommendation not widely adopted.

As is the case with CEA for colon cancer, there is significant evidence that indicates that CA19-9 concentrations are good indicators of prognosis and tumor recurrence. The data concerning preoperative values are somewhat controversial. In one study, preoperative CA19-9 concentrations >200 U/mL were clearly correlated with improved prognosis (28). Median survival was 22 vs 8 mo for patients with preoperative values >200 U/mL. When multivariate analysis was used by Yasue et al. to control for stage of disease, pancreatic resection, and intraoperative radiation, patients with elevated preoperative CA19-9 values had worse prognoses (8). The difference, however, was no longer statistically significant. Finally, when a cutoff of 370 U/mL was used, CA19-9 concentrations were only considered to be significant predictors of prognosis in patients with stage II and III disease (29).

The weaknesses of preoperative CA19-9 in determining prognosis were not seen when postoperative values were evaluated. Normal postoperative CA19-9 concentrations uniformly predicted improved prognosis. Sperti et al. reported a median survival of 22 mo for 15 patients whose CA19-9 values returned to normal, whereas those ($n = 15$) with a persistently elevated CA19-9 had a median survival of only 7 mo (28). These data have been confirmed by other studies. In the series by Glenn et al., seven of eight patients who showed postoperative normalization of CA19-9 after pancreatic resection survived longer than 18 mo, whereas no patient with persistently elevated CA19-9 values survived more than 1 yr (26). In the series by Berretta et al., all of the patients with normal postoperative CA19-9 values survived more than 7 mo, and no patient with elevated postoperative CA19-9 values survived longer than 7 mo (30). There is some evidence that postoperative CA19-9 in combination with CEA may predict survival more accurately (8). In all studies, significant elevations in CA19-9 following postoperative normalization correctly predicted tumor recurrence or metastases prior to radiological evidence.

Serum CA19-9 determinations are commonly used at our institution, both as a diagnostic tool and as an indicator of prognosis and tumor recurrence. Several pitfalls, however, have been identified. Many patients with suspected malignancies present with obstructive jaundice, and the resultant inflammation in the biliary tree presumably results in elevated CA19-9 values. This may be true even in cases of benign obstruction. Additionally, any infection within the biliary tree, even a low-grade, subclinical cholangitis, can cause marked increases in serum CA19-9 values. This becomes important in the evaluation of patients with obstructive jaundice and elevated CA19-9 values. After decompression of the biliary tree, even without surgical resection, CA19-9 values may return to normal.

Nonspecific elevations of CA19-9 may be seen in patients following surgical resection in cases of low grade cholangitis or partial biliary obstruction. These increases may not be related to tumor recurrence and normalize with appropriate antibiotic treatment. Consequently, one must be cognizant of nonspecifically elevated CA19-9 values secondary to cholangitis or biliary obstruction when following patients who have had surgical resections for pancreatic cancer.

Early studies examining the use of CA19-9 determinations in pure pancreatic juice indicated a possible role in augmenting the diagnosis of pancreatic cancer and differentiating pancreatic cancer from chronic pancreatitis. Malesci et al. showed that pancreatic juice CA19-9 concentrations were significantly higher in patients with pancreatic cancer than in normal controls or patients with chronic pancreatitis *(31)*. When the ratio of CA19-9 to protein concentration of pancreatic juice was calculated, 21 of 22 patients had values >2.5 U/μg. Other studies, however, have shown that pancreatic juice CA19-9 is nonspecific. In the study by Yuan-fang et al., pancreatic juice CA19-9 concentrations were also significantly elevated in patients with ampullary carcinoma, choledochal carcinoma, and benign choledochal lithiasis *(32)*. Unlike serum concentrations, pancreatic juice CEA values were later shown to be superior to CA19-9 in differentiating early pancreatic cancer from chronic pancreatitis *(33)*. Regardless, the collection of pure pancreatic juice is not a routine clinical practice.

CA-50 AND CA-195

CA-50 is an antigen characterized by a MAb that binds to both the sialylated Lewis[a] antigen (like CA19-9) and a nonfucosylated sialosyl-lacto-tetraose, which is present in Le[a](–), Le[b](–) individuals *(16)*. Because of the similar epitope recognition, CA-50 serum concentrations in patients with pancreatic cancer show close correlation with those of CA19-9. CA-50 values may be measured immunoradiometrically, using antibody immobilized on polystyrene beads, or by chemiluminescence with antibody immobilized in a microtiter well *(34)*. The same MAb is used in each assay, and the upper range of normal for the two assays is 20 and 14 U/mL, respectively. Up to 50% variations in CA-50 concentrations have been demonstrated in identical samples depending on the methodology used. In one immunoradiometric assay study, serum CA-50 concentrations demonstrated a sensitivity of 96% and specificity of 56% in differentiating pancreatic cancer from other disorders of the upper GI system. The sensitivity and specificity were 95 and 67% when the chemiluminescent assay was used on specimens from the same patients *(34)*. The variation in found concentrations with varying methodologies makes clinical usefulness of CA-50 serum determinations difficult. Most of the studies reviewed here use the immunoradiometric assay.

In retrospective analyses, CA-50 concentrations demonstrate sensitivities of 64.9–96% and specificities of 56–84% in differentiating pancreatic cancer from other gastrointestinal disorders, both benign and malignant *(34–36)*. These results were equal to or worse than those of CA19-9 in all cases. In addition, CA-50 concentrations correlated highly with those of CA19-9. It has been postulated that CA-50 may be superior to CA19-9 in detecting pancreatic cancer in Le[a](–), Le[b](–) patients because of the ability to detect the nonfucosylated sialosyl-lacto-tetraose epitope present in these individuals. When the two were compared in relation to Lewis blood cell status, however, CA-50 and CA19-9 values were shown to correspond closely regardless of Lewis blood type *(37)*.

Antibodies to CA-195 (upper normal 14 U/mL), like CA-50, react with both the sialylated Lewis[a] antigen and related isotopes lacking fucosyl residues *(34)*. Serum values are measured using an immunoradiometric assay with antibody immobilized on polystyrene beads. In a study of 97 patients with pancreatic cancer and 93 patients with benign pancreatic disease or other disorders of the upper abdomen, serum CA-195 concentrations demonstrated 96% sensitivity in detecting pancreatic cancer and 73% specificity in differentiating pancreatic cancer from other upper GI disorders *(34)*. These concentrations were not considered to be statistically different from those of CA19-9. Data from Banfi et al. confirm the high correlation between CA-195 and CA19-9 *(38)*.

In summary, serum CA-50 and CA-195 determinations do not confer any advantage over CA19-9 in the diagnosis of pancreatic cancer. In addition, little to no information can be gained when multiple tests are combined. Consequently, there are no clinical indications for serum CA-50 or CA-195 determinations in the diagnosis of pancreatic cancer at the present time.

Span-1

The Span-1 antigen is recognized by a murine MAb produced against a human pancreatic cancer cell line *(39)*. The antibody has been shown to recognize sialylated Lewis^a antigen as well as its nonfucosylated precursor, sialyllact-*N*-tetraose *(14)*. In this regard it is similar to both CA-50 and CA-195. Serum Span-1 antigen concentrations are measured by radioimmunoassay with an upper range of normal of 30 U/mL *(40)*. A number of studies have demonstrated improved sensitivities over CA19-9 determination in diagnosing pancreatic cancer. For example, in the study by Kiriyama et al., elevated Span-1 values were present in 81.3% of patients with pancreatic cancer, whereas CA19-9 was elevated in only 73.4% *(39)*. Clinical usefulness is limited, however, by a high rate of FPs. Abnormal elevations (>30 U/mL) of Span-1 occurred frequently in hepatocellular carcinoma (62.5%), biliary cancer (51.1%), and colorectal carcinoma (41.1%).

Because the Span-1 antigen is present in Lewis^a (–) individuals, Span-1 may play a role as an adjunct to CA19-9. In fact, Kawa et al. have demonstrated significantly elevated Span-1 concentrations in two Lewis^a (–) pancreatic cancer patients with normal CA19-9 concentrations *(14)*. Overall, the diagnostic accuracy of the two tests is comparable, and there are no large series comparing their efficacy in relation to Lewis blood cell status. The role of serum Span-1 determination in the diagnosis of pancreatic cancer, therefore, remains unclear.

DU-PAN-2 and CAR-3

DU-PAN-2 is an antigen also recognized by a mouse MAb to a human pancreatic cancer cell line. The antibody recognizes the nonfucosylated sialyllact-*N*-tetraose Lewis^a precursor also recognized by Span-1 *(14)*. Antibodies to DU-PAN-2 do not, however, react with the Lewis^a antigen. Serum DU-PAN-2 concentrations are determined by enzyme-linked immunoassay with an upper normal of 400 U/mL.

In their series, Satake et al. demonstrated a relatively low sensitivity for DU-PAN-2 (47.7%) in detecting pancreatic cancer, but the specificity (85.3%) was the highest of all markers studied *(35)*. DU-PAN-2 values were elevated in only 1.8% of benign pancreatic diseases and 12.5% of benign hepatobiliary diseases. Sensitivities for malignant hepatobiliary disease were high, however, with elevated concentrations in 27.4% of hepatocellular carcinomas and in 41% of biliary tract cancers. Other studies have shown that DU-PAN-2 determinations are clearly inferior to CA19-9 *(41)* and Span-1 *(39)* in the diagnostic accuracy for pancreatic cancer.

Because the DU-PAN-2 antigenic epitope is present in Lewis^a (–) individuals, DU-PAN-2 concentrations may be more sensitive in these patients. Overall, it seems that Span-1 would be more useful because its antibody recognizes both epitopes. The future role of serum DU-PAN-2 may have more significance in differentiating malignant upper GI lesions from benign ones, rather than differentiating pancreatic cancer from other types of cancer.

Serum CAR-3 determinations are made using immunoradiometric techniques employing a MAb and have an upper normal of 19.5 U/mL. Limited data indicate that CAR-3 is inferior to CA19-9 in the differential diagnosis of pancreatic cancer with elevated concentrations in 39% of patients with pancreatic cancer as opposed to 83% for CA19-9. In addition, CAR-3 values seem to be highly correlated with indicators of cholestasis and jaundice (i.e., serum bilirubin and alkaline phosphatase) indicating nonspecificity *(41)*.

CA-242, CA-494, AND CAM-43

The MAb to CA-242 recognizes an antigenic epitope residing on the same macromolecule as the CA-50 antigen, although these are not identical *(42)*. Serum CA-242 determinations are made using a dissociation-enhanced lanthidine fluoroimmunoassay with an upper normal of 30 U/mL *(36)*. When receiver operator characteristic curves were used to determine optimal cutoff values, CA-242 determinations demonstrated 86% diagnostic accuracy in diagnosing pancreatic cancer as opposed to 84% for CA19-9. In this study, CA-242 and CA19-9 concentrations correlated highly with each other. In vitro, CA-242 antigen demonstrated significant crossreactivity with antibody to CA19-9, indicating that the antigens are very similar *(42)*. CA-242 antibody, however, does not bind with sialylated Lewis^a (CA19-9) antigen *(43)*. Other studies, utilizing multivariate analysis, have demonstrated that CA-242 is inferior to CA-50 in the differential diagnosis of pancreatic cancer *(36)*.

CAM-43 is defined by reactivity with MAbs CT43 and CT66 of which only CT66 binds sialylated Lewis^a antigen *(44)*. Serum concentrations are measured with an immunoenzymometric assay with an upper normal of 10 U/mL. When compared with CA19-9 in patients with pancreatic cancer and benign GI disease, CAM-43 elevations demonstrated 60% sensitivity and 94.7% specificity in diagnosing pancreatic cancer. The values for CA19-9 were 79 and 60%, respectively *(37)*. The increase in specificity was offset by a corresponding decrease in sensitivity, and CAM-43 determinations were not believed to be an improvement over CA19-9.

CA-494 is a recently described tumor-associated antigen that is defined by reactivity with the MAb BW 494. This antibody was initially raised against a human colorectal cancer cell line. The antibody identified in a large number of grade I and II pancreatic cancers by immunohistochemical techniques and was initially utilized as passive immunotherapy for the treatment of pancreatic cancer. A prospective trial demonstrated no significant survival advantage for those treated with BW 494 *(45)*. The exact CA-494 epitope has not been identified, but is thought to belong to a family of blood group precursor type-1 chain-related structures that includes the β-linked Thomsen-Freidenreich-disaccharide *(46)*. In addition, CA-50 and CA19-9 antibodies react with CA-494 antigen. CA-494 concentrations are determined by enzyme-linked immunoassay with an upper normal of 40 U/mL. Serum CA-494 determination is as specific as CA19-9 (sensitivity of 90% each), and CA-494 has increased specificity in differentiating pancreatic cancer from chronic and acute pancreatitis as well as other benign conditions *(46)*. CA-494 concentrations are elevated in other gastrointestinal cancers, notably gastric cancer (sensitivity 61%). CA-494 may be one of the few mucin-directed tumor-associated antigens superior to CA19-9 in the differential diagnosis of pancreatic cancer.

TUMOR-ASSOCIATED TRYPSIN INHIBITOR (TATI), TISSUE POLYPEPTIDE ANTIGEN, AND TISSUE POLYPEPTIDE-SPECIFIC ANTIGEN

TATI is a 6000-Dalton peptide isolated from the urine of a patient with ovarian cancer *(47)* and has been shown to share homology with pancreatic secretory trypsin inhibitor (PSTI). Because both of these peptides have been found in pancreatic tumors as well as adjacent normal pancreatic tissue *(48)*, it has been postulated that serum concentrations of TATI may prove useful as a tumor marker for pancreatic cancer. Several studies utilizing radioimmunoassays for TATI in pancreatic cancer patients and controls have demonstrated poor sensitivities and specificities in comparison with CA19-9 *(34,49)*. TATI, therefore, is of no use in the diagnosis or management of pancreatic cancer.

Tissue polypeptide antigen (TPA) is a protein produced by rapidly growing tissues *(50)*. Because TPA values reflect tumor proliferation as opposed to tumor burden, serum TPA determinations have been proposed as an adjunct to serum mucin antigen measurements in diagnosing pancreatic cancer. Serum TPA concentrations are measured by radioimmunoassay. In studies utilizing cutoff values of 150 U/mL, TPA concentrations are highly sensitive (97%) indicators of pancreatic malignancy. However, inadequate specificities (37%) preclude their clinical usefulness *(51)*. When cutoff values are raised to 320 U/mL, elevated TPA concentrations demonstrate 52% sensitivity and 85% specificity in diagnosing pancreatic cancer *(36,52)*. TPA elevations were equally specific, but less sensitive than mucin antigen in all cases, negating their usefulness as an independent indicator of pancreatic cancer. The authors believed that TPA was useful when used in combination with CA-50 or CA-242 by significantly improving the diagnostic efficiency of either test alone. It should be noted, however, that there was some decrease in sensitivity.

Tissue polypeptide specific antigen (TPSA) is defined by reactivity with a MAb to the M3 epitope of TPA. Although TPSA determinations have been speculated to achieve improved specificity over TPA in detecting pancreatic cancer, this was proven to be untrue in various studies *(36,38)*. For example, in the study by Banfi et al., TPSA concentrations were elevated in 98% of patients with pancreatic cancer, but demonstrated only 22% specificity in differentiating pancreatic cancer from benign pancreatic diseases *(38)*. TPSA values correlate well with those of TPA, but TPSA is, in fact, highly nonspecific (Fig. 1).

OTHER TUMOR-RELATED ANTIGENS

Numerous other tumor markers, including POA and pancreas cancer-associated antigen (PCAA), have been studied. Although elevated concentrations are seen in patients with pancreatic cancer, they are also nonspecific *(7)*. In the leukocyte adherence inhibition (LAI) assay, results are considered positive when the subject's leukocytes demonstrate loss of glass adherence properties in the presence of tumor leukocyte extract *(7)*. This test has been reported to have superior sensitivity when compared to both CA19-9 and TPA in the detection of early lesions *(51)*. Sensitivity decreases with tumor stage, indicating that this test should be used in conjunction with other tumor markers with adequate sensitivities for advanced disease. However, the LAI assay has

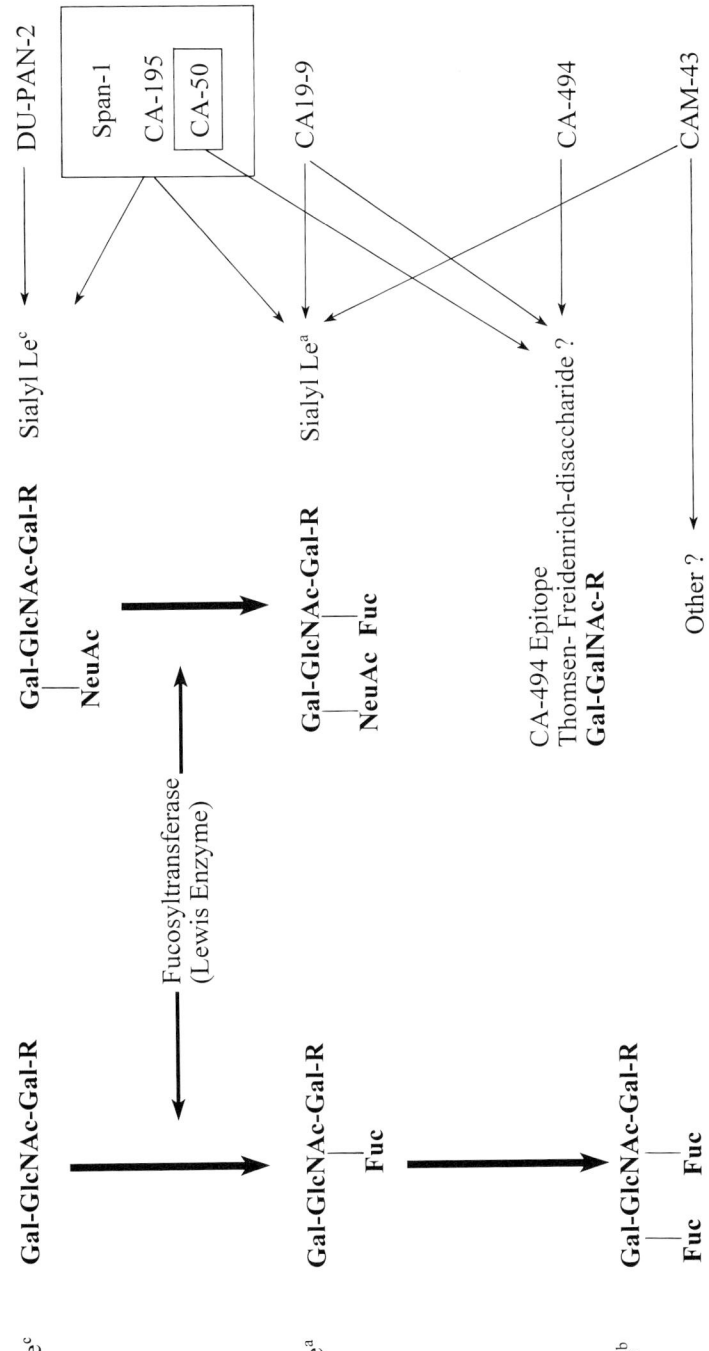

Fig. 1. Tumor-related antigens and the carbohydrate determinants recognized by their corresponding MAbs.

numerous technical flaws, including the requirement for subjective visualization of specimens when performing the test, a lack of uniform standardization measures, and poor reproducibility in different laboratories.

Serum Enzyme Activities

Serum amylase and lipase activities may be elevated in patients with pancreatic cancer, but are more commonly associated with pancreatitis and usually reflect its presence when elevated in patients with pancreatic cancer. Pancreatitis is recognized in approx 80% of pancreatic cancer patients at the time of their diagnosis, and pancreatic cancer may present as pancreatitis. One should, therefore, be cognizant of the possibility of underlying malignancy in these patients. Nonetheless, serum amylase and lipase activities do not play a role in the differential diagnosis of pancreatic cancer because of their nonspecificity. Numerous other pancreatic enzymes exist, and it has been postulated that serum concentrations of these may be more specific indicators of pancreatic malignancy. These include elastase 1, ribonuclease, and galactosyltransferase isoenzyme II.

Serum elastase 1 concentrations are measured by radioimmunoassay, and the usual upper limit of normal is 400 ng/dL. In the study by Satake et al., for all tumor stages, elastase 1 determinations demonstrated only 51.1% sensitivity in detecting pancreatic cancer, and 75.6% specificity in differentiating its presence from other GI malignancies and benign diseases *(35)*. Its specificity was comparable to that of CA19-9, but sensitivity was clearly inferior (51.1 vs 72.5%). Other studies have shown serum elastase 1 to be frequently elevated in benign pancreatic disease, other nonpancreatic GI malignancies, and benign disorders *(7)*.

In the above study, CA19-9 and Span-1 were superior to elastase 1 in detecting early pancreatic tumors. These data conflict with the findings of Chang et al. *(53)*, in which serum elastase 1 elevations were present in 62% of T1 lesions and 67% of T2 lesions. Hayakawa et al. confirmed the finding that serum elastase 1 elevations occur at earlier stages *(54)*. In addition, elevated serum elastase 1 values were found more frequently in prognostically favorable lesions of the pancreatic head. Both studies indicate that serum elastase 1 may be useful in diagnosing pancreatic cancers that are more amenable to surgical treatment. Elevated CA19-9 values are clearly correlated with unfavorable outcomes.

As stated previously, screening with CA19-9, serum elastase 1, and abdominal ultrasound is cost-effective in diagnosing pancreatic cancer and other GI malignancies in symptomatic patients, but not in the general population *(25)*. In another prospective trial utilizing serum elastase 1 determinations and abdominal ultrasound, serum elastase 1 values were not shown to add any benefit to the use of ultrasound alone in detecting pancreatic cancer in symptomatic patients *(55)*. In fact, of 19 patients ultimately found to have pancreatic cancer, none had elevated serum elastase 1 values in the presence of a normal ultrasound examination.

Galactosyltransferase is an enzyme involved in the synthesis of membrane glycoproteins and is detectable in serum *(56)*. The galactosyltransferase II (GTII) isoenzyme was first identified by Podolsky et al. using serum electrophoresis from patients with neoplasms. GTII concentrations were subsequently shown to be elevated in patients with various cancers, particularly pancreatic cancer *(57)*. When combined with ultrasound, Podolsky demonstrated 100% sensitivity in detecting pancreatic cancer. However, results have not been confirmed by other investigators. In addition, the technique is expensive and difficult to perform, limiting its availability. A radioimmunoassay utilizing an MAb to GTII exists, but results from this test demonstrated poor specificity *(58)*.

Serum ribonuclease activity has been proposed as an indicator of pancreatic disease; activities are measured by comparing ribonuclease activity on *Escherichia coli* tRNA or synthetic oligoribonucleotides with known standards. Studies of patients with benign and malignant pancreatic diseases indicate that it is useful only in detecting pancreatic necrosis in the absence of coexisting renal dysfunction *(59)*. Nonspecific elevation in the presence of acute pancreatitis, renal failure, and in healthy controls severely limits its use in the differential diagnosis of pancreatic cancer.

In summary, serum elastase 1 determinations may be useful in detecting early malignancies when combined with other tumor markers. GTII data are limited, but there is evidence that serum determinations may improve the diagnostic efficiency of imaging studies. In general, however, all serum pancreatic enzymes are nonspecific and do not currently play a role in the routine diagnosis and management of pancreatic cancer.

Hormonal or Oncofetal Products

Hormonal or oncofetal products produced by tumors constitute another set of tumor markers with proposed value in diagnosing pancreatic cancer. As will be discussed below, hormone determinations play a pivotal role in the diagnosis of endocrine tumors of the pancreas. The use of the oncofetal protein, AFP, in the diagnosis of hepatocellular carcinoma is an example of the significant potential these substances may play in the diagnosis of various malignancies. Unfortunately, extensive investigations have shown that serum hormonal and oncofetal protein determinations are not beneficial in the diagnoses of pancreatic cancer because of their nonspecificity.

β-2-microglobulin is an HLA-associated protein produced by all nucleated cells and platelets. In one study, elevated values were found in 85.0% of patients with pancreatic cancer *(60)*. They were also elevated, however, in 32.0% of patients with chronic pancreatitis, in 56.3% of benign nonpancreatic GI diseases and in 100.0% of nonpancreatic GI malignancies. It is now thought that serum β-2-microglobulin elevation is a result of immune system activation and that it is not produced by tumor cells. This would explain its presence in nonmalignancies and consequent nonspecificity.

The role of serum AFP determination in diagnosing hepatocellular carcinoma (and embryonal carcinoma) is well established. Elevated concentrations have been reported in numerous GI malignancies, including pancreatic cancer, but have not approached the sensitivities and specificities demonstrated by the mucin tumor-associated antigens *(7)*. There are reports that serial AFP concentrations may be useful markers for the treatment and follow-up of pancreatic cancer patients when preoperative values are elevated *(61)*, but these are based on an extremely small numbers of patients. The use of CEA and CA19-9 in this fashion is much better documented. Data on the use of serum and urine concentrations of human choriogonadotropin and its β-subunit (βHCG) are limited, but they do indicate approximately equivalent sensitivities and specificities to CA19-9 in detecting pancreatic and biliary malignancies *(62)*.

Multivariate Analysis

No single marker alone has been shown to be an adequate test to provide significant aid in the diagnosis of pancreatic cancer. There are a few studies that examine the use of a battery of serum tests in this regard. Because it is reasonable to assume that by combining tumor markers, especially ones that measure unrelated antigens, improved diagnostic accuracy may be obtained, so their existence bears mentioning here. It should be noted that improvements in accuracy would have to outweigh the cost of additional testing. In a prospective study of patients presenting with symptoms suspicious for pancreatic cancer, Pasanen et al. utilized a computer-aided scoring system to predict the presence of pancreatic malignancy. Serum measurements included CA-50, CA-242, CEA, TPA, and TPSA. The sensitivity obtained in their analysis was 36% with a specificity of 90% and an efficiency of 82% *(36)*. Although specificity was superior to that of the individual tests, the authors believed that this method was inadequate because of corresponding decreases in sensitivity and increased cost. In another study by Kuno et al. *(63)*, a computer-aided analysis was developed that used a total of nine serum markers. These included CA19-9, DU-PAN-2, TPA, elastase 1, γ-glutamyltranspeptidase, lactate dehydrogenase, lipase, amylase, and alkaline phosphatase. The battery, called CAMPAS-PX1, demonstrated marginally improved specificity (94.1 vs 81.9% for CA19-9) over CA19-9 alone while maintaining sensitivity (80.9 vs 87.2%). Again, the improvement was not considered cost-effective, and the authors could not recommend its use over that of CA19-9 alone. Reference was also made to a battery known as CAMPAS-PX2 that in preliminary studies demonstrated a sensitivity of 100% (42/42) and a specificity of 96.7% (292/303) in detecting pancreatic cancer. These results were obtained retrospectively, however, and it remains to be seen whether similar results will be obtained when the battery is used in a prospective fashion.

In summary, there are promising data concerning the use of computer-aided analyses of serum tumor marker batteries for the diagnosis of pancreatic cancer. This technique is still in its infancy, and it is unknown whether these batteries will significantly contribute to the diagnosis of pancreatic cancer in the future.

TUMORS OF THE ENDOCRINE PANCREAS

Each year only five of every million people are diagnosed with a pancreatic endocrine tumor *(64)*. Endocrine tumors of the pancreas are named after the peptides they secrete, and include insulinoma, gastrinoma, vasoactive intestinal peptide (VIP)-oma, glucagonoma, somatostatinoma, pancreatic polypeptideoma (PPoma), and nonfunctional islet-cell tumors.

All endocrine tumors of the pancreas have a similar light microscopic appearance, so most routine histologic examination does not predict the biologic behavior or endocrine manifestations of these neoplasms. Malignancy is generally determined by the presence of local invasion, a spread to regional lymph nodes, or the existence of hepatic or distant metastases. Special stains (immunofluorescence) allow the identification of specific hormones within tumor cells. The goals of surgery are primarily to control excess hormone secretion, and prevent or at least prolong recurrence by excising the maximal amount of tumor possible.

The clinical laboratory plays a unique and prominent role in the diagnosis of pancreatic endocrine tumors. Three-fourths of the endocrine tumors of the pancreas are functional and elaborate one or more hormonal products into the bloodstream. The diagnosis hinges on recognition of the characteristic clinical syndrome, and detection of elevated serum hormone concentrations by radioimmunoassay or other methods (Table 2). Once this is done, preoperative localization is accomplished in 80% by CT scanning and selective use of angiography, and rarely, portal venous sampling *(64)*. In the remaining patients where the primary tumor cannot be localized, exploratory surgery is indicated solely on the basis of the biochemical diagnosis.

Insulinoma

The most common endocrine tumor of the pancreas is the insulinoma, accounting for one case per million population annually *(65)*. Insulinomas originate from the β-cells of the pancreatic islets; they synthesize and secrete insulin autonomously. In 1927, Wilder et al. reported the first description of the insulinoma syndrome *(66)*. Whipple and Frantz described diagnostic criteria that have since been referred to as "Whipple's triad" *(67)*. That consists of symptoms of hypoglycemia with fasting or exercise, a plasma glucose of <50 mg/dL and relief of symptoms with oral or iv glucose. Hypoglycemia causes a whole host of symptoms, including hunger, irritability, weakness, headaches, blurry vision, incoherence, abnormal behavior, personality change, mental confusion, amnesia, and psychosis, as well as the more obvious obtundation, and finally seizure and coma. The associated catecholamine release is responsible for symptoms, such as palpitations, diaphoresis, and tremors. The clinical syndrome caused by insulinoma can be misleading in that patients are often labeled with psychiatric conditions until the true cause of their problem is found.

The laboratory diagnosis of insulinoma is made during a monitored 72-h fast. Plasma concentrations of glucose and insulin are determined every 4–6 h until symptoms of hypoglycemia develop. An inappropriately elevated insulin (>5 mU/mL) in the presence of low glucose (<40 mg/dL) during fasting establishes the diagnosis. A more sensitive test is the insulin-to-glucose ratio with values being <0.3 in normal individuals and >0.4 after an overnight fast in patients with insulinoma *(64)*. An amended ratio, calculated as (insulin × 100)/(glucose − 30), that is ≥50 has been found in virtually all patients with organic hyperinsulinism *(68)*. In a review of 43 patients with insulinoma, Grama et al. reported that the average delay in diagnosis was 15 mo from the onset of symptoms *(69)*. Diagnosis was made within 24 h of fasting in 88% and only 10% had to fast 72 h. Three patients could not undergo fasting, because they required a continuous glucose infusion to prevent severe hypoglycemia. One caveat is that a radioimmunoassay with polyclonal rather than the newer monoclonal anti-insulin antibodies is a better screening test for insulinoma *(70)*. In normal subjects, the insulin concentrations are similar with poly- and monoclonal tests. However, patients with insulinoma have values three times higher with the polyclonal antibody test than with the newer MAb assay. This is explained by the fact that high concentrations of proinsulin in insulinoma patients are detected by the polyclonal, but not the monoclonal assay. The monoclonal test is reserved for tumor-localization tests where low basal values increase the sensitivity.

Provocative testing for insulinoma has also been used for diagnosis. Tolbutamide tolerance testing relies on the ability of tolbutamide to cause release of endogenous

Table 2
Endocrine Tumors of the Pancreas: Clinical Syndromes, Hormone Concentrations, and Provocative Testing

Tumor/syndrome	Primary symptoms	Normal fasting range[a]	Suggestive pathologic range[a]	Provocative testing
Insulinoma	Hypoglycemia	<30 μ U/mL	>30U/mL with prolonged hypoglycemia	72-h fast tolbutamide
Gastrinoma	Recurrant peptic ulcer	<150 pg/mL	>150 pg/mL with gastric pH <2.0	Secretin
Zollinger-Ellison	Gastric hypersecretion			Somatostatin suppression
VIPoma	Secretory diarrhea	<190 pg/mL	>200 pg/mL	Pentagastrin
Verner-Morrison	Hypocalemia			Somatostatin suppression
	Hypochlorhydria			
	Hypercalcemia with hypophosphatemia			
Glucagonoma	Mild diabetis	<120 pg/mL	>1000 pg/mL	Tolbutamide
	Dermatitis			Arginine
	Deep vein thrombosis			
Somatostatinoma	Impairment of carbohydrate metabolism	<100 pg/mL	>150 pg/mL	Pentagastrin
	Cholelithiasis			Tolbutamide
	Diabetes			
	Steatorrhea			
PPoma	Often secondary marker for other tumors	na	na	na

[a]Concentrations are highly dependent on assay used.

insulin from β-cells. After a fasting blood sample has been obtained, 1 g of tolbutamide is given as a rapid iv bolus. Blood samples are obtained at 3, 5, 10, 15, 30, 45, 60, 120, and 180 min for glucose and insulin quantitation. Early samples are necessary to observe the immediate release of tumor insulin, whereas later samples are used to monitor the degree and duration of the resulting hypoglycemia. Peak insulins of >150 U/mL with resulting hypoglycemia are usually diagnostic. In most cases of insulinoma, the hypoglucemia can be severe, and require immediate and extended iv administration of glucose to reverse the symptoms. Other agents (glucose, glucagon, leucine, calcium) have been used to stimulate the release of insulin from tumors, but are mainly of research interest *(71)*.

A number of other diagnoses that are associated with an elevated plasma insulin need to be ruled out in the laboratory diagnosis of insulinoma, and include reactive hypoglycemia, functional hypoglycemia, chronic adrenocortical insufficiency, hypopituitarism, extensive hepatic insufficiency, and surreptitious administration of insulin or sulfonlyureas. Historically, surreptitious administration of insulin was detected by characterizing the insulin species using high-performance liquid chromatography. Although the malingerer using animal-derived insulin can still be detected by this method, the development of recombinant human insulin for medical use made measurement of C-peptide and proinsulin concentrations necessary. These are synthesized in excess along with insulin by insulinoma cells, and are thus usually elevated in true cases of insulinoma, but are low in patients with administered insulin. Lebowitz and Blumenthal reported that the molar ratio of insulin to C-peptide was more sensitive in the diagnosis of surreptitious or inadvertent insulin administration *(72)*. They reasoned that although insulin and C-peptide are secreted into the portal vein in a 1:1 molar ratio, the liver clears insulin, but not C-peptide. Thus, the molar ratio of insulin to C-peptide in peripheral venous blood is normally <1.0, but is >1.0 when exogenous insulin is introduced. The ingestion of sulfonylureas, a class of oral hypoglycemic agents that stimulate insulin release, can be ruled out by serum and urine screening for metabolites of these drugs.

Insulinomas behave in a clinically benign manner in 90% of patients and are evenly distributed throughout the pancreas. If the tumor is not in proximity to the pancreatic duct, simple enucleation is performed. If at the time of exploration no tumor is identified, a blind distal pancreatectomy is recommended. To avoid this scenario, aggressive attempts to localize the tumor preoperatively and intraoperatively are warranted. If CT and arteriography fail to localized the tumor, portal venous sampling is a sensitive test, but requires considerable expertise to cannulate the small veins draining the pancreas. Selective injection of calcium gluconate into the arteries feeding the pancreas, and sampling for insulin gradients in the hepatic veins is technically easier to perform and has been reported to be a reliable method of determining the region of the pancreas within which the insulinoma lies *(73)*, although it is obviously invasive and is only recommended sparingly.

Gastrinoma

Gastrinoma, the second most common pancreatic endocrine neoplasm, occurs only half as frequently as insulinoma *(64)*. Gastrinomas are non-β-cell tumors that secrete gastrin, and arise from the pancreas in about 75% of cases or are found close to the pancreas in the duodenal wall, antrum, or hepatoduodenal ligament *(74)*. Ninety percent of gastrinomas are found in the anatomic area described by Stabile et al. as the "gastrinoma triangle," the apices of which are defined by the junctions of the cystic and common bile duct, the second and third portions of the duodenum, and the neck and body of the pancreas *(75)*. In 1955, Zollinger and Ellison were the first to describe the triad of peptic ulcerations in unusual locations, gastric hypersecretion despite therapy, and an islet-cell tumor of the pancreas *(76)*. They hypothesized that an "ulcerogenic factor" secreted by the tumor caused the associated syndrome. Gastrin was subsequently isolated from tumor extracts, and pathophysiologic proof of its role as the proposed factor was provided *(77)*. Hypergastrinemia causes peptic ulceration of the upper GI tract in about 60% of the patients; it is commonly recurrent and occurs in atypical locations *(68)*. Diarrhea is present in about half of the patients, and 10% present with diarrhea as the only manifestation of the syndrome. Clinical situations that should prompt a search for gastrinoma are recurrent peptic ulcer disease despite adequate medical treatment or operation, postbulbar ulcers, prominent gastric rugal folds on upper endoscopy, peptic ulcers with diarrhea, a family history of peptic ulceration, or the multiple endocrine neoplasia type 1 (MEN-1) syndrome.

The laboratory diagnosis of gastrinoma is made by the quantitation of serum gastrin. An elevated fasting serum gastrin level >150 pg/mL provides the diagnosis most of the time, as long as the patient has not been taking antacids, H_2 blockers, or antisecretory medications. A fasting serum gastrin level >1000 pg/mL with the presence of gastric hyperacidity is usually diagnostic, and concentrations >1500 pg/mL suggest metastatic disease *(78)*. However, many patients with a gastrinoma have concentrations between 200 and 1000 pg/mL. Other conditions where elevated gastrin concentrations can occur are retained antrum, gastric outlet obstruction, G-cell hyperplasia, pernicious anemia (achlorhydria, atrophic gastritis), postvagotomy state, short gut syndrome, and renal failure. These must be excluded before the diagnosis of gastrinoma can be made. Sometimes measurements of gastric acid secretion assist in making the diagnosis. A fasting plasma gastrin >100 pg/mL and a basal acid output (BAO) >15 mEq/h are characteristic. A BAO >5 mEq/h in patients with previous acid-reducing operations is suggestive. A ratio of BAO/MAO (pentagastrin stimulated) in excess of 0.6 also supports the diagnosis *(64)*. If a laboratory diagnosis of gastrinoma still cannot be made, provocative testing is indicated. Intravenous secretin results in a paradoxical rise in serum gastrin in patients with gastrinoma. A 200 pg/mL rise in serum gastrin over baseline with provocative testing (secretin, 2 U/kg, iv) is diagnostic of gastrinoma (Fig. 2). Provocative testing with calcium is no longer routinely done, because secretin is safer and more reliable *(79)*. However, in cases that remain equivocal after the secretin-stimulation test, a combined secretin-calcium stimulation test has been reported to be more sensitive *(80)*.

After diagnosis, acid hypersecretion is often controlled medically, whereas attempts at tumor localization are made. Preoperative localization has traditionally relied on CT scan, although 70% of primary tumors and 44% of metastases may be missed using this technique *(81)*. Approximately 75% of neuroendocrine gastroenteropancreatic tumors are identifiable by scintigraphy utilizing Indium-111-pentetreotide (octreotide), a somatostatin analog, as a probe. Identification has been shown to be secondary to somatostatin receptor subtype 2 expression in these tumors *(82)*. Octreotide scanning

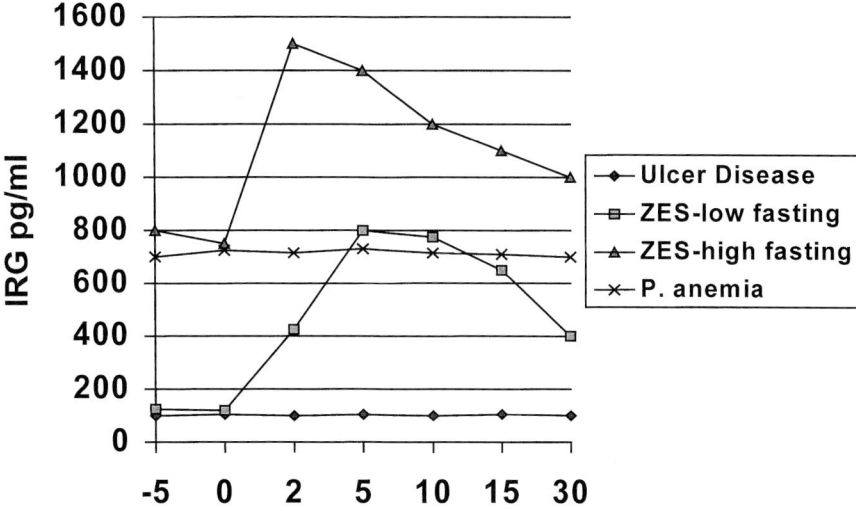

Fig. 2. Serum gastrin response to iv secretin administation (2 U/kg) in patients with benign ulcer disease, Zollinger-Ellison Syndrome (low and high fasting serum gastrin concentrations), and pernicious anemia.

is particularly helpful in identifying small tumors. In one study, octreotide scanning was positive in four of seven tumors smaller than 1 cm, including one 4-mm tumor. In the same group of patients, no lesions <1 cm in size were identified by CT scan (81). In cases where tumor cannot be localized preoperatively, surgical exploration is still warranted. At our institution, various methods are utilized to localize gastrinomas intraoperatively. These include direct visualization, intraoperative ultrasound, and radioimmune-guided surgery utilizing octreotide probe. Patients with potentially resectable lesions undergo resection with the intent for cure. Pancreatic gastrinomas are enucleated or removed by partial pancreatectomy, duodenal tumors are resected with a narrow margin of duodenum around the tumor, and parietal cell vagotomy is added in selective cases. In a recent review of our institution's 40-yr experience with gastrinomas, complete surgical resection was shown to reduce mortality regardless of other factors (83). Blind pancreatic resection for unlocalized tumors has not proven to be efficacious.

VIPoma

A VIPoma is a less common pancreatic endocrine tumor with an annual incidence of about 1/10 million population (84). The tumor, which is usually located in the pancreas, secretes VIP. In 1958, Verner and Morrison described a syndrome that consisted of large volumes (1–3 L/d) of watery diarrhea, hypokalemia, and achlorhydria associated with an islet-cell tumor (85). The syndrome has thus been called "WDHA Syndrome" as well as "Verner-Morrison Syndrome" and "pancreatic cholera." The diarrhea is secretory, which means that it is not relieved by nasogastric suction as in the diarrhea of Zollinger-Ellison Syndrome. The hypokalemia is caused by loss of potassium in the stool, and the hypochlorhydria or achlorhydria is caused by the inhibitory effect of VIP on gastric acid secretion (86). A few patients may have flushing caused by the vasodilatory effects of VIP (86).

The laboratory diagnosis of VIPoma is made by detection of fasting plasma VIP concentrations >200 pg/mL. The normal fasting VIP is 0–190 pg/mL, and in 29 patients with VIPoma, the mean level was 956 pg/mL with a range of 225–1850 pg/mL *(86)*. Administration of iv pentagastrin has been reported to stimulate the release of VIP and neurotensin in patients with VIPoma *(87)*. The long-acting somatostatin analog, octreotide, is useful for reducing circulating VIP concentrations, controlling symptoms, and allowing more rapid preparation for operation *(88)*. Whereas VIP is elevated in all patients with the syndrome and is generally accepted as the pathophysiologic agent responsible for the syndrome, increased concentrations of other peptides, like pancreatic polypeptide, neurotensin, peptide-histidine-methionine, calcitonin, and prostaglandin E, are also frequently found *(89)*.

Ninety percent of VIPomas are located in the body and tail of the pancreas *(90)*. Because extrapancreatic VIPomas occur along the autonomic nervous system and in the adrenal medulla, if no tumor is found, a careful exploration of the retroperitoneum, including the adrenals, is done. If the tumor still cannot be localized, a distal pancreatectomy is considered. Manifestations of VIPoma are clearly ameliorated by debulking procedures *(91)*.

Glucagonoma

A glucagonoma is an even less common pancreatic endocrine tumor with an annual incidence of about 1/20 million population *(92)*. Glucagonomas arise from the α-cells of the islets, are usually large tumors (>5 cm), and are usually (80%) located in the body or tail of the pancreas *(92)*. The typical clinical syndrome caused by excess glucagon secretion, sometimes referred to as the "4-D Syndrome," includes mild diabetes, a pathognomonic dermatitis (migratory necrolytic erythema), deep venous thrombosis, and depression. The rash, demonstrated by Norton et al. to be caused by amino acid deficiency, is perhaps the clinical key to the diagnosis, and typically appears in the perioral area and on the distal extremities, perineum, and thighs *(93)*. The lesions begin as red erythematous blotches followed by central erosions and vesicopustules that desquamate white flakes leaving an area of central clearing and brown pigmentation.

Normal serum glucagon values are 0–120 pg/mL and the laboratory diagnosis of glucagonoma is made by demonstrating values >1000pg/mL. Most patients have concentrations >150 pg/mL. One caveat, however, is that patients with a glucagonoma may have infrequent episodic hypersecretion of glucagon that can lead to sampling errors *(94)*. Provocative testing with secretin, as in gastrinoma, may be helpful, but is usually not necessary *(95)*. An elevated level of CEA, βHCG, or CA 19–9 may be present in some cases, and confirms the malignant nature of glucagonomas *(89)*. A resection for cure is possible in the minority, since most present with metastatic disease making debulking the more common procedure. Patients should be given prophylaxis for thromboembolism and pulmonary embolism, because these are common complications after surgery for glucagonoma *(93)*.

Somatostatinoma

Somatostatinomas are among the rarest of the pancreatic endocrine tumors with an annual incidence of 1 in 40 million population *(96)*. Somatostatinomas arise from the somatostatin-producing δ-cells of the pancreatic islets and GI tract. The "somatostatinoma syndrome," first described by Ganda et al. in 1977, is associated with somatostatinomas arising from the pancreas and consists of cholelithiasis, type II diabetes, and steatorrhea *(97)*. Somatostatinomas arising from the duodenum are usually not associated with hypersomatostatinemia and do not produce the syndrome. In a recent review, Dayal and Ganda found only 80 cases reported in the literature with the most common location being in the head of the pancreas (68%) and less commonly the duodenum (19%), often with liver metastases present at exploration *(98)*. Resection for cure has been rare, but safe debulking procedures including pancreaticoduodenectomy are indicated to manage the manifestations of hypersomatostatinemia.

The laboratory diagnosis of somatostatinoma is difficult, because the tumor is rare and the early findings are nonspecific. In the rare case where the diagnosis is entertained preoperatively, confirmation is obtained by demonstrating an elevated fasting somatostatin concentration by radioimmunoassay (normal, <100 pg/mL). Most patients with pancreatic somatostatinomas have markedly elevated fasting somatostatin values. One series reported a mean level 50 times greater than normal *(99)*. Other studies have reported concentrations ranging from 160 pg/mL to 107 ng/mL (107,000 pg/mL) *(92,99)*. However, the patients with duodenal somatostatinomas rarely have the syndrome, and none have had abnormal somatostatin concentrations *(100)*. No provocative tests are available, although tolbutamide has recently been reported to increase somatostatin concentrations in patients with somatostatinomas, but not in normal control patients *(101)*.

PPoma

Pancreatic polypeptide (PP) is normally secreted from the F-cells, which are most prominently found in the periphery of the islets in the head of the pancreas *(102)*. PP binds to specific receptors, inhibits exocrine pancreatic secretion of enzymes, bicarbonate, and water, and suppresses gastric and small intestinal motility *(103)*.

Since there is no clinical syndrome described for PP secreting tumors, many PPomas are considered to be nonfunctional pancreatic endocrine tumors. In addition, since PP is frequently secreted in small amounts by the more common endocrine pancreatic tumors, by definition, a tumor must have at least 50% PP-secreting cells to classify it as a PPoma *(88)*. As with all pancreatic endocrine tumors, surgical resection is the treatment of choice, and debulking of large metastatic lesions may be palliative.

The laboratory diagnosis of PPoma can be established by measuring fasting concentrations of PP by radioimmunoassay. Values in patients with PPoma are usually four times the normal in age-matched controls, and concentrations >300 pmol/mL are considered diagnostic regardless of age *(104)*. To assist in the diagnosis of borderline or difficult cases, administration of atropine is suggested; it reduces PP concentrations in normal persons, but not in patients with a PPoma *(105)*. Also, provocative testing with secretin may improve diagnostic accuracy. It is interesting that as many as two-thirds of patients with "nonfunctioning" islet-cell tumors have an exaggerated response to secretin when tested, indicating that many of the tumors previously considered to be nonfunctioning tumors are actually PPomas *(88)*.

Nonfunctioning Islet-Cell Tumors

The majority of pancreatic endocrine tumors are functional, but 15–25% do not secrete islet peptide products and, thus, are not associated with a clinical syndrome (106). These patients present with abdominal pain, weight loss, and jaundice similar to patients with pancreatic adenocarcinoma. However, even patients with surgically incurable disease may benefit from primary tumor debulking, because 5-yr survival is possible even without curative resection. Neuron-specific enolase has been proposed as a possible serum marker for nonfunctioning islet cell carcinomas (107). Recent studies also suggest that plasma marker 7B2 may be a good indicator of nonfunctioning pancreatic islet cell tumors (108). Because of the absence of a clinical syndrome, diagnosis is difficult prior to histologic confirmation.

CLINICAL CONSIDERATIONS IN EXOCRINE PANCREATIC TUMORS

Since the majority of all tumors of the pancreas are adenocarcinomas, the following sections will deal exclusively with an overview of the epidemiology, etiology, diagnosis, prognosis, and management of these exocrine tumors of the pancreas.

Epidemiology and Etiology

Incidence and Mortality

An estimated number of 26,300 cases of pancreatic cancer will be diagnosed in 1996 (109). The grim prognosis of pancreatic cancer is exemplified by the fact that the incidence rates are essentially equal to the mortality rates. Pancreatic cancer is the fifth leading cause of death from cancer in the United States exceeded only by cancer of the lung, colon and rectum, breast, and prostate. Approximately 26,000 Americans died as a result of pancreatic cancer in 1992, and it is estimated that this number will increase to 27,800 in 1996. Age-adjusted mortality rates increased steadily from 2.9/100,000 in 1920 to 9/100,000 in 1970 (110). Mortality rates have slowly decreased since that time in White men, whereas in Black women, they have slowly increased. (Updated data not available at time of publication.)

Because of its high prevalence, pancreatic cancer has become a major health concern in the United States. The significance of pancreatic cancer is heightened when its poor prognosis is considered. In a review of 61 clinical studies, representing approx 15,000 patients (111), Gudjonsson et al. calculated the absolute 5-yr survival rate to be 0.4% for patients diagnosed with pancreatic cancer. The mean survival is reported to be 2–3 mo from the time of diagnosis. Pancreatic cancer is usually diagnosed at a relatively late stage in its progression with 90% of patients having regional nodal metastases at the time of diagnosis and 80% having liver metastases. The high mortality for pancreatic cancer is presumed to be because of the late diagnosis of most patients. Radical surgery is indicated for cure in cases where the tumor is deemed resectable and remains the cornerstone of treatment. Most patients are not surgical candidates, but 5-yr survival rates of up to 30% have been reported following surgical resection. In addition, surgery has proven to be good palliative treatment for patients with unresectable tumors in cases of biliary or duodenal obstruction.

Demographic and Geographic Patterns

Incidence and mortality rates for pancreatic cancer vary widely in countries throughout the world. Age-adjusted rates are lowest in Japan and Italy and highest in Western and industrialized nations *(112)*. Studies of Japanese immigrants to the United States and their descendants have demonstrated a higher rate of pancreatic cancer among Japanese immigrants than either their children or US Whites *(113)*. These data are puzzling and suggest the influence of some environmental factor in the cause of pancreatic cancer.

Pancreatic cancer has traditionally been more prevalent in males than females. According to the Surveillance, Epidemiology, and End Results program, the male/female ratio was 1.55 among Whites and 1.48 among Blacks in the United States *(114)*. In another study by Grieve *(115)*, the gender ratios were examined for different tumor locations, and found to be 1.5 for carcinoma of the head of the pancreas and 0.6 for carcinomas of the body and tail of the pancreas. The gender ratio seems to have reversed in recent years with 13,399 female deaths in 1992 as opposed to 12,672 male deaths *(112)*, a result of the changing distribution of mortality rates in Black females and White males.

In the United States, mortality rates for Blacks are higher than in any other ethnic group except Japanese *(116)*. The mortality rates for US Blacks are higher than those for African Blacks. Once again, this suggests environmental factors. Pancreatic cancer incidence rates increase steadily with age, and 80% of cases occur between the ages of 60 and 80. Cases below age 40 are rare, but do occur *(117–119)*. Studies of the effect of socioeconomic status on incidence rates have not shown any statistically significant relations, except that of a higher incidence in white woman in the highest category for each socioeconomic variable studied *(114)*. There are no significant differences among rural and urban populations.

Possible Etiologic Factors

It has been firmly established for over 60 yr that diabetes mellitus occurs more frequently in patients with pancreatic cancer than in the general population. Some argue that pancreatic cancer causes diabetes, whereas others believe that diabetes represents a true risk factor for the development of pancreatic cancer. Diabetes has been shown to increase the risk of subsequent pancreatic cancer in many studies even when cases of diabetes of 2-, 5-, or even 10-yr duration are excluded. This is not true in all studies, however, leading some authors to conclude that diabetes of recent (2–10 yr) onset is caused by the tumor. Whether one sets the exclusion at 2, 5, or 10 yr of pre-existing diabetes is arbitrary. In many of these cases, the conclusion that the cancer preceded the diabetes is tenuous, because the duration of diabetes is difficult to determine, especially in retrospective studies. Given the known association between diabetes and pancreatic cancer, the recent diagnosis of diabetes in the patients with pancreatic cancer could have been owing to a search for diabetes after the diagnosis of pancreatic cancer. In addition, reliance on recall of subjects is likely to result in a considerable underestimation of the incidence of diabetes. Perhaps most importantly, the true time of onset of diabetes is difficult to determine. NIDDM may be present for more than 7 yr before the clinical diagnosis is made. Undiagnosed diabetes may have preceded the pancreatic cancer for many years. "Recent-onset diabetes" may actually represent a recent exacerbation of long-standing subclinical diabetes by the occult malignancy.

In prospective cohort studies, the existence of diabetes is defined at the start of the study, and those who are going to develop pancreatic cancer are unknown. Thus, the issue of whether the diabetes preceded the pancreatic cancer is known, and a more definitive statement about diabetes and the subsequent development of pancreatic cancer can be made. In a recent meta-analysis of a number of such studies, Everhart and Wright concluded that the pooled relative risk of pancreatic cancer for diabetics of five or more years of duration relative to nondiabetics was 2.0 (95% CI, 1.2–3.2) *(120)*.

Cigaret smoking appears to increase the risk of pancreatic cancer. According to the American Cancer Society Survey, the relative risk of pancreatic cancer in males aged 45–64 was estimated to be 2.69 and 2.17 in males aged 65–79 *(121)*. Consumption of diets high in meat and fat has also been shown to be associated with pancreatic cancer. Coffee consumption also has been correlated with an increased risk of pancreatic cancer. There has been some controversy over this issue because coffee drinkers tend to smoke more, although MacMahon et al. *(122)* demonstrated that the relationship is still significant when cigaret smoking was accounted for. Alcohol consumption has also been shown to be associated with pancreatic cancer. In studies where smoking was taken into account, this relationship was not found to be significant *(123)*.

Current data indicate that a relationship exists between chronic pancreatitis and pancreatic cancer, but these data continue to be controversial. Many patients with pancreatic cancer are found to have foci of pancreatitis at the time of autopsy. In many cases, this is thought to be owing to an inflammatory response secondary to ductal obstruction. A much stronger relationship exists with so-called hereditary pancreatitis and tropical pancreatitis. Hereditary pancreatitis has been described in numerous lineages *(124–128)* and approx 30% of patients in these families will develop pancreatic cancer. Interestingly, the risk of pancreatic cancer is the same for all members of these families whether or not they have pancreatitis.

No relationship exists between pancreatic adenocarcinoma and radiation exposure in human or animal studies. In addition, no evidence exists to support an infectious etiology in pancreatic cancer. As far as chemical exposure is concerned, numerous chemicals are known to produce pancreatic tumors in animal models. The majority of these are nitrosamine compounds. N-nitosobis(2-hydroxypropylamine) (or BOP) is frequently used to produce pancreatic ductal adenocarcinomas in the Syrian Golden Hamster model, and azaserine treatment consistently induces pancreatic acinar tumors in rats *(129)*. In humans, increased pancreatic cancer rates have been found in workers exposed to coal gas, coal tar pitch derivatives, β-naphthylamine, and benzidine, as well as those who operate pile-drivers in wood-related occupations *(112)*.

Diagnosis and Management

Clinical Presentation

The fact that pancreatic cancer presents at such a late stage in its progression is most likely owing to the relatively inaccessible, retroperitoneal location of the pancreas. Patients usually present with epigastric pain, jaundice, or both *(3)*. Those who do not present with these symptoms frequently present with weight loss, nausea and vomiting, or other, vaguer, symptoms. It should be noted that lesions in the head of the pancreas usually present with jaundice because of close proximity to the common bile duct, whereas lesions in the tail present with more vague symptoms.

Pancreatic cancer may present as acute pancreatitis in 14% of patients *(130)*. Findings on physical examination may include hepatomegaly, jaundice, guaiac-positive stools, abdominal mass, or ascites.

Conventional Diagnostic Modalities

As previously discussed, the diagnosis of pancreatic carcinoma has been traditionally based on abdominal ultrasound, CT scan, ERCP, and angiography, as well as surgical or percutaneous biopsy. In recent years, various modalities, such as endoscopic and intraoperative ultrasound, measurement of pancreatic exocrine secretion, and cytologic analysis of duodenal aspirate, or pancreatic juice obtained at ERCP, have been developed to augment accurate and early diagnosis in suspected cases.

In institutions with access to skilled and experienced ultrasonographers, ultrasound has become the preferred initial study performed in the workup of pancreatic cancer. Hepatic metastases, common bile duct dilatation, and intraparenchymal pancreatic masses as small as 1.0–1.5 cm are all findings consistent with pancreatic cancer identifiable by ultrasound examination *(7)*. In addition, other lesions, such as pancreatic cystadenomas and cystadenocarcinomas, can be identified. Current data indicate that ultrasound has at least a sensitivity of 76% and a specificity of 90% in diagnosing pancreatic cancer *(131)*.

In cases where ultrasound is negative or nondiagnostic, CT scan of the abdomen should be performed. A CT scan improves sensitivity by approx 10% over ultrasound *(7)* and can be used to determine tumor resectability. Invasion of adjacent vascular structures or organs, as well as distant metastases, are usually contraindications to resection of the primary tumor in hopes of cure.

ERCP with cytology is indicated if either ultrasound or CT scan is consistent with pancreatic cancer, or if there is a strong clinical suspicion for pancreatic cancer. Advantages include 92% sensitivity in detecting pancreatic cancer, as well as >95% specificity *(132)*, and the ability to confirm diagnosis by tissue sample. In a prospective analysis of various modalities in the early diagnosis of pancreatic cancer by Moossa and Levin, ERCP demonstrated the highest diagnostic accuracy of all tests studied (89%) *(133)*. Disadvantages include a 15% technical failure rate *(133)*, and a small but significant risk of complications compared with other noninvasive studies. Because of cost and technical difficulty, ERCP remains an uncommon clinical test except in a relatively few centers.

Prior to the widespread availability of the above-mentioned techniques, angiography was the primary diagnostic modality in the workup of pancreatic cancer. Because of a low sensitivity of 60% *(134)*, high cost, and the risk of possible complications, angiography should no longer be used as a primary study in the diagnosis of pancreatic cancer. It should, instead, be reserved for determining vascular invasion and resectability in cases where resection for cure is being considered and CT evidence of resectability is unclear.

At the time of presentation to the surgeon, a pancreatic mass, with or without jaundice, is the most common finding in pancreatic cancer. When a small mass with no evidence of metastatic disease is identified, diagnosis is difficult. Serum markers may be of some benefit, but histological confirmation is often necessary. In patients with large masses or evidence of metastatic disease, percutaneous needle biopsy may be performed. This is not routinely recommended, however, in patients with small, potentially resectable lesions. A FN rate of 20–30% has been reported, and a negative diagnostic biopsy does not exclude malignancy. Additionally, the added risk of seeding the peritoneum and needle tract with malignant cells exists, and may contribute to mortality.

Patients with small pancreatic lesions require surgical exploration, and laparoscopy may be a useful tool in the initial part of the exploration. A significant number of hepatic and peritoneal metastases are not detected by conventional imaging studies, and these may be identified at the time of laparoscopy. If such is the case, the surgeon may elect not to proceed with laparotomy, thus avoiding the considerable morbity and mortality associated with major abdominal surgery in these patients. Additional tools, such as laparoscopic ultrasound, are valuable in evaluating the local extent of pancreatic lesions.

In the absence of metastatic disease, open surgical exploration is necessary for diagnosis in most patients with a mass in the head of the pancreas. Determination of resectability is based on the clinical suspicion of malignancy and technical factors, including local invasion of the pancreatic mass. Routine intraoperative biopsies are not performed, since their accuracy is not reliable. Surgical resection may occasionally be required in order to provide histologic confirmation of malignancy.

Pathology

There have been numerous attempts to classify tumors of the exocrine pancreas by histological criteria. These have been complicated by the coding of specimens at many institutions into broad categories, such as "adenocarcinoma" or "adenocarcinoma NOS" *(1)*. Accurate classification is necessary, however, in order to identify those patients with more favorable tumor types. This is despite the fact that 75–90% of these tumors are duct-cell adenocarcinomas with poor prognoses.

As discussed previously, the vast majority of pancreatic tumors are of ductal origin, with ductal adenocarcinomas accounting for 75–90% of all exocrine tumors. Benign adenomas and papillomas have been described *(134)*, but are exceedingly rare. Mucinous cystadenomas and cystadenocarcinomas may be differentiated on a histological basis, but in practice should be treated as the same entity, by surgical excision. This is because of the high rate of malignant transformation in "benign" mucinous cystadenomas and difficulty in differentiating these lesions preoperatively. In fact, when extensively sampled, most mucinous cystadenomas demonstrate focal areas of atypia *(135)*. Serous cystadenomas are truly benign, in contrast to the mucinous type, and should be treated conservatively in the absence of symptomatology *(136,137)*. Mucinous cystadenomas and cystadenocarcinomas comprised only 0.8% of pancreatic tumors in the series by Baylor and Berg *(1)*, and accounted for <10% of cystic lesions of the pancreas (the majority are benign pseudocysts) *(137)*. Despite their low incidence, it is vital to differentiate these lesions from benign pseudocysts and serous cystadenomas to treat them properly. The use of cyst fluid analysis in the differential diagnosis of cystic pancreatic lesions has traditionally relied on cytology, fluid viscosity, and pancreatic enzyme concentrations. Recent reports indicate that elevated concentrations of tumor markers (CEA, CA19-9, and so forth) in cyst fluid accurately differentiate mucinous cystadenomas and cystadenocarcinoma from pseudocysts and benign serous cystadenomas *(136,138,139)*. These data are encouraging, but their use has not yet gained wide clinical acceptance.

Duct-cell adenocarcinomas are the underlying lesion in the majority of "pancreatic cancers." Pathological characteristics include an intense desmoplastic stromal response that gives the tumor a firm, fibrous consistency *(135)*. Needle aspirate or biopsy specimens subsequently demonstrate a high rate of sampling error, making diagnosis difficult. Approximately 65% of tumors arise in the head of the pancreas, 10–15% arise in the body, and 5–10% arise in the tail. The remainder are more diffuse in location *(140)*. Histologically, ductal adenocarcinomas demonstrate invasion of stromal elements by individual or small clusters of cells that have enlarged hyperchromatic nuclei, and densely eosinophilic or coarsely granulated cytoplasm. Poorly differentiated specimens exhibit mitotic figures and a high nuclear-to-cytoplasmic ratio, as well as perineural invasion demonstratable on laminin staining.

Squamous and adenosquamous carcinomas of the pancreas are rare, and comprise approx 0.9% of pancreatic cancers *(135)*. These are often classified together because of their similar biologic and prognostic characteristics. The two are differentiated by the presence of glandular elements in the adenosquamous type, although some investigators believe that all tumors of the exocrine pancreas contain glandular components. Their prognosis is similar to that of ductal adenocarcinoma with a reported 1-yr survival of 4.8%. Papillary neoplasms of the pancreas are even rarer, occurring in an estimated 0.17% of cases *(141)*. They are significant, however, because of an prognosis; the 1-yr survival is 30% and 5-yr survival is 4%. They are also unique in that they are more common in woman and they usually present at a later age than most forms of pancreatic cancer *(1)*. Giant-cell or pleomorphic carcinomas of the pancreas exhibit striking histological similarity to other tumors such as malignant melanoma, choriocarcinoma, and hepatocellular carcinoma. These tumors have been reported to comprise 2% of pancreatic adenocarcinomas and exhibit an extremely aggressive clinical course *(142)*. Most patients do not survive more than a few months. The cellular origin of giant-cell carcinomas is unknown, and they are therefore listed as being of both ductal and acinar origin in the proposed classification.

As is the case with ductal adenomas, acinar-cell adenomas, although described, are an exceedingly rare entity. Acinar adenocarcinomas are thought to comprise 1–2% of carcinomas of the exocrine pancreas *(140)* and their behavior closely approximates that of ductal adenocarcinomas. There are some data to indicate that these tumors may be more prevalent in children with pancreatic cancer and have a more favorable prognosis in these cases *(143)*.

Microcystic adenomas or serous cystadenomas are significant because of their benign behavior. They are relatively common and often asymptomatic. Ten cases in a review of 34 by Oertel et al. were diagnosed incidentally at autopsy *(144)*. It is important to differentiate these tumors from others, because they may be treated nonoperatively in older, asymptomatic patients. Surgery is usually reserved for patients who become symptomatic from tumor invasion into surrounding structures. Solid and papillary epithelial neoplasms of the pancreas are extremely rare (0.17% of cases) *(141)*, affect women more frequently, and are of low-grade malignant potential. Tumor-related deaths are extremely rare *(144)*. Pancreatoblastomas are a rare pancreatic neoplasm of infancy whose variable tissue elements suggest oncogenesis very early in embryonic life and are highly malignant *(145)*.

Treatment and Prognosis

Surgery has traditionally been the mainstay of both treatment and palliation for pancreatic adenocarcinoma. For stage I disease involving the head of the pancreas, pancreaticoduodenectomy or the "Whipple" procedure should be performed. Tumors involving the body and tail of the pancreas are extremely morbid, and resection has improved survival; almost all of these tumors are widely disseminated by the time they are diagnosed. The number of patients found to have resectable tumors at the time of exploration varies from study to study, but is thought to be around 5–10%. This number approaches 10–20% today with more accurate methods of preoperative staging. Mean survival following surgical resection is approx 18–20 mo, and 5-yr survival rates range from 5–18% *(2)*. The Japanese Pancreatic Cancer Register has further classified primary adenocarcinomas of the pancreas according to size. Tumors <2 cm in size were found to be resectable in 91.8% of cases with a 5-yr survival rate of 37.5%, whereas tumors between 2 and 4 cm were resectable 80% of the time with a 5-yr survival of 15.9%. Tumors between 4 and 6 cm and >6 cm were resectable in only 45.3 and 20.5% of cases, respectively, with 5-yr survival rates of 13.1 and 8.1%. There were no 5-yr survivors in patients with tumors >2 cm in size who did not undergo surgical resection *(25)*.

Overall, the prognosis for pancreatic cancer is poor. As stated previously, when all patients are considered, the 5-yr survival is ~0.4% despite all treatment. It is still unknown whether resection results in improved overall survival. Surgery, however, is the only hope for cure, and the significantly improved survival advantage in patients with small tumors confined to the pancreas emphasizes the need for aggressive management in all cases where resection is a possibility. Surgical exploration should be undertaken for all patients in whom distant spread or local invasion precluding resection has not been ruled out. In addition, pancreaticoduodenectomy is recommended for patients with suspicious masses in the head of the pancreas, even in the absence of tissue diagnosis. A significant number of these tumors may be other periampullary cancers, such as distal cholangiocarcinoma. Patients with these tumors demonstrate improved survival after resection, and failure to treat a nonpancreatic periampullary cancer would be unfortunate.

Pancreaticoduodenectomy is the most common operation, and historically, it has been associated with significant morbidity and perioperative mortality. Modern data suggest that pancreaticoduodenectomy can be performed with minimal in-hospital mortality, an acceptable complication rate, and good long-term results. Some authors now even suggest pancreaticoduodenectomy in the face of metastatic disease as an effective technique of palliation for biliary and duodenal obstruction. The morbidity and mortality for pancreaticoduodenctomy approaches that of a palliative surgical procedure when performed in an institution where pancreaticoduodenectomy is relatively common. At the current time, the decision for surgical resection must be based on the intraoperative findings of the surgeon.

Our institution's experience parallels these results. Clearly, accurate techniques for the preoperative diagnosis of pancreatic cancer would exclude those patients with benign pancreatic head lesions from unnecessary surgical resection. In fact, 25% of patients undergoing pancreaticoduodenectomy may have benign disease when final histology fails to confirm a malignancy. Overall, the decision for surgical exploration and resection should be based on the patient's overall clinical condition, the clinical suspicion of a malignancy, and the ability of the treating institution and physicians to offer the patient a chance at cure and good, long palliation.

For patients with advanced disease, surgical resection is not performed with the intent to cure. Indeed, mean survival for patients with unresectable disease is probably only 2–3 mo. Surgical palliation may be necessary in cases of biliary or duodenal obstruction, however, the availability of nonsurgical biliary drainage procedures, such as percutaneous transhepatic biliary drainage (PTBD) and endoscopic biliary stent placement, is rapidly increasing. Options for palliation depend on many factors and are beyond the scope of this discussion.

Chemotherapy and radiation have proven to be of little benefit in advanced disease, although 5-Fluoro-Uracil (5-FU) in combination with radiation has been shown to improve the dismal prognosis slightly *(146)*. These treatments are often withheld because of their limited value in patients with advanced disease and poor quality of life. Recent data indicate that gemcitabene, a nucleoside analog, may provide subjective relief of symptoms in 23.8% of patients with advanced pancreatic cancer. In addition, 1-yr survival rates following gemcitabine treatment have been shown to be 18% compared to 2% for those receiving 5-FU *(147)*.

Chemotherapy and radiation are of of some benefit, in combination with surgery, as adjuvant therapy for resectable disease. Data concerning their use are still incomplete, and these approaches should be employed only as part of experimental protocols. Studies employing the use of hormonal or immunotherapy are currently under way, but they are still in the very early stages. It is unclear what role these modalities, if any, will play in the future for the treatment of pancreatic cancer. It should be noted that considerable recent interest has been given to the use of the gastrointestinal hormone, somatostatin. Our laboratory has shown that somatostatin treatment inhibits the growth of human pancreatic cancer tumor cells expressing the somatostatin receptor subtype-2 gene when planted subcutaneously in nude mice *(148)*. Clinical trials utilizing somatostatin as a treatment for pancreatic cancer are currently under way.

SUMMARY

Neoplastic disorders of the pancreas run the gamut of indolent, slow-growing endocrine tumors producing distinct clinical syndromes that persist for decades to quickly metastasizing, occult adenocarcinomas that kill within months of the initial diagnosis. The causes for this spectrum of diseases remain hidden, but are under intense study throughout the medical community. Surgical and medical treatment modalities for adenocarcinoma of the pancreas are mainly palliative, whereas those for endocrine tumors can be truly curative.

Pancreatic ductal adenocarcinoma is a significant health problem with considerable mortality. The diagnosis of pancreatic cancer continues to rely on clinical presentation, conventional imaging studies, surgical exploration, and histologic confirmation.

A large amount of research has been conducted in recent years concerning the use of laboratory tests for the diagnosis and management of pancreatic cancer. These have been shown, at best, only to augment other diagnostic modalities. Serum CA19-9 determinations are currently the most useful test in this regard. The use of CA19-9 assays is limited by nonspecificity and, in fact, is probably of no value for diagnosis in jaundiced patients. In contrast to diagnosis, management and, to a lesser extent, prognosis can be optimized by utilizing various tumor markers, specifically CA19-9 and CEA. Other tumor-related antigens, such as CA50, CA242, and so on, recognize the same or similar epitopes and are not superior to CA19-9. Serum enzyme activities and hormonal or oncofetal antigens alone are basically not helpful in the diagnosis of pancreatic cancer, and their use has been abandoned. Active research continues on techniques to develop a noninvasive technique to identify and correctly diagnose pancreatic cancer in high-risk populations. Detection of genetic mutations, such as k-*ras*, in peripheral blood or even in the stool would be ideal and is currently being evaluated.

In contrast to pancreatic adenocarcinoma, endocrine tumors of the pancreas lend themselves to definitive diagnosis through quantitation of tumor-specific hormones, except in cases of nonfunctioning tumors. Mortality from these tumors rarely results from the clinical syndromes caused by overproduction of these hormones.

REFERENCES

1. Baylor SM, Berg JW (1973) Cross-classification and survival characteristics of 5,000 cases of cancer of the pancreas. J Surg Oncol 5(4):335–358.
2. Warshaw AL, Swanson AS (1988) Pancreatic cancer in 1988. Possibilities and probabilities. Ann Surg 208(5):541–553.
3. Go VLW. Editorial. Pancreas 1994;9(6):673.
4. Ho JCL, Kim YS (1992) Serological pancreatic tumor markers and the MUC1 apomucin. Pancreas 9(6):674–691.
5. Martin EW, James KK, Purtubise PE, et al. (1977) The use of CEA as an early indicator for gastrointestinal tumor recurrence and second look procedures. Cancer 39: 440–46.
6. Steinberg WM, Gelfand R, Anderson KK, Glenn J, Kurtzman SH, Sindelar WF, et al. (1986) Comparison of the sensitivity and specificity of the CA19-9 and carcinoembryonic antigen assays in detecting cancer of the pancreas. Gastroenterology 90:343–9.
7. Niederau C, Grendell, JH (1992) Diagnosis of pancreatic carcinoma: Imaging techniques and tumor markers. Pancreas 7(1):66–86.
8. Yasue M, Sakamoto J, Teramukai S, Morimoto T, Yasui K, Kuno N, et al. (1994) Prognostic values of preoperative and postoperative CEA and CA19-9 levels in pancreatic cancer. Pancreas 9(6):735–740.
9. Okai T, Sawabu N, Takemori Y, Ohta H, Motoo Y, Kidani H (1992) Levels of carcinoembryonic antigen and carbohydrate antigen (CA19-9) in pure pancreatic juice and sera in a patient with occult pancreatic cancer. J Clin Gastroenterol 15(2):162–164.
10. Matsumoto S, Harada H, Tanaka J, Ochi K, Seno T, Tsurumi T, et al. (1994) Evaluation of cytology and tumor markers of pure pancreatic juice for the diagnosis of pancreatic cancer at early stages. Pancreas 9(6):741–747.
11. Koprowski H, Steplewski Z, Mitchell K, Herlyn D, Fuhrer JP (1979) Colorectal carcinomas detected by hybridoma antibodies. Somatic Cell Genet 5:957–972.
12. Atkinson BF, Ernst CS, Herlyn M, Seplewski Z, Sears HF, Koprwoski H (1982) Gastrointestinal cancer-associated antigen in immunoperoxidase assay. Cancer Res 42: 4820–3.

13. Magnani JL, Milsson M, Brockhaus D, Zopf Z, Steplewski Z, Koprowski H (1982) A monoclonal antibody-defined antigen associated with gastrointestinal cancer is a ganglioside containing sialylated lacto-N-fucopentanose II. J Biol Chem 257:14,365–14,369.
14. Kawa S, Tokoo M, Oguchi H, Furuta S, Homma T, Hasegawa Y, et al. (1994) Epitope analysis of Span-1 and DUPAN-2 using synthesized glycoconjugates sialyllact-N-fucopentaose II and sialyllact-N-tetraose. Pancreas 9(6):692–697.
15. Koprowski H, Blaszczyk M, Steplewski Z, Brockhaus D, Magnani JL, Ginsberg V. (1982) Lewis blood-type may affect the incidence of gastrointestinal cancer. Lancet i:1332–1333.
16. Von Rosen A, Linder S, Harmenberg U, Pegert S (1993) Serum levels of CA19-9 and CA 50 in relation to Lewis blood cell status in patients with malignant and benign pancreatic disease. Pancreas 8(2):160–165.
17. Schmeigel W (1989) Tumor markers in pancreatic cancer—current concepts. Hepatogastroenterology 36:446–449.
18. Safi F, Beger HG, Bittner R, Buchler M, Krautzberger W (1986) CA19-9 and pancreatic adenocarcinoma. Cancer 57:779–783.
19. Farini R, Fabris C, Bonvicini P, Piccoli A, DelFavero G, Venturini R, et al. (1985) CA19-9 in the differential diagnosis between pancreatic cancer and chronic pancreatitis. Eur J Cancer Clin Oncol 21(4):429–432.
20. Safi F, Roscher R, Bittner R, Schenkluhn B, Dopfer HP, Beger HG (1987) High sensitivity and specificity of CA19-9 for pancreatic carcinoma in comparison to chronic pancreatitis. Serological and immunohistochemical findings. Pancreas 2(4):398–403.
21. Malesci A, Montorsi M, Mariani A, Santambrogio R, Bonato C, Bissi O, et al. (1992) Clinical utility of the serum CA19-9 test for diagnosing pancreatic carcinoma in symptomatic patients: A prospective study. Pancreas 7(4):497–502.
22. Malesci A, Tommasini M, Bocchia P, et al. (1984) Differential diagnosis of pancreatic cancer and chronic pancreatitis by a monoclonal antibody detecting a new cancer associated antigen (CA19-9). Ric Clin Lab 14:303–306.
23. Ritts RE, Nagorney DM, Jacobsen DJ, Talbot RW, Zurawski VR (1994) Comparison of serum CA19-9 levels with results of diagnostic imaging modalities in patients undergoing laparotomy for suspected pancreatic or gallbladder disease. Pancreas 9(6): 707–716.
24. Satake K, Chung Y, Umeyama K, Takeuchi T, Kim YS (1991) The possibility of diagnosing small pancreatic cancer (less than 4.0 cm) by measuring various serum tumor markers. Cancer 68:149–152.
25. Satake K, Takeuchi T, Homma T, Ozaki H (1994) CA19-9 as a screening and diagnostic tool in symptomatic patients: The Japanese experience. Pancreas 6:703–6.
26. Glenn J, Steinberg WM, Kurtzman SH, Steinberg SM, Sindelar WF (1988) Evaluation of the utility of a radioimmunoassay for serum CA19-9 levels in patients before and after treatment of carcinoma of the pancreas. J Clin Oncol 6(3):462–468.
27. Forsmark CE, Lambaise L, Vogel SB (1994) Diagnosis of pancreatic cancer and prediction of unresectability using the tumor-associated antigen CA19-9. Pancreas 9(6): 731–734.
28. Sperti C, Pasquali C, Catalini C, Cappellazzo F, Bonadimani B, Behboo R, et al. (1993) CA19-9 as a prognostic index after resection for pancreatic cancer. J Surg Oncol 52:137–141.
29. Lundin J, Roberts PJ, Kuusela P, Haglund C (1994) The prognostic value of preoperative serum levels of CA19-9 and CEA in patients with pancreatic cancer. Br J Cancer 69:515–519.
30. Berretta E, Malesci A, Zerbi A, Mariani A, Carlucci M, Bonato C, et al. (1987) Serum CA19-9 in the postsurgical follow-up of patients with pancreatic cancer. Cancer 60: 2428–2431.

31. Malesci A, Tommasini MA, Bonato C, Bocchia P, Bersani M, Zerbi A, et al. (1987) Determination of CA19-9 antigen in serum and pancreatic juice for differential diagnosis of pancreatic adenocarcinoma from chronic pancreatitis. Gastroenterology 92:60–67.
32. Yuan-fang C, Can-rong M, Zhen-jun T, Zi-tan F, Jie Z, Xing-hua L, et al. (1989) The diagnostic significance of carbohydrate antigen CA19-9 in serum and pancreatic juice in pancreatic carcinoma. Chinese Med J 102(5):333–337.
33. Matsumoto A, Tommasini MA, Bonato C, Bocchia P, Bersani M, Zerbi A, et al. (1987) Determination of CA19-9 antigen in serum and pancreatic juice for differential diagnosis of pancreatic adenocarcinoma from chronic pancreatitis. Gastroenterology 92:60–67.
34. Masson P, Palsson B, Andren-Sandberg A (1991) Evaluation of CEA, CA 19–9, CA-50, CA-195, and TATI with special reference to pancreatic disorders. Int J Pancreatol 8: 333–344.
35. Satake K, Takeuchi T (1994) Comparison of CA19-9 with other tumor markers in the diagnosis of cancer of the pancreas. Pancreas 9(6):720–724.
36. Pasanen PA, Eskelinen M, Partanen K, Pikkarainen P, Pentilla I, Alhava E. (1994) A prospective study of serum tumor markers carcinoembryonic antigen, carbohydrate antigens 50 and 242, tissue polypeptide antigen and tissue polypeptide specific antigen in the diagnosis of pancreatic cancer with special reference to multivariate diagnostic score. Br J Cancer 69:562–565.
37. Von Rosen A, Linder S, Harmenberg U, Pegert S (1993) Serum levels of CA19-9 and CA 50 in relation to Lewis blood cell status in patients with malignant and benign pancreatic disease. Pancreas 8(2):160–165.
38. Banfi G, Zerbi A, Pastori S, Parolini D, DiCarlo V, Bonini P (1993) Behavior of tumor markers CA19-9, CA195, CAM43,CA242, and TPS in the diagnosis and follow-up of pancreatic cancer. Clin Chem 39(3):420–423.
39. Kiriyama S, Hayakawa T, Kondo T, Shibata T, Kitagawa M, Ono H, et al. (1990) Usefulness of a new tumor marker, Span-1, for the diagnosis of pancreatic cancer. Cancer 65:1557–1561.
40. Takeda S, Nakao A, Ichihara T, Suzuki Y, Nonami T, Harada A, et al. (1991) Serum concentration and immunohistochemical localization of Span-1 antigen in pancreatic cancer. A comparison with CA19-9 antigen. Hepato-Gastroenterology 38:143–148.
41. Ferrara C, Basso D, Fabris C, Malesci A, Fogar P, Meggiato T, et al. (1991) Comparison of two newly identified tumor markers (CAR-3 and DU-PAN-2) with CA19-9 in patients with pancreatic cancer. Tumori 77:56–60.
42. Plebani M, Basso D, Navaglia F (1995) Is CA 242 really a new tumour marker for pancreatic adenocarcinoma? Oncology 52:19–23.
43. Haglund C, Lindgren J, Roberts PJ, Kuusela P, Nordling S (1989) Tissue expression of the tumor associated antigen CA242 in benign and malignant pancreatic lesions. A comparison with CA50 and CA19-9. Br J Cancer 60:845–51.
44. Banfi G, Parolini D, Murone M, Bonini PA (1990) CAM43 in the diagnosis of pancreatic cancer: preliminary results. J Nucleic Med Allied Sci 34(Suppl 3):203.
45. Buchler M, Friess H, Schultheiss KH, Gebhardt C, Kubel R, Muhrer KH, et al. (1991) A randomized controlled trial of adjuvant immunotherapy (murine monoclonal antibody 494/32) in resectable pancreatic cancer. Cancer 68:1507–1512.
46. Friess H, Buchler M, Auerbach B, Weber A, Malfertheiner P, Hammer K, et al. (1993) CA 494-A new tumor marker for the diagnosis of pancreatic cancer. Int J Cancer 53:759–763.
47. Stenman UH, Huhtala ML, Koistinen R, Steppala M (1982) Immunochemical demonstration of a ovarian cancer associated urinary peptide. Int J Cancer 30:53–57.
48. Haglund C, Huhtala ML, Halila H, Nordling S, Roberts P, Scheinin T, et al. (1986) Tumour-associated trypsin inhibitor, TATI, in patients with pancreatic cancer, pancreatitis and benign biliary disease. B J Cancer 54:297–303.

49. Aroasio E, Piantino P (1991) tumor-associated trypsin inhibitor in pancreatic diseases. Scand J Clin Lab Invest 51(Suppl 207):71–73.
50. Bjorkland B, Bjorkland V (1957) Antigenicity of pooled human malignant and normal tissues by cyto-immunological techniques: presence of an insoluble, heatlabile tumor antigen. Int Arch Allergy 10:153–184.
51. Meduri F, Doni MG, Merenda R, Bizzarini M, Neri D, Gerunda GE, et al. (1989) The role of the leukocyte adherence inhibition (LAI), CA19-9, and tissue polypeptide antigen (TPA) tests in the diagnosis of pancreatic cancer. Cancer 64:1103–1106.
52. Pasanen PA, Eskelinen M, Partanen K, Pikkarainen P, Pentillla I (1993) Clinical evaluation of tissue polypeptide antigen (TPA) in the diagnosis of pancreatic carcinoma. Anticancer Res 13:1883–1888.
53. Chang JM, Takeuchi T (1990) Clinical significance of measurement of serum Spar-1 antigen in the diagnosis of pancreatic cancer. J. Jpn Pancreas Soc 5:80–88.
54. Hayakawa T, Kondo T, Shibata T, Hamano H, Kitagawa M, Sakai Y, et al. (1988) Sensitive serum markers for detecting pancreatic cancer. Cancer 61:1827–1831.
55. Nakaizumi A, Tatsuta M, Uehara H, Iishi H, Yamamura H, Okuda S, et al. (1992) A prospective trial of early detection of pancreatic cancer by ultrasonographic examination combined with measurement of serum elastase 1. Cancer 69:936–940
56. Basso D, Fabris C, Panucci A, Del Favero G, Agonese C, Plebani M, et al. (1988) Tissue polypeptide antigen, galactosyltransferase isoenzyme II and pancreatic oncofetal antigen serum determination: role in pancreatic cancer diagnosis. Int J Pancreatol 3: S95–S100.
57. Podolsky DK, McPhee MS, Alpert E, Warshaw AL, Isselbacher KJ (1981) Galactosyltransferase isoenzyme II in the detection of pancreatic cancer: comparison with radiologic, endoscopic and serologic tests. N Engl J Med 304:1313–1318.
58. Podolsky DK, Isselbacher KJ (1984) Characterization of monoclonal antibodies to serum galactosyltransferase. Proc Natl Acad Sci USA 81:2529–2533.
59. Kemmer TP, Malfertheiner P, Buchler M, Kemmer ML, Ditschuneit H (1991) Serum ribonuclease asctivity in the diagnosis of pancreatic cancer. Int J Pancreatol 8(1):23–33.
60. Pezzilli R, Billi P, Fiocchi M, Beltrandi E, Cappelletti O, Sprovieri G, et al. (1995) Serum β-2 microglobulin in chronic disease of the pancreas. Int J Pancreatol 17(2):161–166.
61. Kawamoto S, Hiraoka T, Kanemitsu K, Kimura M, Miyauchi Y, Takeya M (1992) Alpha-fetoprotein-producing pancreatic cancer—a case report and review of 28 cases. Hepato-Gastroenterology 39:282–286.
62. Alfthan H, Haglund C, Roberts P, Ulf-Hakan S (1992) Elevation of free β subunit of human choriogonadotropin and core β fragment of human choriogonadotropin in the serum and urine of patients with malignant pancreatic and biliary disease. Cancer Res 52:4628–4633.
63. Kuno N, Kurimoto K, Fukushima M, Hayakawa T, Shibata T, Suzuki T, et al. (1994) Effectiveness of multivariate analysis of tumor markers in diagnosis of pancreatic carcinoma: a prospective study in multiinstitutions. Pancreas 9(6):725–730.
64. Norton J (1994) Neuroendocrine tumors of the pancreas and duodenum. Curr Probl Surg 31(2):79–156.
65. Buchanan KD, Johnston CF, O'Hare MMT, et al. (1986) Neuroendocrine tumors: A European view. Am J Med 86 (Suppl 6B):14–23.
66. Wilder RM, Allan FN, Power, MH, Robertson HE (1927) Carcinoma of the islets of the pancreas: hyperinsulinism and hypoglycemia. JAMA 89:348–355.
67. Whipple AO, Frantz VK (1935) Adenoma of islet cells with hyperinsulinism: A review. Ann Surg 101:1299.
68. Fajans SS, Vinik AI (1989) Insulin-producing islet cell tumors. Endocrinol Metab Clin North Am 18:45–74.
69. Grama D, Eriksson B, Martensson H, et al. (1992) Clinical characteristics, treatment and survival in patients with pancreatic tumors causing hormonal syndromes. World J Surg 16:632–639.

70. Shimizu T, Sasakuma F, Ishikawa O, et al. (1994) Assessment of immunoassays for insulin in diagnostic tests for insulinoma. Diabetes Res and Clin Prac 26:149–154.
71. Field JB (1993) Insulinoma. In: Endocrine tumors, Mazzaferi EL, Samaan NA, eds, Boston: Blackwell Scientific, pp. 504–506.
72. Lebowitz MR, Blumenthal SA (1993) The molar ratio of insulin to C-peptide. An aid to the diagnosis of hypoglycemia due to surreptitious (or inadvertant) insulin administration. Arch Intern Med 153:650–655.
73. Doppman JL, Miller DL, Chang R, et al. (1993) Intraarterial calcium stimulation test for detection of insulinomas. World J Surg 17:439–443.
74. Rothmund M, Stinner B, Arnold R (1991) Endocrine pancreatic carcinoma. Eur J Surg Oncol 17:191–199.
75. Stabile BE, Morrow DJ, Passaro E Jr (1984) The gastrinoma triangle:operative implications. Am J Surg 147:25–31.
76. Zollinger RM, Ellison EH (1955) Primary peptic ulcerations of the jejunum associated with islet cell tumors of the pancreas. Ann Surg 142:709–728.
77. Gregory RA, Tracy HJ, French JM, et al. (1960) Extraction of a gastrin-like substance from a pancreatic tumor in a case of Zollinger-Ellison syndrome. Lancet 1:1045–1048.
78. Stabile BE, Morrow DJ, Passaro E Jr (1980) Serum gastrin and human chorionic gonadotropin in the Zollinger-Ellison syndrome. Arch Surg 115:1090–1095.
79. Passaro E Jr. Basso N, Walsh JH (1972) Calcium challenge in the Zollinger-Ellison syndrome. Surgery 72:60–67.
80. Norton JA, Doppman JL, Collen MJ, et al. (1986) Prospective study of gastrinoma localization and resection in patients with Zollinger-Ellison syndrome. Ann Surg 204:468–479.
81. Schirmer WJ, Melvin WS, Rush RM, O'Dorisio TM, Pozderac RV, Olsen JO, Ellison EC. (1995) Indium-111–pentetreotide scanning versus conventional imaging techniques for the localization of gastrinoma. Surgery 118(6):1105–13.
82. John M, Meyerhof W, Richter D, Waser B, Schaer JC, Scherubl H, et al. (1996) Positive somatostatin receptor scintigraphy correlates with the presence of somatostatin receptor subtype two. Gut 38(1):33–9.
83. Ellison EC (1995) Forty-year appraisal of gastrinoma. Back to the future. Ann Surg 222(4):511–24.
84. Gower WR and Fabri PJ (1990) Endocrine neoplasms (non-gastrin) of the pancreas. Semin Surg Oncol 6:98–109.
85. Verner JV, Morrison AB (1958) Islet cell tumor and a syndrome of refractory watery diarrhea and hypokalemia. Am J Med 29:529.
86. O'Dorisio TM, Mehkjian HS, Gaginella TS (1989) Medical therapy of VIPomas. Endocrinol Metab Clin North Am 18:545.
87. Brunt LM, Mazoujian G, O'Dorisio TM, Wells SA, Jr (1994) Stimulation of vasoactive intestinal peptide and neurotensin secretion by pentagastrin in a patient with VIPoma syndrome. Surgery 115:362–369.
88. Maton PN, Gardner JK, Jensen TR (1989) The use of the long acting somatostatin analogue 201–995 in patients with pancreatic endocrine tumors. Dig Dis Sci 34:29–37S.
89. Delcore R, Friesen S (1994) Gastrointestinal neuroendocrine tumors. J Am Coll Surg 178:187–211
90. Bloom SR, Long RG, Bryant MG, et al. (1980) Clinical, biochemical and pathological studies on 62 VIPomas. Gastroenterology 78:1143A.
91. Nagorney D, Bloom S, Polak J, et al. (1983) Resolution of recurrent Verner-Morrison syndrome by resection of metastatic vipoma. Surgery 93:348–353.
92. Mozell E, Stenzel P, Woltering E, et al. (1990) Functional endocrine tumors of the pancreas: Clinical presentation, diagnosis, and treatment. Curr Probl Surg 27:303–386.
93. Norton JA, Kahn CR, Schiebinger R, et al. (1979) Amino acid deficiency and the skin rash associated with glucagonoma. Ann Intern Med 91:213–215.

94. Bloom SR, Polak JM (1987) Glucagonoma syndrome. Am J Med 82(5B):25–36.
95. Stacpoole PW (1981) The glucagonoma syndrome: clinical features, diagnosis and treatment. Endocr Rev 2:347.
96. Krejs GJ, Collins SM, McCarthy D, et al. (1986) Follow-up of a patient with somatostatinoma [Letter]. N Engl J Med 315:1295.
97. Ganda OP, Weis GC, Soeldner A (1977) Somatostatinoma: A somatostatin-containing tumor of the endocrine pancreas. N Engl J Med 296:963.
98. Dayal Y, Ganda OP (1991) Somatostatin-producing tumors. In: Endocrine pathology of the gut and pancreas, Dayal Y, ed., Boca Raton, FL: CRC, pp. 241–277.
90. Vinik AJ, Strodel WE, Eckhauser FE, et al. (1987) Somatostatinomas, PPomas, neurotensinomas. Semin Oncol 14:263–281.
100. Vinik AI and Moattari AR (1989) Treatment of endocrine tumors of the pancreas. Endocrinol Metab Clin North Am 18:45–74.
101. Pipleers D, Couturier E, Gepts W, Somers G (1983) Five cases of somatostatinomas: clinical heterogeneity and diagnostic usefulness of basal and tolbutamide-induced hypersomatostatinemia. J Clin Endocrinol Metab 56:1236–1242.
102. Hazelwood RL (1989) Biosynthesis, chemistry and storage of islet (endocrine) products. In: The Endocrine Pancreas, Hadley ME, ed. Englewood Cliffs, NJ: Prentice Hall, Chapter 3, pp. 27–48.
103. Grossman MI, Brown JC, Said S, et al. (1974) Candidate hormones of the gut. Gastroenterology 67:730–755.
104. Adrian T, Uttenthal LO, Williams SJ, et al. (1986) Secretion of pancreatic polypeptide in patients with pancreatic endocrine tumors. N Engl J Med 315:287–291.
105. Schwartz TW (1978) Atropine suppression test for pancreatic polypeptide. Lancet 2: 43–44.
106. Solcia E. Sessa F, Rindi G, et al. (1991) Pancreatic endocrine tumors: general concepts; nonfunctioning tumors and tumors with uncommon function. In: Endocrine pathology of the gut and pancreas, Dayal Y, ed., Boca Raton, FL, CRC, pp. 105–132.
107. Prinz RA, Marangos PJ (1983) Serum neuron specific enolase: a serum marker for nonfunctioning pancreatic islet cell carcinoma. Am J Surg 145:77–81.
108. Iguchi H, Yasuda D, Yamada Y, et al. (1991) 7B2, a possible marker for nonfunctioning pancreatic islet cell tumor. Horm Metab Res 23:486–489.
109. American Cancer Society (1996) Cancer facts and figures—1996. New York, American Cancer Society.
110. Gordis L, Gold EB (1986) Epidemiology and etiology of pancreatic cancer. In: Go VLW, et al., eds. The exocrine pancreas: Biology, pathobiology and diseases, New York: Raven, pp. 621–35.
111. Gudjonsson B, Livstone EM, Spiro HM (1978) Cancer of the pancreas: Diagnostic accuracy and survival statistics. Cancer 42:2494–2506.
112. Gordis L, Gold EB(1984) Epidemiology of pancreatic cancer. World J Surg 8:808–821.
113. Haenszel W, Kurihara M (1968) Studies of Japanese migrants I. Mortality from cancer and other diseases among Japanese in the United States. J Nat Cancer Inst 40:43.
114. Levin DL, Connelly RR, Devesa SS (1981) Demographic characteristics of cancer of the pancreas: Mortality, incidence and survival. Cancer 47:1456–1468.
115. Grieve DC (1973) Adenocarcinoma of the pancreas (a review of 100 cases). J R Coll Surg 18:221.
116. Fraumeni JF (1975) Cancers of the pancreas and biliary tract: Epidemiological considerations. Cancer Res 35:3437.
117. Moynan RW, Neerhour RC, Johnson TS (1964) Pancreatic carcinoma in children: Case report and review. J Pediatr 65:711.
118. Tsukimoto I, Watanabe K, Lin JB, Nakajima T (1973) Pancreatic carcinoma in children in Japan. Cancer 31:1203.

119. Taxy JB (1976) Adenocarcinoma of the pancreas in childhood. Cancer 37:1508.
120. Everhart, J, Wright D (1995) Diabetes mellitus as a risk factor for pancreatic cancer. A meta-analysis. JAMA 273:1605–1609.
121. Hammond EC (1966) Smoking in relation to the death rates of one million men and women. In: Epidemiological approaches to the study of cancer and other chronic diseases, Haenszel W, ed. US Public Health Service, National Cancer Institute Monograph 19, Bethesda, MD: U.S. Government Printing Office, p. 126.
122. MacMahon BY, Trichopoulos D, Warren K, Nardi G (1981) Coffee and cancer of the pancreas. N Engl J Med 304:630.
123. Wynder EL, Mabuchi K, Maruchi N, Fortner JG (1973) Epidemiology of cancer of the pancreas. J Natl Cancer Inst 50:645.
124. Gross JB, Bambill EE, Ulrich JA (1962) Hereditary pancreatitis. Description of a fifth kindred and summary of clinical features. Am J Med 33:358.
125. Whitten DM, Feingold M, Eisenklam EJ (1968) Hereditary pancreatitis. Am J Dis Child 116:426.
126. Davidson P, Costanza D, Swieconeck JA, Harris JB (1968) Hereditary pancreatitis. A kindred without gross aminoaciduria. Ann Intern Med 68:88.
127. Lapey A, Kattwinkel J, DiSant Angese PA, Laster L (1971) Hereditary pancreatitis (HP) without aminoaciduria: Two new kindred. Pediat Res 5:389.
128. Appel MF (1974) Hereditary Pancreatitis: Review and presentation of an additional kindred. Arch Surg 108:63.
129. Longnecker DS, Memoli V, Pettengill OS (1992) Recent results in animal models of pancreatic carcinoma: Histogenesis of tumors. Yale J Biol Med 65:457–464.
130. Kohler H, Lankisch PG (1987) Acute Pancreatitis and hyperamylasemia in pancreatic carcinoma. Pancreas 2:117–119.
131. Campbell JP, Wilson SR (1988) Pancreatic neoplasms: how useful is evaluation with US? Radiology 167:341–4.
132. Freeny PC, Ball TJ (1981) Endoscopic retrograde cholangiopancreatography in the diagnosis of pancreatic disease: a comparative study. Cancer 47:1666–78.
133. Moossa AR, Levin B (1981) The diagnosis of "early" pancreatic cancer: The University of Chicago experience. Cancer 47:1688–1697.
134. Glenner GG, Mallory GK (1956) The cystadenoma and related nonfunctional tumors of the pancreas. Cancer 9:980–986.
135. Lack EE (1989) Primary tumors of the exocrine pancreas: Classification, overview and recent contributions by immunohistochemistry and electron microscopy. The Am J Surg Pathol 13(Suppl 1):66–88.
136. Sperti C, Cappellazzo F, Pasquale C, Militello C, Catalini S, Bonadimani B, et al. (1993) Cystic neoplasms of the pancreas: Problems in differential diagnosis. The Am Surg 59(11):740–5.
137. Taft DA, Freeny PC (1981) Cystic neoplasms of the pancreas. Am J Surg 142:30–5.
138. Lewandroski KB, Southern JF, Pins MR, Compton CC, Warshaw AL (1993) Cyst fluid analysis in the differential diagnosis of pancreatic cysts. A comparison of pseudocysts, serous cystadenomas, mucinous cystic neoplasms, and mucinous cystadenocarcinomas. Ann Surg 217:41–47.
139. Pinto MM, Meriano FV (1991) Diagnosis of cystic pancreatic lesions by cytologic examination and carcinoembryonic antigen and amylase assays of cyst contents. Acta Cytologica 35(4):456–463.
140. Cubilla AL, Fitzgerald PJ (1984) Tumors of the exocrine pancreas. In: Atlas of tumor pathology, 2nd ser, fasc 19, Washington, DC: Armed Forces Institute of Pathology, pp. 1–287.
141. Cubilla AL, Fitzgerald PJ (1980) Cancer (non-endocrine) of the pancreas. A suggested classification. In: The pancreas, Fitzgerald PJ, Morrison AB, eds., Baltimore: Williams and Wilkins, pp. 82–110.

142. Webb JN (1977) Acinar cell neoplasms of the exocrine pancreas. J Clin Pathol 30:103–112.
143. Lack EE, Levey R, Cassady JR, Vawter GF (1983) Tumors of the exocrine pancreas in children and adolescents. A clinical and pathological study of eight cases. Am J Surg Pathol 7:319–327.
144. Oertel JE, Mendelsohn G, Compagno J (1982) Solid and papillary epithelial neoplasm of the pancreas. In: Pancreatic tumors in children, Humphrey GB, Grindley GB, Dehner LP, Acton RT, Pysher TJ, eds. The Hague: Martinus Nijhoff, pp. 161–71.
145. Horie A, Yano Y, Kotoo Y, Miwa A (1977) Morphogenesis of pancreatoblastoma, infantile carcinoma of the pancreas. Report of two cases. Cancer 39:247–54.
146. Beazley RM, Cohn I (1991) Tumors of the pancreas, gallbladder, and pancreatic ducts. In: American Cancer Society textbook of clinical oncology. Holleb AI, Fink DJ, Murphy GP, eds., Atlanta, The American Cancer Society, pp. 219–236.
147. Eli Lilly and Company (1994) Treatment IND of gemzar (gemcitabine) for patients with pancreatic cancer.
148. Fisher WE, Muscarella P, O'Dorisio TM, O'Dorisio MS, Kim JA, Doran TA, Sabourin CL, Schirmer WJ (1996) Differential expression of the somatostatin receptor subtype-2 gene predicts response of human pancreatic cancer to somatostatin. Surgery 120(2):234–241.

5
Biochemistry, Pathogenesis, and Laboratory Diagnosis of Endocrine Disorders of the Pancreas

Manjula K. Gupta

INTRODUCTION

The endocrine function of the pancreas was first recognized in 1889; in a classic experiment, Von Mering and Minkowski determined the role of the pancreas in the development of diabetes *(1)*. Early in the 20th century, numerous investigators attempted to prepare pancreatic extracts to treat diabetes, but it was almost 35 years later that the successful isolation of insulin was accomplished, and 70 years after that when the structure of insulin was known and insulin was synthesized by Meinhofer et al. in 1963 *(2)*. The endocrine tissue of the pancreas, the islets of Langerhans, accounts for <1% of the total pancreatic mass. The cytochemical differences between the endocrine cells of islets were also observed early in this century *(3)*. This led to the recognition of islets as bihormonal secretory units, which are vital to the hormonal control of plasma glucose primarily by the production and activity of insulin and glucagon.

Diabetes mellitus is the most prevalent disorder of abnormal function of the pancreatic islets. This disease remains the leading endocrine cause of morbidity and mortality in the United States. In contrast to the hyperglycemia of diabetes, hypoglycemia is not a common clinical disorder and is frequently associated with endocrine tumors of the pancreas. Although simply defined on the basis of hyperglycemia, diabetes mellitus today is known to be a highly heterogeneous disease. In the late 1960s, insulin-dependent diabetes mellitus (IDDM, type I) was distinguished from noninsulin-dependent diabetes mellitus (NIDDM, type II).

The incidence of diabetes is rising, and based on the National Health Interview Survey (NHIS, 1993) the prevalence of diabetes is 3.1%, which is three times the prevalence of 0.93% in 1958 *(4)*. In the US, there were 7.8 million diagnosed cases of diabetes in 1993; approx 7% of these are considered IDDM (onset at age <30 yr) and the remaining 90–95% appear to be NIDDM. Thirty thousand new cases of IDDM are diagnosed each year, and there are considerable racial and ethnic differences, with rates being highest for Whites (17.3/p 100,000) as compared to African Americans (12.1/p 100,000) and Hispanics (8.8/p 100,000) *(4)*.

For NIDDM, the prevalence rate increases with age: 1.3% at age 18–44 yr, 6.2% at age 45–64 yr, and 10.4% at age 65 yr or more *(4)*. NIDDM is more common in

From: Clinical Pathology of Pancreatic Disorders *Edited by: J. A. Lott Humana Press Inc., Totowa, NJ*

African Americans, Mexican Americans, Japanese Americans, and native Americans than in non-Hispanic whites. The prevalence rates between men and women do not differ, and an estimated 625,000 new cases of NIDDM are diagnosed annually in the United States *(4)*. In addition to diagnosed cases, probably an equal number are undiagnosed based on oral glucose tolerance test results.

The two technical advancements that have contributed extensively to our current knowledge of the natural history and pathogenesis, as well as to our ability to diagnose pancreatic endocrine disorders, are the development and application of immunochemical and molecular biology techniques. These techniques provide powerful tools for detection, identification, and measurement of pancreatic hormones and autoantigens. The pioneering development of the radioimmunoassay for insulin by Yalow and Berson *(5)* led the way to accurate measurement of most pancreatic polypeptides and hormones. The molecular biology techniques have permitted copy-deoxyribonucleic acid (cDNA) cloning of various autoantigens that provides the basis for the current in vitro translation assays for sensitive detection of autoantibodies. This chapter focuses on the laboratory techniques currently used for evaluating pancreatic islet-cell function, and their role in the diagnosis and management of patients with related disorders.

ISLET ANATOMY AND THE ORIGIN OF ISLET CELLS

To understand the intricacy of the various factors involved in the biosynthesis of multiple hormones by the islets, an understanding of basic islet anatomy and its local implications is necessary. The islets of Langerhans, numbering roughly >1 million, are dispersed in the exocrine pancreas. They are highly vascularized microorgans that are also innervated by sympathetic, parasympathetic, and peptidergic nerves *(6)*. These characteristics point to the remarkable sophistication of these islets, and the complex interactions and communication that occur between different cell types through paracrine mechanisms.

Each islet contains four endocrine cell types designated as beta (β), alpha (α), delta (δ), and PP cells (F) that synthesize insulin, glucagon, somatostatin, and pancreatic polypeptide, respectively. In addition to insulin, β-cells also secrete islet amyloid polypeptide, or amylin. The F-cells secrete PP and are found only in islets located in the posterior head of the pancreas. This portion of the pancreas originates from the primordial ventral bud as opposed to the dorsal bud. These islets contain primarily F-cells (roughly 80%), a lesser number of β-cells, and very few, if any, of the glucagon-producing α-cells. In contrast, islets located in other areas of the pancreas contain predominately insulin-secreting β-cells (roughly 80%) and are surrounded by a smaller number of glucagon-secreting α-cells (roughly 20%), and δ-cells (3%) that produce somatostatin. In addition to these well-recognized hormones, the endocrine cells of the pancreatic islets normally release a number of other amines and polypeptides that coordinate the physiologic processes of digestion and carbohydrate metabolism. Islet cells have been classified as belonging to the amine-precursor uptake and decarboxylation (APUD) series and may arise from neuroblasts. Thus, the APUD concept, formulated in the late 1960s, cytologically and embryologically integrates the neural and endocrine system *(7)*. The evidence in favor of the APUD concept comes from the finding that several characteristics of a neural phenotype are expressed by the islet cells and in a wide variety of tumors of APUD cells, e.g., apudomas in both neural and pancreatic locations. These characteristics include the measurable nerve cell enzymes, neuron-specific enolase *(8)* and synaptophysin *(9)*. Islet cells also express many other antigens normally present in the neuronal cells, including γ-aminobutyric acid (GABA) *(10)* and β-calcitonin gene-related peptide (CGRP) *(11)*. Furthermore, the finding of the catecholamine-synthesizing enzyme, tyrosine hydroxylase, in glucagon precursor cells and insulin precursor cells of the islets strongly supports a neuroectodermal origin for the pancreatic endocrine cells *(12)*. Tyrosine hydroxylase was considered specific for neuroectodermally derived cells. More recently, the autoantigen on β-cells has been identified and characterized as glutamic acid decarboxylase (GAD), an enzyme that controls the biosynthesis of GABA, an inhibitory neurotransmitter, and is expressed both in β-cells and the brain. Autoantibodies reactive to GAD were initially found in the "stiff-man syndrome," and are often associated with IDDM, evidence further supporting a common origin of β-cells and neuronal cells *(13)*.

PANCREATIC HORMONES: PHYSIOLOGIC ROLE, BIOCHEMISTRY, BIOSYNTHESIS, AND MEASUREMENT

Insulin, Proinsulin, and C-Peptide

Physiologic Role of Insulin

Insulin is the major player in maintaining the blood glucose concentrations within a normal range. Glucose is the primary stimulant for insulin release from the β-cells, and insulin concentrations are constantly adjusted to fluctuating blood glucose concentrations to maintain normoglycemia. Although insulin affects every tissue directly or indirectly, the major endocrine sites for insulin action are liver, muscle, and adipose tissue. In addition, its paracrine action on neighboring α-cells and its ability to inhibit glucagon secretion are well documented (Fig. 1).

The liver is the first major organ insulin reaches through the bloodstream. In the liver, insulin promotes glycogen synthesis and storage, inhibits glycogen breakdown, and increases triglyceride synthesis and very low-density lipoprotein formation. It promotes glycolysis by activating glycolytic enzymes, and inhibits catabolism by inhibiting hepatic glycogenolysis, ketogenesis, and gluconeogenesis.

In muscle, insulin promotes protein synthesis by increasing amino acid transport and stimulating ribosomal protein synthesis. By increasing glucose transport, insulin promotes glycogen synthesis. In adipose tissues, insulin promotes triglyceride storage by inducing lipoprotein lipase in endothelial cells, which in turn causes active hydrolysis of triglycerides from circulating lipoproteins. It also inhibits intracellular lipolysis of stored triglycerides by inhibiting intracellular lipoprotein lipase.

In the absence of glucose, essential amino acids (leucine, arginine, and lysine) stimulate insulin secretion *(14)*, suggesting that effects of amino acids are independent of glucose changes. However, these effects are potentiated by the presence of glucose. In contrast to amino acids, various lipids stimulate β-cell secretion of insulin only weakly.

The autonomic neurotransmitters, acetylcholine and norepinephrine, also influence insulin secretion from β-cells *(15)*. They also affect other islet cells, including α-, δ- and F-cells (Fig. 2). Acetylcholine directly stimulates insulin release; the release is blocked by atropine. Both norepinephrine and epinephrine have an insulin-inhibitory

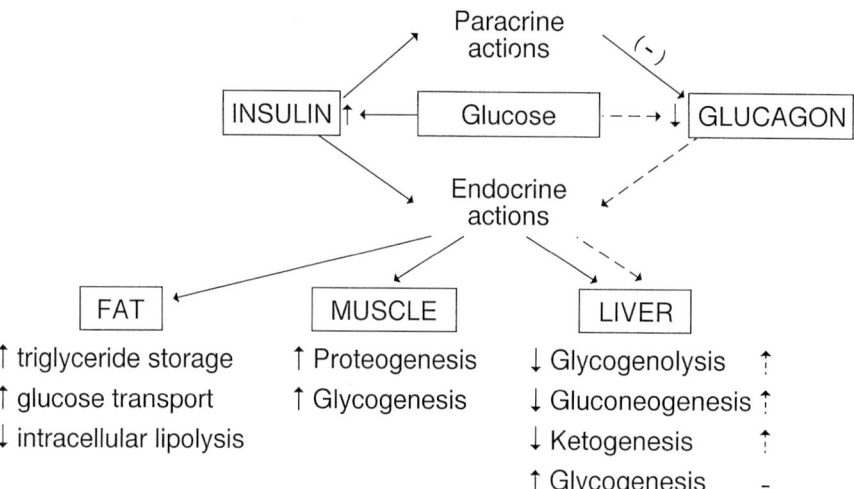

Fig. 1. Illustration of the target organ actions of the two major regulatory hormones of glucose homeostasis: insulin and glucagon. The insulin actions are shown by the solid lines and arrows, and the glucagon actions are shown by dashed lines and arrows.

effect on β-cells that is glucose-dependent. Epinephrine is a more potent insulin inhibitor than norepinephrine, and α-antagonists completely abolish epinephrine's inhibitory effect, suggesting it is mediated via α-receptors.

The β-cell response is also affected by a number of other hormones, including glucagon, somatostatin, and growth hormone. Glucagon and somatostatin may also exert a paracrine effect on β-cells. They have contrasting effects: glucagon stimulates, but somatostatin suppresses insulin release (16,17).

The most important stimulus for insulin release is hyperglycemia, and an increase in blood glucose normally elicits a biphasic insulin release from the β-cells. The first phase lasts 5–10 min and is followed by a progressive increase in insulin release that persists for the entire duration of hyperglycemia. An iv glucose tolerance test detects the initial response and is used frequently to assess β-cell function.

Insulin metabolism has been studied extensively both in vivo and in vitro (18). The liver is the major known site for insulin metabolism, and as much as 50% of insulin delivered to the liver is extracted. The rest is removed predominately by renal clearance (19). Hepatic clearance of insulin is closely related to insulin binding to insulin receptors in the hepatocytes. The glucose concentration has been suggested as an important regulator of hepatic insulin metabolism (20). Other factors that may affect this process include glucagon, somatostatin, and protein ingestion (21). The half-life of insulin in the circulation is approx 3–5 min.

Biochemistry and Biosynthesis of Insulin

Insulin is the major secretory hormone of the endocrine pancreas. It is a 51 amino acid protein (mol wt 5,734 Dalton) composed of two polypeptide chains designated as A and B. The A-chain contains 21 amino acids and is acidic. It is joined by two disulfide bonds to the 30 amino acid B-chain, which is basic. A sequence on the B-chain, amino acids 22–26, is important for biological activity, because cleavage anywhere

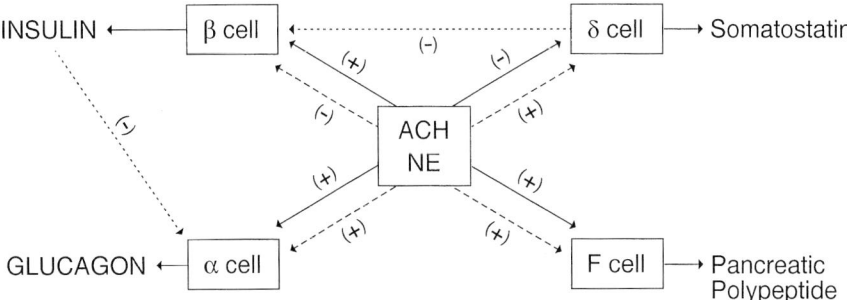

Fig. 2. Schematic presentation of the regulatory role of the neural hormones, acetacholine (ACH) and norepinephrine (NE), on hormonal secretion of various islet cells. The solid lines represent ACH actions, and the dashed lines represent NE actions. Also, the paracrine role of somatostatin on insulin and that of insulin on glucagon secretion are shown with the dotted lines.

between B20 and B23 inactivates insulin. A similar sequence is also found in insulin growth factor-I and may be responsible for its insulin-like activity. Other studies have further delineated the role of the B24 and B25 residues in insulin's interaction with its receptor (22). The human insulin sequence is identical to that of porcine insulin except for one amino acid—threonine instead of alanine at the carboxyl-terminus of the β-chain (B30). Human insulin differs from beef insulin by two additional amino acids on the A-chain (A8 and A10). These structural differences between species are enough to affect the immunologic reactivity of insulin. Whereas porcine insulin appears immunologically identical to human insulin, beef insulin has a variable degree of crossreactivity to insulin antibodies. Both pork and beef insulins are commonly used for insulin-replacement therapy and are responsible for antibody development in patients. Insulin antibodies interfere with most insulin radioimmunoassays, thus making accurate determination of insulin concentration in these patients difficult. The recently available recombinant human insulin has significantly improved insulin-replacement therapy, and it reduces the antibody response.

Figure 3 illustrates the cleavage of proinsulin to insulin and C-peptide by the proteases PC-2 (type II) and PC-3 (type I) and carboxypeptidase H via the production of proinsulin intermediates as reported by Given et al. (23). Insulin is synthesized in the endoplasmic reticulum of β-cells as a larger precursor molecule, pre-proinsulin, of mol wt 11,500 Dalton. Isolating this protein has been difficult, because it is cleaved by microsomal enzymes to become proinsulin almost immediately after its synthesis (24). Proinsulin has a mol wt of 9000 Dalton that is, in turn, converted into insulin by proteolytic cleavage at two sites by removing a 31 amino acid connecting peptide or C-peptide. The latter is removed, and at the same time two dipeptide linkages are removed from either side of the C-peptide molecule (Fig. 3) (25). Thus, insulin and C-peptide are secreted in an equimolar ratio from the β-cells. The human porcine and bovine C-peptide show a roughly 50% amino acid homology that contrasts with the high degree of homology found in insulin. Along with insulin and C-peptide, β-cells also secrete any proinsulin that has escaped cleavage, along with its incomplete (partially cleaved) conversion products (23). Because proinsulin is not removed by the

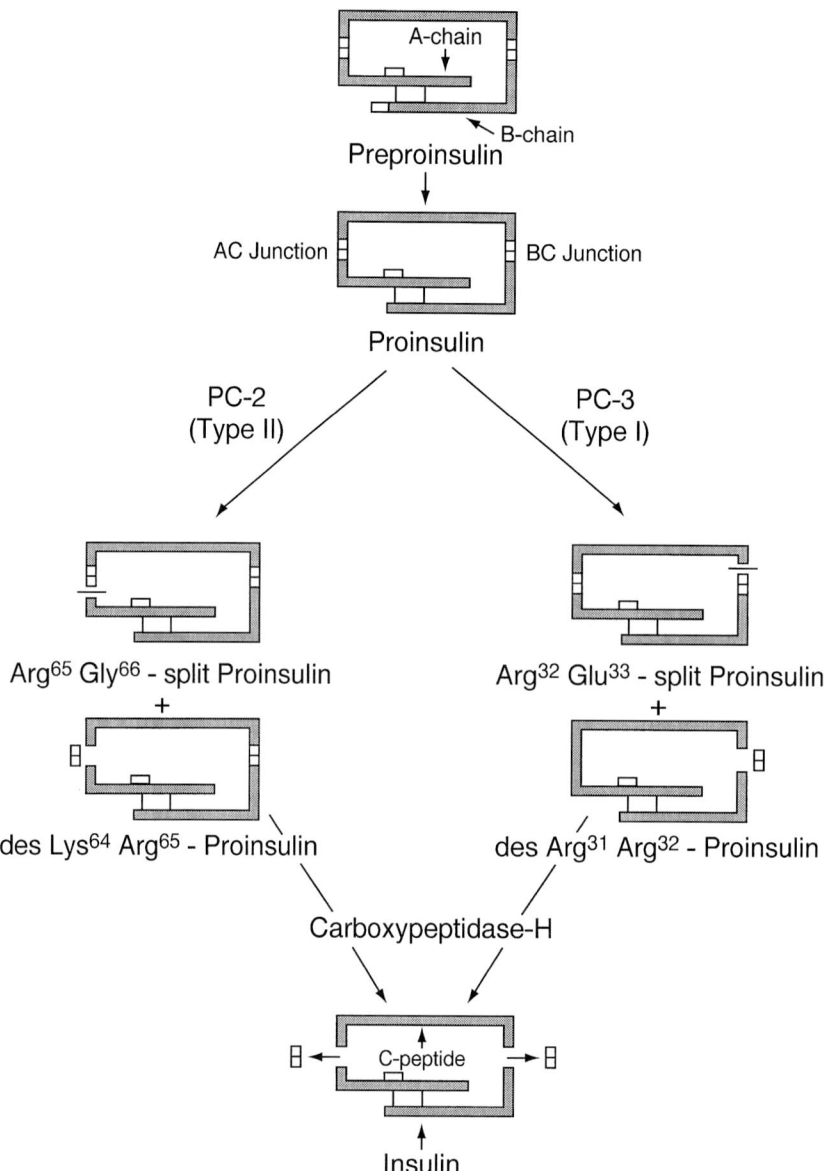

Fig. 3. Diagrammatic presentation of steps involved in biosynthesis of insulin and C-peptide. The various cleavage steps are shown. Proteases PC2 and PC3 cleave proinsulin at the BC and AC junctions to produce partially cleaved products that are further cleaved with carboxypeptidase-H to produce insulin and C-peptide based on refs. *23* and *26*.

liver, its half-life in circulation is about four times that of insulin. The biologic activity of proinsulin is estimated to be about 3–5% of that of insulin. In addition to intact proinsulin, four major proinsulin conversion products, also known as splits products of proinsulin, have been identified in the circulation *(23)*. These products include Arg^{32} Glu^{33} split proinsulin (split 32,33), Arg^{65} Gly^{66} split proinsulin (split 65,66), des Arg^{31} Arg^{32} proinsulin (des 31,32), and des lys^{64} Arg^{65} proinsulin (des 64,65). These products likely result from the different activities of the two conversion enzymes that cleave proinsulin *(26)*.

Measurement of Insulin

In most clinical laboratories, insulin is measured by the radioimmunoassay (RIA) technique. Since the first description of insulin assays by RIA, a number of methods to separate bound and free insulin have been developed *(27–29)*. The most commonly used separation methods are second antibody, dextran-coated charcoal, and polyethylene glycol (PEG) precipitation. RIA in general and insulin assays in particular suffer from poor precision, and in particular demonstrate a nonspecific matrix effect. The basal serum insulin concentrations are in the range of 4–20 mU/L. The lower normal range is within the same range as the detection limit of most assays (2–6 mU/L). Therefore, most insulin assays cannot accurately detect small changes in basal insulin values. The lack of a universally accepted insulin standard also makes the comparison of results between laboratories difficult.

Insulin antisera are generally prepared in guinea pigs, which generate a higher affinity antibody response than rabbits. Most insulin antibodies crossreact substantially with proinsulin. Therefore, most assays measure both insulin and proinsulin, and hence, the term "immunoreactive insulin" is often used to describe insulin immunoreactivity. Such assays result in overestimation of insulin concentrations in patients with NIDDM, because they have a disproportionate increase in proinsulin and proinsulin intermediates *(30,31)*. For specific measurement of insulin, it is necessary to separate insulin from proinsulin.

Insulin has been labeled using chloramine-T *(32)*, a procedure that allows the exchange of a tyrosyl hydroxyl group with ^{125}I. Roughly more than 75% of the ^{125}I is fixed on the A-chain, although the B-chain also contains two tyrosyl groups. With careful control of iodination conditions, it is possible to label only one tyrosyl residue in the A-chain, the so called mono-iodinated insulin *(33)*. This mono-iodination preserves the biologic activity and provides a labeled preparation that is ideal for radioreceptor assays. This method also produces more stable preparations with minimal incubation damage. Nonetheless, solid-phase adsorbents, such as charcoal and talc, are widely used in insulin RIA, but they are subject to interference by the plasma matrix, leading to imprecise results.

In recent years, immunoradiometric and immunoenzymometric assays have been described *(34,35)*. Enzyme-linked immunosorbent assays (ELISA) may be more sensitive and more reproducible than immunoradiometric assays. Monoclonal antibodies (MAbs) offer several advantages in these two-site immunometric assays; however, there are only a few reports on the production of insulin-specific MAbs *(36–38)*. The MAb-based nonisotopic assays include the time-resolved fluoroimmunoassay *(39)* and enzyme immunoassay *(40)*. Both detect insulin in serum in 3–4 h with more analytical sensitivity and precision. More recently, an automated two-site immunometric assay has been made available using the sensitive alkaline phosphatase-labeled tracer antibody and 4-methylumbelliferyl phosphate (4-MUP) as substrate. The assay is based on detection of fluorescent 4-methylumbelliferone as the end product (Tosoh Medics, Foster City, CA). The assay is precise, and the automated system is a true random-access system that generates results within 1 h *(41)*.

Although insulin can be measured with precision in human plasma, its measurement has limited clinical value in the diagnosis of diabetes, because a simple measurement of glucose (glucose tolerance test) may be adequate. Insulin measurements also are limited for assessing β-cell function in diabetic patients. First, the assay does not differentiate between exogenous and endogenous insulin. Second, insulin antibodies are frequently detected in newly diagnosed IDDM patients or in diabetic patients who have been treated with insulin preparations, and these antibodies interfere in insulin RIA. Therefore, it is necessary to screen serum specimens for insulin antibodies. Positive specimens must be processed for free and total insulin measurements as described below.

Free and Total Insulin

The presence of insulin antibodies in patients' sera results in erroneously high or low insulin concentrations, depending on the RIA separation method used. Free insulin and antibody-bound insulin can be measured after extracting the serum with PEG *(42)*. From serum, the immunoglobulins (including antibody-bound insulin) can be precipitated by mixing it with an equal volume of 18% PEG. After centrifugation, the free insulin concentration can be estimated in the supernatant. In a separate aliquot, the antibody-bound insulin can be dissociated with 1 mol/L HCl acid. After 1 h of incubation, the pH is neutralized with 1 mol/L NaOH and followed by immediate precipitation of immunoglobulin with PEG. The total insulin in the supernatant is then measured. The PEG separation is simple and is used in most clinical laboratories. However, in practice, the validity of free-insulin measurments is questionable, because freeze-thawing and other factors during collection may affect binding of antibody to insulin.

Measurement of C-Peptide

The development of an assay for C-peptide has provided an alternative method for studying β-cell function in IDDM; the subject has been extensively reviewed *(43)*. Although both insulin and C-peptide are secreted in equimolar concentrations, this relationship is not maintained in the circulation, because their clearance rates differ. Approximately 50% of insulin is rapidly degraded by the liver, whereas C-peptide degradation is about 12%. In addition, C-peptide is inert and is primarily removed from the circulation by the kidneys. The half-life of C-peptide in the circulation is roughly two to five times longer than that of insulin. All these factors produce a five to six times greater concentration of circulating C-peptide than insulin. Therefore, circulating C-peptide levels are a more accurate measure of insulin secretion than peripheral insulin itself.

The first RIA for C-peptide was described in 1970 *(44)*. However, several technical assay problems hindered its commercial availability and use in clinical laboratories. The C-peptide molecule differs extensively between species in both the number and sequence of amino acids; therefore, human C-peptide is required for the antibody production and for the preparation of radioligand and standards. The iodination of natural human C-peptide is complicated by the absence of the tyrosine residue in the peptide chain, so this amino acid must be added to the synthetic or natural peptide before chloramine-T radioiodination. Tyr-synthetic C-peptide is an important variable in the assay, and differences in C-peptide levels with different labeled preparations in which the same antisera are used have been described *(44)*. Also synthetic C-peptide coupled to albumin is used as the immunogen for raising antibodies. However, various antisera differ in their ability to identify different antigenic determinants *(45)*, and these differences contribute to the variation of C-peptide concentrations as measured by different assays. The crossreactivity with human proinsulin and its intermediates varies among the antisera used to measure C-peptide. Even a minor degree of crossreaction will interfere significantly in C-peptide measurement. This problem is especially of concern in a diabetic patient with residual proinsulin secretion and circulating insulin antibodies. The latter do not react to C-peptide; however, they show a variable degree of crossreactivity to proinsulin *(46)*. When proinsulin binds to insulin antibodies (proinsulin–insulin antibody complexes), proinsulin clearance is reduced, resulting in the accumulation of these immune complexes (proinsulin-like material) in the circulation. The high concentration of the proinsulin-like material produces spuriously high concentrations of C-peptide *(47)*. To obtain accurate results for C-peptide, precipitating these complexes from sera using PEG may be necessary before testing *(48,49)*.

Although using synthetic C-peptide for antisera production and as a standard has reduced many of the problems of C-peptide immunoassays, the variability of the C-peptide immunoassays has not been eliminated. Among the various C-peptide immunoassays, one extensively used procedure is based on commercial C-peptide antiserum (M1230 from Novo Nordisk, Bagsvaerd, Denmark) *(50)*. This antiserum has been extensively characterized with respect to its binding affinity, capacity, and nonspecific binding; it has low (10%) crossreactivity with proinsulin, and the assay itself has been used extensively *(51,52)*. However, recently, Novo Nordisk has replaced this antiserum with a new polyclonal antiserum, M1221. A comparison of the M1230 assay with the assay using M-1221 as well as a number of other commercially available immunoassays has revealed that C-peptide concentration varies depending on the assay method *(53)*. Furthermore, they all show variable decreases in C-peptide levels after PEG treatment of serum samples. The contributing factors may be nonspecific interference, uneven tracer quality, and heterogeneity of C-peptide immunoreactivity. These findings indicate a need for extensive validation of the C-peptide assay before it is used in the clinical laboratory.

As discussed above, C-peptide measurement compared to insulin has a number of advantages, but the most important is its ability to differentiate between endogenous insulin secretion and exogenous injected insulin. Therefore, the C-peptide measurement is valuable in the diagnosis of factitious hypoglycemia *(54,55)*. Another significant advantage of the C-peptide assay is in its urinary clearance and measurement. Urinary measurement of C-peptide provides an excellent way to get around the rapid secretory fluctuation in plasma insulin levels *(56)*. Urinary values essentially represent an average of plasma concentrations filtered over a prolonged time. However, only some small amounts of the immunoreactive insulin appear in urine, and most insulin assays are not sensitive enough to detect these low concentrations. In contrast, the urinary C-peptide concentration is several fold higher and can be measured accurately. Urinary C-peptide, measurement thus is a simple noninvasive procedure to assess β-cell function *(57,58)*.

Measurement of Proinsulin

Accurately measuring proinsulin has been difficult because the polyclonal antibodies used in RIA crossreact with insulin and C-peptide. Also, the circulating concentrations of proinsulin are low and require high-sensitivity assays. Over the years, a number of RIAs, both indirect and direct, have been developed. Indirect RIAs require separation of proinsulin from insulin before measurement with crossreactive insulin antibodies. These separation methods include gel chromatography and enzymatic degradation of insulin or immunoprecipitation of proinsulin. In gel chromatography, the proinsulin elutes before insulin and represents approx 15–20% of the immunoreactivity of insulin *(59,60)*. Extensive studies were performed using these techniques, all concluding that the proinsulin-to-insulin ratios remained unchanged in healthy subjects, normal pregnancy, and gestational diabetes. However, an increased proinsulin-to-insulin ratio has been detected in hyperglycemia associated with hypoinsulinemia (i.e., in IDDM), in obese patients with NIDDM, and in patients with chronic renal failure *(61–63)*. These increased levels in proinsulin-like material suggest that proinsulin and its intermediates may be useful predictive markers for the manifestation of diabetes and signify the importance of proinsulin measurement.

Although gel-chromatography studies provide important data, the technique has several drawbacks. It is cumbersome to use routinely, and most insulin assays are not sensitive enough to measure directly the low concentrations of proinsulin immunoreactivity. Thus, proinsulin levels must be calculated by subtracting the specific insulin fraction from the total immunoreactive insulin in plasma. In addition, gel chromatography separates proinsulin incompletely from its intermediates. To solve this problem, high-performance liquid chromatography (HPLC) has been applied *(64)*. Reverse-phase HPLC in combination with ELISA has shown that intact proinsulin and des 31, 32 proinsulin are present in normal subjects *(65,66)*. Intact proinsulin is roughly two-thirds of the total concentrations of proinsulin-like material. These reverse-phase HPLC studies have also revealed the substantial heterogeneity of proinsulin-like material in sera from normal and NIDDM patients. The data obtained with this technique suggest that the major portion of the circulating proinsulin-like material in NIDDM patients consists of proinsulin metabolites. Data also suggest that the heterogeneity of proinsulin may be genetically determined and may relate to variations in enzymes responsible for conversion of proinsulin to insulin.

The indirect RIA method includes enzymatic degradation of insulin using an insulin-specific protease that selectively destroys insulin, but not proinsulin *(67)*. However, the enzymatic degradation of insulin usually is not complete, and hence, this method gives imprecise results *(68)*. Because C-peptide is present only in proinsulin and not in insulin, C-peptide or insulin antibodies have been used to immunoprecipitate proinsulin, and then proinsulin is measured as either insulin or C-peptide immunoreactivity in the immunoprecipitates *(69)*. Nonetheless, most of these assays suffer from poor sensitivity and specificity.

Direct RIAs are based on the use of specific polyclonal antibodies to proinsulin. Cohen et al. first used biosynthetic human proinsulin in a direct assay *(70)*. It was based on a polyclonal antibody raised primarily toward the B-chain and C-peptide (BC) junction of the proinsulin molecule. This assay detected intact proinsulin as well as its 65, 66 split. Using antibodies against both BC and A chain C-peptide (AC) junctions simultaneously in a proinsulin RIA assay, Cohen et al. also reported that the dominant conversion product in humans is the AC intermediate, i.e., 32, 33 split of proinsulin *(71)*. The results obtained with specific RIA convincingly demonstrate that proinsulin is disproportionately more elevated than insulin in NIDDM patients compared with the nondiabetics *(30,31)*.

To overcome some problems associated with RIA, immunoradiometric assays employing antibodies to insulin and C-peptide permit direct measurement of proinsulin *(72,73)*. These assays use both polyclonal antibodies and MAbs, and have improved the sensitivity and specificity of proinsulin measurements. Carefully selecting MAb has improved the measurement of proinsulin and the 65, 66 and 32, 33 proinsulin splits with an analytical sensitivity of 1 pmol/L. Also, ELISAs using antibodies to insulin and C-peptide have improved sensitivity *(65)*. With these assays, a preferential appearance of an intermediate cleaved at the B-chain junction (32,33 and des 31,32 proinsulin) in sera from NIDDM patients has been found. More recently, an immunoradiometric assay using commercially available MAbs reactive to intact proinsulin HP-1-005 (from Novo, Bagsvaerd, Denmark) has been described *(74)*. The MAb recognizes the epitope at the B-chain and C-peptide junction. The antibody cross-reacts with the proinsulin splits 65,66 and des 64,65 but does not react with the proinsulin split 32,33, or des 31,32 or with insulin or C-peptide. For the assay, the antibody is used as a labeled localizing antibody along with another MAb used as a capture antibody that crossreacts with insulin and proinsulin. This antibody combination allows specific measurement of intact proinsulin, since the concentrations of splits 65,66 and des 64,65 proinsulin are very low in the circulation. The assay has an analytical sensitivity of 0.4 pmol/L and allows the detection of proinsulin in healthy, fasting subjects where the range is 1.0–9.1 pmol/L.

More recently, a two-step, time-resolved fluoroimmunoassay for proinsulin has been developed *(75)* that also uses commercial MAb HP1-005, which is coated on microtiter wells and allows specific capture of proinsulin. After the initial incubation with HP1-005 and a wash step, the proinsulin reacts with a biotin-labeled polyclonal anti-insulin antibody (guinea pig antiporcine insulin). This reaction is followed with the addition of europium-labeled streptavidin and has a sensitivity for proinsulin of 1 pmol/L. However, the concentrations measured in healthy subjects with this assay are lower than reported with the assay using the same MAb as a localizing antibody; the difference cannot be explained based on proinsulin reference preparations, since both assays use synthetic proinsulin as a standard. Regardless of the methodology differences, both studies found that basal proinsulin levels significantly increase in NIDDM patients, therefore confirming the pioneering work of Rubenstein and coworkers *(60)* who used crude gel chromatography and RIA procedures.

Islet Amyloid Polypeptide

Physiologic Role

Another recently discovered cosecretory product of β-cells is a neuropeptide-like molecule called islet amyloid polypeptide (IAPP) or amylin. Its structure, biology, and disease relevance have been reviewed recently *(76)*. This peptide was first discovered as a major constituent of amyloid deposits, usually present to a great extent in the islets of patients with long-standing NIDDM and in benign insulinomas (77). Although the exact in vivo role of IAPP is not clearly understood, recent in vitro studies have shown that it inhibits glucose uptake and glycogen synthesis in muscle. In this respect, it is similar to CGRP. Studies so far have suggested that IAPP may have some insulin-antagonistic activity primarily in skeletal muscle (78,79). However, the physiologic significance of this activity remains to be determined. Glucose stimulates IAPP secretion in vitro, in isolated pancreatic islets or in islet β-cell lines, and in in vivo systems. Also, in vivo circulating IAPP concentrations increase after oral or iv glucose administration; however, this increase is modest (two- to threefold) compared to the increase in insulin (four- to eightfold) (80).

Certain diseases are associated with abnormal concentrations of IAPP, as determined in studies in animal models as well as humans. In IDDM, IAPP is deficient as a consequence of a loss of β-cells; this deficiency could contribute to insulin-induced hypoglycemia. It has been postulated that the hyperglycemia of NIDDM is largely caused by the decreased uptake of glucose in skeletal muscle, and that IAPP may be the primary factor causing this reduced uptake and thus contributing to the pathogenesis of insulin resistance in NIDDM (77). Increased IAPP production by the β-cells may be an early event and may precede the onset of overt NIDDM. Circulating IAPP concentrations may be modestly increased in NIDDM patients compared to normal controls (80). Whether this modest elevation is enough to cause insulin resistance is still debated, primarily because the degree of ligand-mediated receptor desensitization is unknown. Furthermore, IAPP in high doses inhibits glucose-stimulated insulin release from rat islets, suggesting a possible role for IAPP in the impaired insulin release of NIDDM (81). However, a study failed to support such a role for IAPP in normal subjects (82).

Early deposition of amyloid may further contribute to NIDDM by disrupting the function or damaging the islet cells. IAPP is elevated in human obesity and chronic renal failure. The cause of amyloid deposition in diabetes remains unclear, but may be related to the hypersecretion of IAPP that is associated with hyperglycemia along with unknown factors that may enhance amyloid β fibril formation.

Biochemistry and Biosynthesis

Although amyloid-like material was first described in 1901, it was not successfully solubilized until 1986 (83). Analysis of this solubilized material revealed that it was solely composed of a single peptide, IAPP. It is a 37 amino acid peptide that has a theoretical molecular mass of 3859 Dalton. Sequence analysis of this peptide showed close homology with the two CGRPs 1 and 2 having 43 and 48% homology, respectively. The nonhomologous region of the molecule is the amino acid sequence between residues 20 and 29, which is related to the amyloidogenicity as well as to the immunogeneic specificity of IAPP. Also, synthetic peptide that corresponds to this region spontaneously aggregates and forms amyloid-like fibrils in vitro. The gene that codes for IAPP is located on the short arm of chromosome 12.

Like insulin, IAPP is derived from a larger mol-wt 89 amino acid precursor molecule, the pre-pro-IAPP, that contains a signal peptide ending in lysine and arginine at the N-terminus (84). The IAPP is represented by amino acid residues 34–70 in the pre-pro-IAPP sequence, and is flanked by short amino-terminal and carboxyl-terminal propeptides. IAPP also has a carboxyl-terminal amine that is characteristic of many neuropeptides. The IAPP precursor is likely transported with proinsulin to Golgi vesicles, where it is processed into a mature 37-residue carboxyl-amidated peptide and is cosecreted with insulin.

Measurement

IAPP is measured with an RIA described in 1989 *(85)*. The antiserum is raised in the rabbits by immunizing with the 24–37 peptide sequence coupled to bovine thyroglobulin. There is no crossreactivity with β-calcitonin gene-related protein, insulin, or PP. The purified human IAPP labeled with ^{125}I is used as the ligand. The IAPP from plasma samples is extracted with SepPak (C-18) cartridges (Millipore Corp, Milford MA), and antibody-bound antigen is separated using second antibody precipitation. The assay is specific and sensitive enough to detect circulating IAPP levels. In one study, the fasting normal IAPP levels ($n = 18$) were 4.5 ± 0.7 pmol/L and increased to 14 ± 1.7 pmol/L at 60 min after oral glucose administration *(86)*. Glucose-stimulated IAPP secretion increases in obese subjects, but decreases in those with NIDDM *(87)*. Percy et al. recently reported a sensitive sandwich enzyme immunoassay for the measurement of IAPP in plasma *(88)*. The assay detection limit is 2 pmol/L, which is significantly lower than that found by RIA and allows direct measurement of IAPP in a small sample volume. Using their assay, these investigators confirmed the low fasting IAPP concentrations in patients with IDDM. Furthermore, they demonstrate that a glucose challenge caused higher IAPP concentrations in patients with impaired glucose tolerance than in healthy subjects. The pathophysiological significance of this finding remains unclear and of glucose-stimulated IAPP secretion measurement has no defined clinical value at present.

Glucagon

Physiologic Role

Glucagon and insulin jointly regulate glucose, amino acid, and fatty acid metabolism. Glucagon secretion is negatively controlled by glucose. It is not clear at present whether this control is a direct effect of α-cells or is mediated indirectly via release of insulin and somatostatin from the neighboring β-cells that inhibit α-cell secretion. In contrast to insulin, which promotes energy storage, glucagon makes energy available to tissues between meals. The liver is the major target organ of glucagon action. At physiologic concentrations, glucagon has no known effect on tissues other than liver. It stimulates the breakdown of stored glycogen, maintains hepatic gluconeogenesis, and promotes hepatic production of ketone bodies (ketogenesis) (Fig. 1). Glucagon's action is mediated via its binding to glucagon receptors on hepatocytes that activates adenylate cyclase and the generation of cyclic AMP, both of which promote glycogenolysis and gluconeogenesis.

In view of the regulatory roles of insulin and glucagon, it is understandable that full metabolic expression of insulin deficiency in IDDM may require glucagon and may not occur if both glucagon and insulin are deficient *(89)*. In the latter situation, the hepatic production of glucose and ketones is only slightly greater than that expected when both hormones are under the normal physiologic control. Thus, the metabolic expression will depend only on glucose use by other tissues. Therefore, glucagon blockade or suppression may help maintain near-normal hepatic glucose and ketone production despite the insulin deficiency. Such an approach may be beneficial in managing IDDM patients. The coordinated secretion of insulin and glucagon in response to various stimuli efficiently controls glycemic fluctuations below or above the normal range. Decreasing glucose causes an instantaneous islet response, i.e., reduction in the insulin-to-glucagon ratio. In simple terms, the fed state is characterized by a relatively high insulin-to-glucagon ratio, whereas the fasting state is characterized by a relatively lower insulin-to-glucagon ratio.

Biochemistry and Biosynthesis

Glucagon, a factor in hyperglycemia, was isolated, purified, and crystallized in 1955 by Staub et al. from a crude fraction obtained during commercial preparation of insulin *(90)*. Two years later, the amino acid sequence of glucagon was known *(91)*. It is a 29 amino acid, single-chain peptide that is structurally related to other neurohormonal peptides, including secretin, vasoactive intestinal peptide, gastric inhibitory peptide, and growth hormone-releasing factor. The structural similarity among these peptides suggests a common ancestral origin. All these hormones, including glucagon, are expressed in the gut, pancreas, and central nervous system. Furthermore, glucagon is a highly conserved molecule and shows close homology between species. The amino acid sequence of all mammals, except guinea pigs, is identical. Chicken and turkey glucagon differs from human by only one amino acid. This strong evolutionary conservation indicates that multiple structural features of the molecule contribute to its biologic activity. Glucagon fragments of <25 amino acids lose substantial receptor binding ability. Also, deletion of the N-terminal histidyl residue or C-terminal dipeptide sequence markedly reduces its receptor binding activity *(92)*.

The knowledge of the glucagon structure led to the chemical synthesis of glucagon analogs specifically designed to prepare potent glucagon antagonists. These studies showed that loss of histidyl-1 and replacement of ASP-9 with other amino acids are crucial for the dissociation of the biologic activity and receptor binding activity *(93)*. These changes result in potent antagonistic activity. These glucagon antagonists have potential therapeutic utility in diabetes, because they decrease hyperglycemia.

Like insulin, glucagon is derived from a higher-mol-w precursor molecule, the pre-proglucagon that contains the characteristic hydrophobic signal sequence. Pre-proglucagon is rapidly processed to proglucagon, an 18-kDa protein, as estimated by SDS gel electrophoresis. In its sequence, proglucagon contains a 30 amino acid glucagon-related peptide (GRP), a lysine-arginine doublet, a 29 amino acid glucagon sequence, an arginine-arginine doublet, a hexapeptide (an intervening peptide, IP1) followed by another arginine-arginine doublet, IP2, and two glucagon-like peptides (GLP): GLPI and GLP2 *(94)*.

The proteolytic processing of proglucagon occurs at pairs of basic amino acid residues and can produce six different peptides (Fig. 4). These include a 30 amino acid terminal peptide, GRP, glucagon, GLP1, GLP2, IP1, and IP2. However, the processing of proglucagon differs between the α-cells of the islets and the glucagon cells of the intestine. This difference in processing more likely may be the result of differences in the processing enzymes that are expressed in these tissues. Islet α-cells primarily release the 29 amino acid residue glucagon, whereas GLP-1 and GLP-2 are

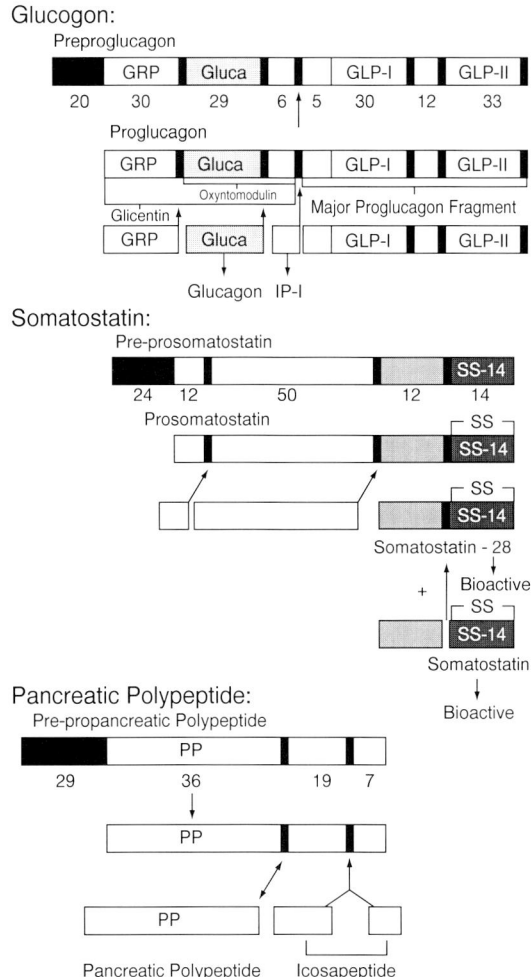

Fig. 4. Diagrammatic presentation of the biosynthesis of glucagon, somatostatin, and pancreatic polypeptide. For proglucagon only tissue-specific processing in α-cells is depicted.

released mainly in the form of the 10-kDa major proglucagon fragment (Fig. 4). The reverse occurs in the ileal region of the small intestine where glucagon is not produced and remains as an incompletely processed peptide, such as glicentin, that contains the GRP and glucagon sequences or oxyntomodulin, which contains a glucagon sequence along with an IP1 sequence. The major secretory products are GLP1 and GLP2 *(94)*. The physiologic importance of these intermediate peptides remains unclear at present.

Measurement

Glucagon is measured by RIA *(95)*. Most assays using polyclonal antibodies show variable crossreactivity with GLP-1 and related molecules. For specific assays, an antiserum directed at the C-terminal segment of pancreatic glucagon is required. These antisera do not crossreact with oxyntomodulin, perhaps because of its C-terminal extension *(95)*. However, they do show some crossreactivity with high-mol-wt glucagon with an N-terminal extension and with the so-called big plasma glucagon. The presence of this glucagon-like immunoreactive material makes it difficult to measure basal glucagon levels accurately in the circulation *(96)*. Because of these difficulties and the fact that glucagon measurement is of little value in clinical conditions other than in the differential diagnosis of glucagon-secreting pancreatic tumors, the glucagon assays are still used primarily for research.

Recently, measurement of the glucagon response to acute insulin administration has revealed that α-cell hyperfunction in diabetes can be completely suppressed and that such hyperfunction is not autonomous *(97)*. Also near-normal glucagon regulation is maintained in IDDM after 4–5 wk of glucoregulation with insulin infusion pumps, thus confirming that adequate insulin therapy can overcome inappropriate glucagon secretion *(98)*.

Somatostatin

Physiologic Role

Somatostatin was first identified in the hypothalamus as an inhibitor of growth hormone. It has also been identified in other tissues, including pancreas, the gastrointestinal tract, and central nervous system. Later studies revealed that somatostatin has a much broader spectrum of inhibitory actions *(99)*. It inhibits many pituitary, pancreatic, and gastrointestinal polypeptide hormones. In islet cells, it is produced solely by the δ-cells and inhibits insulin and glucagon secretion by the neighboring α- and β-cells *(100)*. Most likely this inhibition is mediated via the paracrine pathway. Practically all known stimulators causing insulin release from β-cells also release somatostatin from δ-cells. This pattern is true for glucose, arginine, gastrointestinal hormones, and tolbutamide. The metabolic clearance of somatostatin is extremely rapid, and the half-life in circulation is <2 min *(101)*. Therefore, biochemical research has focused on synthesis of analogs with an increased half-life in circulation and the potency to inhibit peptide hormone synthesis. Some of these synthetic analogs and derivatives inhibit glucagon more than insulin. Such preferential inhibition is reflected in their ability to prevent the hyperglycemia and ketogenesis of IDDM. Therefore, these compounds may have the therapeutic potential of reducing the blood glucose concentration and ketogenesis.

Biochemistry and Biosynthesis

Somatostatin is a 14 amino acid cyclic polypeptide with a mol wt of 1640 Dalton and an internal disulfide bridge. In spite of many technical difficulties, work in the last decade suggests that it is initially synthesized as a high-mol-wt precursor molecule *(100,101)*. In rat islets, somatostatin is derived from a 12.5-kDa precursor peptide that contains a somatostatin moiety at the C-terminus. Subsequent cloning of cDNA from humans and angler fish confirms these findings. Both somatostatin and its precursor structure are well conserved in vertebrate evolution. Although little is known about the processing of the prosomatostatin molecule, recent studies have identified two distinct proteases that are involved in the generation of two molecular forms of somatostatin, 28 amino acid (SS-28) and 14 amino acid (SS-14) peptides *(102)* (Fig. 4). The generation of SS-14 from SS-28 occurs at a site having paired basic residues. Much still remains to be learned regarding the biosynthesis of somatostatin at both the transcriptional and translation levels.

Measurement

Because of its extremely short half-life in the circulation, the accurate measurement of somatostatin is difficult. Plasma somatostatin values as measured by RIA by different investigators show different values in normal subjects *(103–105)* possibly because different RIAs detect different forms. Somatostatin S-14, as well as a somatostatin complex consisting of somatostatin and a larger binding protein, has been identified. In addition, direct assays suffer from nonspecific interference that gives falsely high values. Methods using an extraction step also detect primarily larger species *(106)*. This difference may be the result of fast clearance of somatostatin 14 and accumulation of the larger forms. Circulating forms with somatostatin-like immunoreactivity have been found using several tedious chromatographic steps and HPLC analysis *(107)*. The three forms with somatostatin-like immunoreactivity are present in plasma: SS-28, SS-14, and SS-13 *(108)*. The pathophysiologic significance of somatostatin in the circulation remains uncertain.

Pancreatic Polypeptide

Physiologic Role

Originally identified as a contaminant of some insulin preparations, PP is a 36 amino acid peptide. It is synthesized by a distinct cell type in islet, the F-cells, that are located primarily in the posterior head of the pancreas. The physiologic action of PP is unknown. Its secretion is primarily under vagal control, and it does not appear to regulate carbohydrate metabolism *(109)*. Although the circulating levels of PP increase in response to a meal, it appears to regulate gastrointestinal functions primarily, such as exocrine pancreatic secretion and gallbladder emptying *(109,110)*.

Biochemistry and Biosynthesis

Structurally, PP is related to carboxyl-amidated neuropeptides that include neuropeptide Y. It is derived from a 9–10 kDa precursor from which a second cosecretory product has been derived, the so-called icosapeptide, which are found in human, canine, and bovine forms. In comparison to PP, which is highly conserved, the sequence of icosapeptide is less conserved. The biosynthesis of PP appears to follow that of other islet hormones *(111)*. After removal of the prepeptide sequence in the endoplasmic reticulum, a pro-PP is localized in the Golgi bodies, packaged in presecretory granules, and processed by enzymes similar to proinsulin and proglucagon. Because PP is located in the N-terminus of pro PP, only a single site must be cleaved for its release. The sequence at this site is gly-lys-arg, and cleavage likely requires at least three enzymes: endopeptidase, which recognizes lysine and arginine; carboxyl peptidase (PC2 or PC3) to remove the C-terminal lysine residue; and an amidating enzyme system for additional cleavage to produce an icosapeptide (Fig. 4).

Measurement

RIA is used to detect plasma PP *(112)*; its concentrations increase in response to a meal; however, it does not increase in response to iv glucose and increases only modestly in response to iv amino acid administration. The pathophysiologic significance of circulatory PP measurement remains unclear, and its measurement has no defined clinical value in the diagnosis of pancreatic disorders.

PATHOGENESIS AND DIAGNOSIS OF PANCREATIC ENDOCRINE DISORDERS

Clinically, diabetes is characterized as a syndrome of deranged carbohydrate metabolism with hyperglycemia. Endocrinologically, hyperglycemia may occur because insulin secretion is completely absent or a biologic response to insulin is lacking. Based on this distinction, diabetes is classified in two major categories: insulin-dependent (type I) or noninsulin-dependent (type II).

Insulin-Dependent Diabetes Mellitus

Pathogenesis

IDDM is characterized by the complete absence of insulin, elevated glucagon levels, and the inability of β-cells to respond to any known insulinogenic stimuli. Clinically, it is the most severe form of diabetes and leads to ketosis if not treated. Patients with IDDM require exogenous insulin to maintain normoglycemia. However, many may experience a brief period of return of insulin secretion (the so-called honeymoon period) after diagnosis and initiation of therapy. This return of secretion is somewhat prolonged by early and effective insulin therapy. Nonetheless, it is usually short, and most patients become insulin-dependent within 2 yr.

Today, IDDM is considered to be a chronic autoimmune disease. The autoimmune aspects of IDDM have been reveiwed extensively *(113)*. It is believed that the autoimmune insult to β-cells is triggered by environmental factors in genetically susceptible individuals and is mediated by the immune system effector cells. The disease has a prolonged course, suggesting that β-cell destruction proceeds at a subclinical level for years before the onset of overt diabetes. The natural history of IDDM is summarized in Table 1. The prediabetic phase can roughly be divided into a number of different stages *(114)*. Stage I is genetic susceptibility, in which an individual may have genetic susceptibility, but requires an additional triggering event to initiate the process. Stage II involves the triggering event that gives rise to active autoimmunity. Stage III is characterized with multiple immunologic markers with a progressive decrease in insulin release that leads to stage IV, in which disease is clinically evident; however, some β-cell function still remains. Stage V is characterized by the complete loss of β-cell function and overt diabetes.

IDDM is an immunologic disease; hence, immune intervention should alter the natural history of the disease and potentially arrest the process. In fact, immune intervention does prevent disease in the BB rat and NOD mouse models *(115)*. Investigation with immunosuppressive agents in animal models and in humans indicates that suppressing immune cell activation effectively blocks the ongoing immune insult to β-cells, and can delay or prevent the development of IDDM *(116,117)*. Initial studies have suggested that immunosuppressive therapies (cyclosporin-A and azathioprine) are more effective when started early. Early treatment with cyclosporin in children with recent-onset IDDM can induce remission from insulin dependence *(118)*. Recently, interventional therapies using an antigen-mediated tolerance have further generated optimism

Table 1
Natural History of the Development of IDDM[a]

Stage	Markers[b]	β-cell function	
		Insulin secretion	% β-cell function[c]
I. Genetic predisposition	HLA DR3/DR4+ HLA DQβ$_1$(57ASP−)	Normal	100%
II. Initiation	Triggering event (environmental factors)		
III. Active autoimmunity	Autoantibodies (+) ICA(+) and/or IAA(+) GAD65 and/or IA-2(+)	Normal	80%
IV. Disease onset	Autoantibodies (+) First phase IR(−) C-peptide present	Subnormal	10%
V. Clinical disease	Hyperglycemia No C-peptide	Absent	0%

[a]Based on ref. *114*.

[b]ASP, aspartic acid; GAD65, glutamic acid decarboxylase; HLA, Human leukocyte antigen, IAA, insulin autoantibodies; IA-2, islet autoantigen; ICA, islet-cell antibodies; IR, insulin response.

[c]Estimate based on insulin release.

in disease prevention protocols. In the presence of certain T-cells, tolerance to self-antigens results from anergy, which is defined as the inability of autoreactive T-cells to produce IL-2 in response to specific antigens. Indeed, administering insulin before IDDM develops can prevent or delay disease onset, and can allow β-cells to rest and reduce the expression of activation antigens on the surface *(119)*. The growing knowledge of the mechanisms of peripheral T-cell tolerance has also led to new immunologic intervention strategies, such as T-cell vaccination and antigen vaccination. Vaccination with the autoantigen GAD in susceptible mice prevents the development of IDDM *(120)*. Oral administration of insulin in IDDM is currently being investigated. However, the success of these trials depends on accurately identifying individuals who are at risk for IDDM, and this requires extensive laboratory evaluation; this is the subject of the following discussion.

Human Leukocyte Antigen (HLA) Tests in Assessing Genetic Risk

Family and population studies suggest that predisposition to IDDM is polygenic. Certain HLA types occur with greater frequency in patients with IDDM. Initially, IDDM was found to be associated with B8 and B15 class I antigens. Later studies, however, have indicated a stronger association with DR3 and DR4 (positive association) and DR2 (negative association) antigens (*see* ref. *119* for a review). It is well documented that more than 90% of patients with IDDM are positive for HLA DR3, DR4, or both alleles *(121)*. The relative risk for IDDM in a DR3-positive individual is 3.3, and for a DR4-positive individual, it is 6.4 over non-DR3, non-DR4 subjects. Also, additive risk occurs when both HLA-DR3 and HLA-DR4 are present. However, in an individual with no known family member with diabetes, the presence of this gene does not ensure development of diabetes. The contrary is also true—there are patients with IDDM who have neither the DR3 nor DR4 allele. These findings suggest that another IDDM gene or genes may reside in close association with DR3 and DR4, and they are in linkage disequilibrium with DR antigens.

Subsequent reports have shown that IDDM is more strongly associated with the class II region antigen, HLA-DQ-β1. The α- and β-chains of HLA-DQ contribute the most to a person's susceptibility to IDDM. The presence of the aspartic acid residue at position 57 of the HLA-DQ β-chain decreases susceptibility to IDDM, and its substitution with a noncharged amino acid (alanine, valine, or serine) correlates with increased susceptibility *(122)*. Several studies confirm that the order of degree of susceptibility is HLA-B < HLA-DR < HLA-DQ. Although the HLA-DQ-β1 gene is the most prevalent gene for IDDM susceptibility, its presence is not sufficient to precipitate the disease. Also, the fact that the risk for siblings sharing no HLA haplotype is greater than the risk in the general population indicates that additional factors must be involved in disease predisposition. A genetic link to chromosome 11 in IDDM has also been reported *(121)*. The insulin gene on chromosome 11 shows 5'-releasing flanking polymorphism. This polymorphic locus may represent a marker for a linked gene that also influences the susceptibility to IDDM. Although the predisposition to IDDM may be genetically determined, in some individuals with diabetes, nongenetic factors are equally or more important, for example, viral infections and toxins. The environmental factors maybe obligate cofactors in initiating the pathogenic process.

Modern molecular technologies for analyzing of HLA genes and gene products have been used to study the role of DQ-β1 in diabetes. For large sample analysis, the second exon on the DQ-β1, gene that codes for the first domain of the β-chain and contains the hypervariable segment is amplified with the polymerase chain reaction (PCR). The variations involving the region centered on codon 57 are then recognized by hybridizing the amplified material with the radiolabeled allele-specific oligonucleotides and using dot-blot analysis *(122)*. More recently, a digestion method using restriction enzyme-generated fragments from PCR amplification has been described for studying IDDM susceptibility. The procedure can be completed within 24 h and is simpler than the hybridization method *(123)*.

Cellular Immunity in IDDM

The pathogenic role of T-lymphocytes in the development of IDDM is supported by the predominance of T-cells found within the β-cell insulitis area and also by the efficacy of the T-cell-directed immunosuppression. The infiltrating T-cells in insulitis express activation markers, such as major histocompatibility complex class II antigens and high-affinity IL-2 receptors *(124)*. Suppressor/cytotoxic (CD8+) T-cells predominate in insulitis and may reflect the late phase of the disease process. In NOD mice, a sequential analysis of insulitis before the development of hyperglycemia showed that the predominant T-cell population was the helper/inducer, or CD4+, T-cells *(125)*. Several reports have shown the increase in the ratio of CD4+ to CD8+ T-cells and an absolute increase in circulating T-cells expressing activation markers *(126)*. In a recent study, autoreactive HLA-DR-restricted T-cells that are specific for β-cell antigens have been cloned *(127)*. These reports, along with a vast amount of data from animal studies (BB rat model), provide fairly conclusive evidence for the pathogenetic role of T-cells (CD4+) in anti-islet-cell immunity. Nonetheless, routine T-cell analysis (by flow cytometry) shows that T-cell populations significantly overlap in normal glycemic IDDM and normal nondiabetic subjects. This and the fact that the T-cell analysis remains rather complex precludes the use of these techniques for screening purposes.

Autoantibodies as Predictors of IDDM

Humoral autoimmunity is the most extensively studied autoimmune phenomenon in IDDM. Sera from these patients contain antibodies to multiple islet-cell antigens, and these autoimmune responses have been found as long as 8–12 yr before the onset of clinical symptoms *(114)*, indicating the disease develops slowly *(114)*. Three antibodies are found in high frequency in diabetic patients and their relatives: islet-cell antibodies (ICAs), insulin autoantibodies (IAA), and an antibody reactive to 64 K autoantigen (glutamic acid decarboxylase), all of which have been studied extensively *(113,121)*. More recently, a new autoantigen has been identified and its cDNA isolated by antibody screening of a human islet cDNA expression library using a pool of sera from a patient with newly diagnosed IDDM *(128)*. This antibody was termed ICA-512, and this diabetes autoantigen has been recently identified as IA-2. It is related to protein-tyrosine phosphatase and is an important member of the panel of auto-antibody markers *(129)*.

ISLET-CELL ANTIBODIES

ICA in the serum of IDDM patients were first described in 1974 *(130)*. These antibodies were detected by an indirect immunofluorescent technique using cryostat sections of fresh postmortem human pancreas from blood group O donors. Since then, they have been referred to as cytoplasmic ICAs, because they bind to cytoplasmic antigens in human islet cells. Over the years, this immunohistochemical procedure has undergone numerous improvements and standardization *(131)*. The method was evaluated at the First International Workshop on the Standardization of Islet Cell Antibodies *(132)*. Indirect immunofluorescent techniques showed ICAs were present in 55–80% of patients with recent-onset IDDM *(133)*. The prevalence of ICAs in subjects with other autoimmune endocrine diseases, but without clinical evidence of diabetes is about 6%. The frequency of ICAs decreases with the duration of IDDM, and ICAs are detected infrequently in patients with long-standing IDDM. ICAs are not specific for β-cells, and react with other islet cells even though in IDDM, β-cells are selectively destroyed. The ICAs consist predominately of IgG, are detected in low titers, and can fix complement. Some human sera also have complement-dependent antibody-mediated cytotoxicity toward islet cells *(134)*. The complement fixing ICAs are a subset of ICAs that are referred to as CF-ICA, and are detected by indirect fluorescence with complement and anti-C3 antisera. Both CF ICA and ICA as detected by the protein A assay are comparable in terms of their predictive value for the development of diabetes. The appearance of ICA has been correlated with the deterioration of insulin secretion and is transient. ICAs are more strongly associated with the childhood-onset of IDDM *(133)*. The identity of the antigens responsible for ICA activity has remained elusive. The ICA may not cause β-cell cytotoxicity and may just be a epiphenomenon of the underlying immune response. However, they provide a useful marker for predicting IDDM, and until recently, the analysis of ICA has been the basis for identifying individuals at high risk for IDDM and has been used clinically in the last two decades.

The indirect immunofluorescence technique using human pancreas and fluorescein-labeled protein A is the recommended method for detecting ICA *(132)*. However, the immunofluorescent technique is time-consuming and laborious. In addition, the technique is subject to interpretation bias, has poor reproducibility, and standardization between laboratories has been very difficult. In spite of the use of international reference pool serum to quantify ICA in Juvenile Diabetes Foundation (JDF) units, the test remains semi-quantitative. For these reasons, it is not suitable for large population screening.

INSULIN AUTOANTIBODIES

IAA were first detected in 1983 in the sera of patients with newly diagnosed IDDM before insulin therapy *(135)*. These antibodies suggest that insulin itself is an autoantigen that can induce an immune response. It is possible that β-cell damage caused by T-cell autoimmunity may release insulin, which, in turn, may induce antibody production. IAA have been well documented in the prediabetic phase *(136)*. Direct evidence for their pathogenic role comes from their ability to induce insulitis in normal animals on immunization and from their ability to suppress development of diabetes in NOD mice when administered orally *(119,137)*. This protective effect likely is caused by the immunogenicity of insulin, because a functionally inactive insulin B-chain is as effective as native insulin *(137)*. Results of a pilot trial of low-dose insulin administration to prevent diabetes in relatives of IDDM patients have recently been reported *(138)*.

Currently, IAA are measured by RIA or ELISA. These procedures have different methodologies and varying degrees of sensitivity; therefore, comparing results from different labs has been difficult. A number of factors influence these assays, including the ligand used, incubation time, RIA separation techniques, and the antigen-coating procedure in ELISA. Fluid-phase RIA has been a more sensitive test than solid-phase RIA or ELISA. Also the fluid-phase assay, which uses competition for cold insulin to obtain nonspecific binding as a control, has high specificity and sensitivity. To standardize the measurement of IAA, a panel of coded sera was analyzed by 24 different laboratories; the analytical data varied substantially *(139)*. Fluid-phase assays as a group performed better than ELISAs, showed better specificity, and are currently recommended over ELISAs. With such an assay, elevated IAA levels were found in 100% of children diagnosed with IDDM before age 5 yr, but in fewer than 20% of individuals who developed diabetes after age 15. Patient age and IAA level correlated marginally *(136)*. In this study, the concentration of IAA appeared to be closely linked to the rate of autoimmune β-cell destruction, and so can be helpful in predicting the duration of the prediabetic phase. A number of studies suggest that IAA have little prognostic significance in the absence of ICA *(136)*. However, in combination, they are highly predictive. A family member with an ICA equal or >40 JDF units who is also IAA-positive had a 77% risk of developing diabetes within 5 yr as compared with 42% when ICA was at least 40 JDF units, but IAA was not present *(136)*.

GAD AUTOANTIBODIES

GAD is an enzyme that controls the biosynthesis of the neurotransmitter, γ-aminobutyric acid. In addition to newly diagnosed IDDM patients, GAD antibodies are also found in the absence of diabetes in a rare neurological disorder, stiff-man syndrome *(13)*. It has been identified as a previously described 64-kDa autoantigen in immunoprecipitation experiments with radiolabeled human islet extracts *(13)*. Human islet-cell GAD antigen is an isoform, GAD65. Two isoforms, GAD65 and GAD67, have been cloned from human brain *(140)*. GAD67 shares 65% homology with GAD65, and its gene is located in chromosome 2. The human islet GAD65 has also been cloned and sequenced, and its gene is located on chromosome 10.

Antibodies to the 64-kDa antigen, now known as GAD65, were conventionally detected by immunoprecipitation assays using extracts of radiolabeled human islets *(141)*. Use of more readily available mouse or rat islets resulted in poor sensitivity and required extraction of IgG from the sera before the assay. Using these techniques, GAD antibodies are detected in 60–70% of diabetics and in most ICA-positive prediabetic patients *(141,142)*. An enzyme assay for rat brain GAD has been described and used for clinical studies *(143)*. In this assay, after immunoprecipitation, antibody-bound GAD was detected by determining its enzymatic activity in a CO_2 production assay. The validity of this assay has been questioned compared to the use of human radiolabeled GAD65. First, the rat brain has both GAD65 and GAD67, and after immunoprecipitation, the enzymatic assay detects both forms. Second, the assay is less sensitive and will detect only high-titer antibodies. However, the recent availability of human recombinant GAD65 has radically changed our ability to measure GAD antibodies accurately. Using recombinant human GAD65 expressed in the hamster fibroblast line or other eukaryotic cell systems is superior to animal tissue extracts. The results of the First International Workshop to Standardize GAD Antibodies have confirmed this finding *(144)*. Also, recombinant GAD induces T-cell proliferation in vitro in IDDM patients, leaving little doubt that GAD is one of the major β-cell antigens involved in the pathogenesis of IDDM *(145)*. However, anti-GAD antibodies are not better predictors of IDDM than the ICA *(142,143)*.

More recently, separate GAD65 and GAD67 assays have been described using in vitro synthesized recombinant ^{35}S-methionine-labeled antigen and protein A Sepharose to separate free from antibody-bound ligand *(146,147)*. Using this assay, Grubin et al. *(146)* reported that GAD65 had a diagnostic sensitivity of 77% and specificity of 92% for patients 14 yr old or younger with recent-onset diabetes; in contrast, GAD67 had a sensitivity of only 8% and a specificity of 98% for the same group of patients. This assay is simple, precise, requires a sample size of only 2–4 µL, and is suitable for large-scale screening. However, in the same study, 88% of diabetic patients were positive for ICA, and GAD65 and ICA levels were not correlated. In another study using a similar assay, the prevalence of ICA was significantly greater in younger patients with IDDM (age < 30 yr) than in older patients compared to GAD antibodies; the latter seems to be more prevalent in patients older than >30 yr *(147,148)*. Also, a recent study found that GAD antibody presence at onset predicts the type of diabetes regardless of age and can predict treatment requirements better than the clinical characteristics *(141)*. These differences suggest that antibodies to antigens other than GAD65 may contribute to ICA immunofluorescence. This idea agrees with the observation that GAD does not completely block the majority of ICA-positive sera. The predictive value of GAD alone for IDDM is not higher than the predictive value of GAD and ICA combined.

Antibodies to Tyrosine Phosphatase IA-2/ICA 512

Antibodies reactive to a 64-kDa protein antigen that is distinct from GAD have been described in diabetic patients *(129)*. Trypsin digestion of 64-kDa protein bands obtained by SDS-PAGE results in three major fragments with molecular weights of 50, 40, and 37 kDa *(149)*. Antibodies in diabetic patients that react to the 50-kDa fragment also react to GAD65. On the other hand, there are antibodies that react to the 37- and 40-kDa proteins and do not react with GAD65. Based on these findings, it has been suggested that the 37- and 40-kDa fragments actually originate from an islet antigen that has a molecular mass of 64-kDa, but is distinct from GAD65. Antibodies to these antigens are found in up to 80% of patients with recent-onset IDDM, and are very closely associated with development of IDDM in identical twins and first-degree relatives of IDDM patients *(150)*. These antibodies are also detected in patients with polyendocrine autoimmunity and stiff-man syndrome. Moreover, their presence in conjunction with ICA is associated with a significantly increased risk for the development of IDDM and rapid progression to disease.

Recent attempts to identify these 37- and 40-kDa antigens indicate that 40- and 37-kDa fragments are derived from different, but probably related protein precursors. Furthermore, the 40-kDa fragment is derived from a protein similar or identical to the tyrosine phosphatase-like molecule called IA-2 *(151)*. IA-2 is homologous to protein-tyrosine phosphatase of the receptor-linked family. Also, IA-2 shares sequence homology with another putative islet autoantigen designated ICA 512. The latter was cloned from an islet expression library after screening with human IDDM serum and is related to the protein-tyrosine phosphatases *(128)*. Antibodies to ICA 512 protein are found in 42% of IDDM patients. The predicted size of the IA-2 intracellular segment is 42-kDa, suggesting that IA-2/ICA 512 protein is a precursor of the 40- and 37-kDa islet proteolytic fragment that is immunoprecipitated from IDDM serum.

In a recent study, sera from 51 of 100 patients with new-onset IDDM immunoprecipitated the 37/40-kDa antigen and 53 immunoprecipitated in vitro translated recombinant IA-2 antigen; 49 of these 53 had both reactivities. Also, preincubation of recombinant IA-2 competitively inhibited the binding to the 37- and 40-kDa fragments *(152)*. In the same study, antibody levels reactive to recombinant IA-2 correlated strongly to the presence of the 40- and 37-kDa fragments. Also, IA-2 antibodies correlated with ICA titers in the GAD antibody-negative sera, and preincubation with recombinant IA-2 inhibited ICA immunofluorescence in sera with both ICA and IA-2 antibodies but not in sera that were ICA-positive and IA-2-negative. Results of this study suggested that anti-ICA 512 antibodies contribute to ICA positivity, and these antibodies in combination with GAD can account for most ICA reactivity in IDDM. Nonetheless, these results established the identity of IA-2/ICA 512 as a precursor of the 37- and 40-kDa proteins. In the same study, combined detection of IA-2 antibodies and GAD65 antibodies in a single radiobinding assay using in vitro translated ^{35}S-methionine-labeled proteins (IA-2 and GAD65) had a diagnostic sensitivity of 88% in IDDM patients, whereas GAD alone identified 69% and IA-2 alone identified only 53% of true positive patients. Such an approach provides a single assay for potential population screening for IDDM risk assessment and awaits future studies to confirm these findings.

Environmental Triggers of the Anti-β-Cell Autoimmune Response

Several observations convincingly suggest that environmental factors have a role in the pathogenesis of IDDM in particular and autoimmune diseases in general.

Between identical twins, discordance exceeds 60%. The incidence of disease varies enormously from one country to another *(113)*. Also, there is a north-to-south gradient, i.e., the IDDM incidence is greater in the northern part than the southern part of the world. Several viral infections have been linked to the development of IDDM and probably are significant in its etiology. Support for the role of a virus as cause comes from epidemiological data, particularly the rubella and Coxsackie viruses *(153)*. About one-third of individuals who had rubella *in utero* will develop IDDM. A strain of Coxsackie B virus was isolated from the pancreas of a child who died of recent-onset IDDM *(154)*. The isolated virus induced IDDM in mice. Anti-IgM Coxsackie virus antibodies are detected in a significant percentage of patients with type 1 diabetes. The mechanisms by which the virus influences the development of IDDM are not well understood, but one possible mechanism is related to molecular mimicry. The viral protein conceivably can share sequence homologies with β-cell autoantigens, such as that between coxsackie B virus protein and GAD antigen *(155)*.

Food constituents influence glucose metabolism and, hence, the course of IDDM. It has been recently reported that proteins in cows' milk can accelerate the course of diabetes development in BB rats. In contrast, lactalbumin-free diets are protective if introduced early in life. In a recent study, nearly all patients with newly diagnosed IDDM had IgG antibodies reactive to bovine serum albumin (BSA) as determined using a particle concentration fluoroimmunoassay *(156)*. Anti-BSA antibodies recognize a discrete 17 amino acid region on the BSA molecule that extends from position 152–168. This sequence, called "ABBOS," is the site of a major difference between cow and human, mouse, and rat albumin, being unique to cow BSA. A 69-kDa, interferon-inducible β-cell protein was found to crossreact with anti-ABBOS antibodies, and two laboratories have cloned this 69-kDa autoantigen using anti-BSA or anti-ICA-positive IDDM sera *(156)*. This crossreaction (molecular mimicry) could explain the stimulation of an anti-islet T-cell response by cows' milk during neonatal life in some genetically susceptible infants, especially after a viral infection. Since a viral infection can increase the expression of the interferon-inducible, 69-kDa antigen on β-cells, the cells could become the target of anti-ABBOS antibody-mediated cytotoxicity. It must be noted that recent-onset diabetics do not show T-cell hypersensitivity to BSA or ABBOS *(157)*. Also, some data suggest that breast feeding which delays exposure to cows' milk, significantly reduces the risk of diabetes in children. Confirmation of these data awaits future prospective randomized studies.

A number of drugs and chemicals show selective β-cell toxicity and have the potential to induce IDDM in doses that generally do not cause extra-pancreatic toxicity. Alloxan and streptozotocin are well-known agents that are used to induce IDDM in animal models *(121)*. Streptozotocin has a direct toxic effect and can cause diabetes if given in a large dose. Also, repeated small doses can cause insulitis and β-cell degranulation. The model suggests that subtle chemical injury can activate the immune response. A rodenticide containing *N*-3-pyridylmethyl-*N'*-*p*-nitrophenyl urea (Vacor) can induce IDDM if ingested in large doses *(158)*. Pentamidine, given to patients with acquired immunodeficiency syndrome for prophylaxis of *Pneumocystis carinii* pneumonia, may have a similar toxic effect on the pancreas *(159)*. However, most of these agents probably are not involved in the origin of the common forms of IDDM.

Noninsulin-Dependent Diabetes Mellitus

NIDDM is a highly heterogenous disease, and is characterized by insulin resistance and impaired insulin secretion. Both the impaired insulin secretion and resistance result in decreased glucose clearance and reduced suppression of glucose production, and thus contribute to the development of hyperglycemia. It is a highly prevalent disease, and approx 90% of diabetic patients have NIDDM.

NIDDM, obesity, hypertension, and atherosclerosis are coincident disorders. Many epidemiological studies show a strong association between insulin resistance or compensatory hyperinsulinemia and coronary artery disease *(160)*. These metabolic associations have been variously labeled as "syndrome-X," "insulin-resistance syndrome," coronary artery disease, hypertension, adult-onset diabetes, obesity, stroke ("CHAOS") and glucose intolerance, hypertension, obesity ("GHO").

Pathogenesis

The exact nature of NIDDM pathogenesis is more controversial than that of IDDM. Likely, it is the outcome of the combination of multiple gene defects and environmental factors. Two major pathologic defects have been clearly identified in NIDDM: (1) insulin resistance or decreased insulin action on peripheral tissues, and (2) impaired β-cell function or an inability of the β-cells to produce sufficient insulin to compensate for the insulin resistance. Which of these two factors is the primary abnormality in NIDDM pathogenesis is still controversial. A two-step model of the natural history of NIDDM development has been proposed *(161)*. The first step is the progression from normal glycemia to impaired glucose tolerance, which is primarily influenced by insulin resistance. In the second step, impaired glucose tolerance progresses to NIDDM, which is primarily a result of the β-cell defect and declining insulin secretion. A schematic illustration of the factors likely involved in the pathogenesis of NIDDM is shown in Fig. 5.

INSULIN RESISTANCE

Insulin resistance is difficult to measure in routine clinical settings. Mostly fasting insulin concentrations or insulin responses to glucose are used as an indirect measure of insulin function. Quantitative in vitro measurements of insulin sensitivity, such as the euglycemic insulin-clamp technique or computer model analysis of the glucose response to a bolus insulin, allows the sensitive and accurate assessment of in vivo insulin action. Insulin sensitivity can also be measured with in vitro cell-culture systems. These techniques have been described in detail in a recent review article *(162)*. However, they are complex and time-consuming, and have not yet been adopted for routine clinical analysis.

The clinical spectrum of insulin resistance is broad in NIDDM. It ranges from normal glycemia to hyperglycemia in the presence of a markedly elevated endogenous insulin. Several clinical syndromes are associated with insulin resistance that include type A insulin resistance with acanthosis nigricans and hyperandrogenism, syndrome-X with lipid abnormalities and hypertension, and type B insulin resistance, which is characterized by insulin receptor autoantibodies capable of blocking insulin response. In the last two decades, considerable progress has been made in defining some of the mechanisms involved in insulin resistance.

Endocrine Disorders of the Pancreas

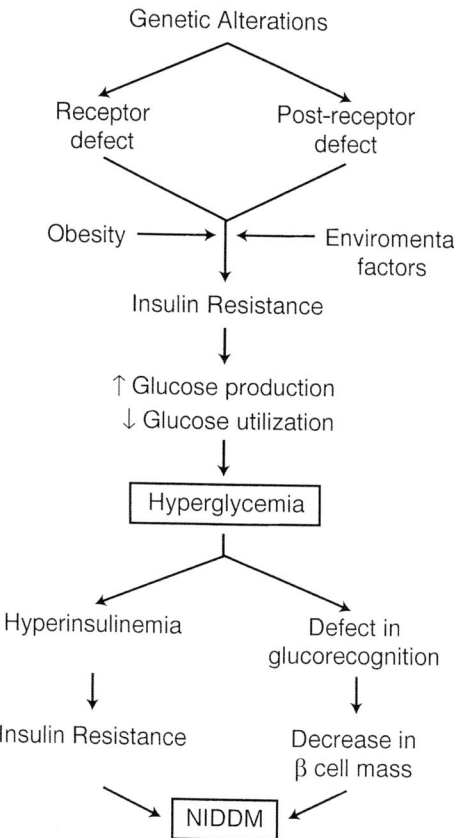

Fig. 5. Schematic presentation of mechanisms responsible for the pathogenesis of noninsulin-dependent diabetes. Likely contributions of genetic susceptibility, obesity, and environmental factors in the development of hyperglycemia and β-cell unresponsiveness are depicted.

The Role of the Insulin Receptor in Insulin Resistance. Recent studies and reviews in diabetes research have focused on the role of the insulin receptor in insulin resistance (163,164). Insulin resistance can be caused by abnormalities at the prereceptor level (before insulin interaction with the cell) or at the postreceptor level (in the signal transduction pathway). Prereceptor abnormalities include the binding of insulin with anti-insulin antibodies or increased degradation of insulin. Decreased insulin receptor binding has also been described in both obese and thin individuals with NIDDM (165). This decrease in binding is attributed to a decrease in the receptor number with minimal or no change in receptor binding affinity. Possibly, this decrease in receptors is secondary to downregulation of the receptor by the elevated basal insulin levels. Early attempts to determine quantitative differences in insulin receptors have used ^{125}I insulin-binding assays, and the patient's lymphocytes or erythrocytes most often are used to assess the receptor binding sites. However, this method has many technical limitations, including the presence of nonspecific binding, and an incubation temperature that causes the bound ligand to be internalized by the cells used in the assay. Also, the number of binding sites that are estimated using erythrocytes cannot be extrapolated to other target tissues in patients. Therefore, at present, measurement of erythrocyte insulin binding has no clinical utility.

The insulin receptor belongs to a family of receptors that have tyrosine kinase activity. It is a heterotetramer consisting of two subunits, α and β, each composed of two polypeptide chains. The α-subunit forms the extracellular membrane portion that binds with insulin, and the β-subunit extends intercellularly through the plasma membrane and contains tyrosine kinase activity. Binding of insulin to the receptor activates tyrosine kinase, which leads to autophosphorylation of the receptor. Also, the insulin receptor catalyzes the phosphorylation of a number of other intracellular proteins. The phosphorylation of these proteins is an essential step for signal transduction. One important substrate protein is insulin receptor substrate 1 (IRS-1). Its phosphorylation leads a cascade of reactions with many intracellular signal transductal proteins that have src homology 2 domain (SH-2) sequences. Differences in the SH-2 domain determine the specificity of binding. Proteins that contain the SH-2 sequence include phosphatidylinositol (PI3) kinase and growth factor receptor binding protein 2 (GRB-2). Both are important in mediating signal transduction *(163)*. In addition to the substrate 1 pathway, the insulin receptor probably activates other pathways, including the glucose transport pathway through an insulin receptor substrate-independent system. Some of these steps are illustrated in Fig. 6.

Several insulin receptor mutations have been identified that can affect its function. One component of a postbinding defect may involve coupling to receptor kinase activation, which decreases the tyrosine kinase activity of the receptor *(163)*. Insulin receptor tyrosine kinase activity has been measured and correlates with insulin resistance in several insulin-resistant states, including NIDDM. Given the complexity of the insulin receptor signal pathway, it is not surprising that insulin binding (as determined by receptor number) or receptor tyrosine kinase activity does not necessarily correlate with insulin resistance. Recent advances in molecular technologies have simplified the detection of point mutations at the gene level. To date, numerous mutations have been identified in the receptor structural gene that cause defects in receptor function *(164,165)*. Many of these mutations reside in the α-subunit and decrease insulin binding, whereas those in the β-subunit produce defective receptor kinase activity. Because multiple mutations are spread out on both α- and β-subunits, the analysis of these mutations in patients so far is too complex a procedure to be used in a clinical setting.

The Role of the Glucose Transport System in NIDDM. One of the best-characterized effects of insulin is its ability to stimulate the glucose transport system *(166)*, which involves the translocation of glucose transporter proteins from an intracellular pole to the cell membrane. Multiple transporter genes have been identified that encode a family of homologous proteins; they exhibit different functional properties and different tissue-specific expression. Five isoforms of these proteins, Glut-1–Glut-5, have been identified. Glut-4 is the major translocating transporter species in human adipose tissue and muscle, and appears to mediate most glucose transport activity. Therefore, glucose resistance at the glucose transport level may be a result of altered Glut-4 function and expression. In pancreatic islet cells, Glut-2 is the major transporter protein that couples plasma glucose to insulin secretion. In obesity and in NIDDM patients, the mechanisms of impaired glucose transport are different between adipocytes and skeletal muscle *(166)*. In adipocytes, a suppressed Glut-4 isoform has been detected, and this suppressed

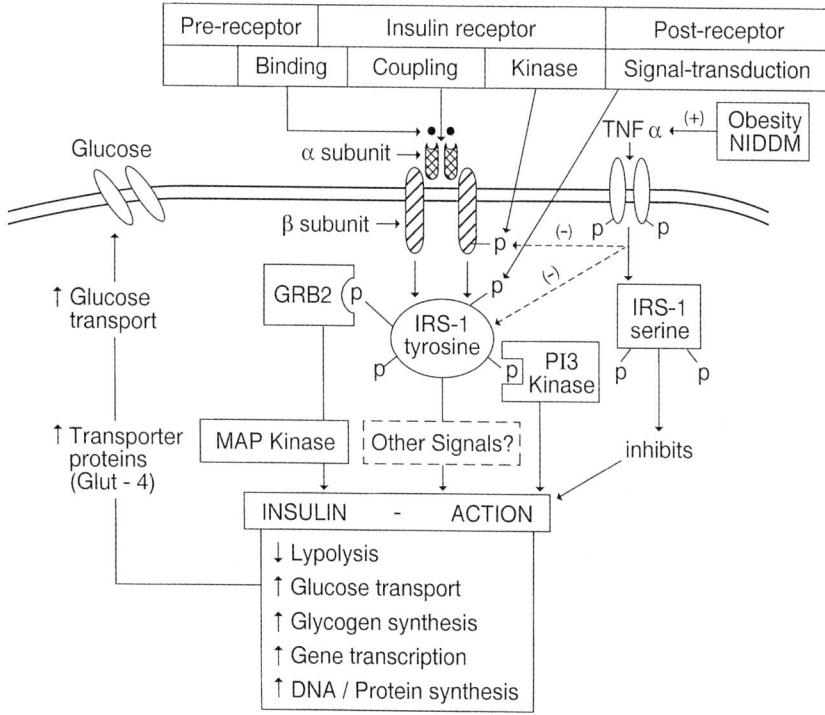

Fig. 6. Illustration of possible sites of insulin resistance at the cell level. Defects at prereceptor, receptor, and postreceptor levels are illustrated. The insulin action involves a cascade of phosphorylation reactions initiated by activation of the insulin receptor (by tyrosine kinase) and its autophosphorylation. Phosphorylation of IRS-1 and subsequent activation of PI3 kinase are depicted. Also, the possible mechanism of TNFα on insulin resistance is illustrated. IRS denotes insulin receptor substrate, P denotes phosphatase, and PI3 denotes phosphatidylinositol. GRB-2 is growth factor receptor binding protein-2, Glut-4 is glucose transport protein-4, and MAP is microtubule-associated protein. Derived from refs. *163* and *171*.

isoform may be the key player for insulin resistance in both obesity and NIDDM *(167)*. In contrast, Glut-4 expression at both mRNA and protein levels in skeletal muscle is normal in both obesity and NIDDM, suggesting that the Glut-4 functional defects or insulin-mediated translocation may not be the cause of insulin resistance in this tissue *(168)*.

Despite considerable investigation to identify the genetic basis for insulin resistance in NIDDM, the genetic defects in insulin receptor or transporter proteins identified so far account for fewer than 5% of patients with NIDDM.

The Role of Tumor Necrosis Factor-α (TNF-α) in Insulin Resistance. Recent studies indicate that TNFα mediates insulin resistance in both obesity and NIDDM. The mRNA expression of TNFα increases in adipose tissues from animals and human patients with obesity and NIDDM *(169,170)*. Also in these animals, TNFα protein is elevated locally and systemically *(169)*. TNFα also decreases tyrosine kinase activity of the insulin receptor. In addition, it induces resistance by phosphorylating the IRS-1 at serine residues. This altered form of IRS-1 inhibits the first step in the insulin pathway, the autophosphorlyation of the insulin receptor after insulin binding *(169)*. Such inhibition has been suggested as the possible mechanism by which TNFα causes insulin resistance in adipocytes and is illustrated in Fig. 6. Also, long-term TNFα treatment of these animals downregulates Glut-4 mRNA *(171)*. TNFα levels correlate with the extent of both obesity and insulin resistance. The role of TNFα is an exciting development in the search for molecular markers of insulin resistance, and future studies are needed to confirm its role at the clinical level.

β-CELL FAILURE IN NIDDM

The increased demand on β-cells caused by insulin resistance may eventually lead to the progressive loss of β-cell function *(172)*. β-cell exhaustion can be demonstrated by using the iv glucose tolerance test, which reveals the absence of the first phase of the insulin response in NIDDM. This loss of insulin release seems to be specific for glucose, because insulin secretion progressively decreases as glucose rises; the insulin response to other secretogog, for example, arginine, remains intact *(172)*. Other insulin secretory abnormalities are the loss of the pulsatility of insulin release and an increased ratio of proinsulin to insulin *(172)*. The mechanisms of the selective β-cell unresponsiveness to glucose are not clear at present. Much existing data indicate that persistent hyperglycemia can make β-cells unresponsive to glucose, a condition frequently termed "glucotoxicity." The level of pancreatic β-cell function seems to correlate with both the level of glucose and the duration of hyperglycemia. Maintenance of nomoglycemia seems to reverse this defect.

Obesity and Development of NIDDM

Approximately 85% of NIDDM patients are obese, and have associated insulin resistance and hyperinsulinemia. Obesity and a family history of diabetes increase the risk of developing NIDDM. The proposed mechanisms of insulin resistance in obesity include hyperinsulinism caused by constant β-cell stimulation as a result of chronic overeating, which can, in turn, downregulate the insulin receptor.

There is evidence that obesity has a strong genetic component. A newly cloned gene called the "OB gene," which encodes the protein leptin, has been associated with the development of obesity *(173)*. The gene is expressed in adipose tissues and may be an important signaling factor in body weight homeostasis. Both eating and insulin administration increases leptin mRNA levels in fasting animals, suggesting potential interactions between leptin and insulin *(174)*. Also, circulating concentrations of leptin increase in diabetic mice. These are preliminary findings, mostly in animals, and future studies are required to elucidate the role of this gene in NIDDM.

Laboratory Tests for Evaluating of Diabetes Mellitus

Glucose Measurement and Glucose Tolerance Tests

The diagnosis of diabetes mellitus (IDDM or NIDDM) can be made on the basis of an elevated fasting glucose level. A fasting glucose concentration of at least 140 mg/dL on more than one occasion is diagnostic. However, in the absence of clinical symptoms, the oral glucose tolerance test may be helpful. For the oral test, although the exact amount of the glucose load is still debated, current recommendations from the National Diabetes Data Group are generally followed *(175)*. The test must be done after 3 d on a diet containing a minimum of 150 g of carbohydrates/d. The following day, after an overnight fast, 75 g of glucose for adults or 1.75 g/kg body wt for children is given in water (≤25 g/dL) and ingested in 5 min. Five samples are generally collected, one before the glucose loading and again at every 30 min up to 2 h after loading. The diagnostic criteria for abnormal glucose tolerance according to National Diabetes Data Group and World Health Organization Expert Committee are a blood glucose level of at least 200 mg/dL at 2 h or at any time during the glucose tolerance. Values between 140 and 199 mg/dL indicate impaired glucose tolerance. This is a heterogenous category that includes many people who may have a subsequent normal oral glucose tolerance test, and almost 30% of patients who develop diabetes may not exhibit impaired glucose tolerance *(176)*. Thus, the oral test results often may be nondiagnostic. Furthermore, in spite of standardization, many factors influence the outcome of the oral glucose tolerance test.

During the oral glucose tolerance test, normally, insulin levels peak at 1 h, reaching 50–130 µU/mL and returning to below fasting concentrations in 2 h. The clinical utility of insulin measurement is limited, primarily because when fasting glucose is elevated, β-cell responsiveness decreases, and when the fasting glucose level is normal, late hyperinsulinism may occur in NIDDM or in the early phase of IDDM.

The iv glucose tolerance test more accurately assesses the rate of glucose disappearance, because it bypasses variations in the absorption rate. The latter is affected in a patient with thyroid disease, malabsorption syndromes, other gastrointestinal diseases, or gastrectomy. For this test, glucose (0.5 g/kg of body wt) is injected intravenously over 1–3 min, and blood is collected at every 10 min for 30 or 60 min. Plasma glucose decreases exponentially, and the glucose disappearance rate can be calculated from this response. The test is valuable in predicting the onset of IDDM, because it evaluates the first phase of the insulin response.

Diabetic Ketoacidosis and Serum Ketone Determination

Diabetic ketoacidosis is the most common cause of mortality in IDDM (*see* ref. *177* for a review). It is a life-threatening complication of uncontrolled diabetes. It occurs more commonly in patients with IDDM; however, stress like trauma, infection, myocardial infarction, or exogenous glucocorticoids can lead to ketoacidosis in NIDDM. Diabetic ketoacidosis is a consequence of an imbalance between insulin action and the counter-regulatory action of hormones that include glucagon, epinephrine, norepinephrine, cortisol, and growth hormone. In the absence of insulin action, excessive lipolysis in adipose tissue releases free fatty acids that are taken up by the liver, and are frequently converted to ketoacids and subsequently to ketone bodies.

Both diagnosis and treatment of diabetic ketoacidosis require laboratory analysis of glucose and ketone levels, acid–base status, and electrolyte balance. In patients with diabetic ketoacidosis, the plasma glucose usually exceeds 500 mg/dL. When insulin is inadequate, three major ketone bodies—acetone, acetoacetate, and β-hydroxybutyrate—are formed in blood and tissues and excreted into the urine. Ketone presence is detected in serum or urine. The test is simple and uses a nitroprusside reaction that measures only acetone and acetoacetate. Therefore, if β-hydroxybutyric acid is the predominate ketone, these tests can be misleading. Specific enzymatic techniques are available to quantify each of ketoacids; however, they are not needed in most clinical situations.

Glycohemoglobin Assays

The term "glycohemoglobin" (previously termed glycosylated hemoglobin or glycated hemoglobin) is applied to a number of chemically distinct hemoglobin components that are generated when glucose binds to hemoglobin. Measurement of glycohemoglobin is an integral part of clinical diabetes management today. The subject has recently been extensively reviewed *(178)*. The test accurately assesses the mean blood glucose level during the preceding 2–3 mo. Therefore, it complements the more traditional measures of glucose control (blood or urine glucose testing).

The glycation of hemoglobin occurs at several amino acid residues, and as a result, several adducts of hemoglobin A (HbA) and various sugars are formed by the nonenzymatic posttranslational glycation process *(179)*. This process involves the formation of a labile Schiff base intermediate followed by the Amadori rearrangement. The reaction is slow, continuous, and irreversible, and the reaction rate depends on the ambient glucose concentration. Minor components of HbA were first recognized because of differences in their electrical charges and were called "fast hemoglobin," since they migrated at a faster rate than an entire HbA molecule when placed in an electrical field. These minor components were labeled in order of elution from a ion-exchange column as $HbA1_a$, $HbA1_b$, and $HbA1_c$. The most important HbA component in diabetes is $HbA1_c$, which has glucose attached at the N-terminal-amino groups of both β-chains of hemoglobin.

Various methods for the measurement of $HbA1_c$ have been described and recently been reviewed *(180)*. They include ion-exchange chromatography, HPLC, colorimetry, spectrometry, electrophoresis, affinity chromatography, and ion-capture chromatography. Immunoassays for HbA1c also have been described *(181)*. Among the methods, HPLC, because of its superior precision and accuracy, has been recommended as a reference method. However, ion-exchange chromatography remains the most widely used, primarily because it is simple and inexpensive. A variety of factors affect ion-exchange chromatographic results, including temperature, pH, ionic strength, and column size. In addition, sample handling and storage conditions affect the analysis. Also, labile intermediates coelute with glycohemoglobin A and may give falsely elevated values. These difficulties indicate the need for careful standardization of assay conditions during ion-exchange chromatography.

Ion-exchange HPLC has been automated to allow processing of a large number of samples. However, hemoglobin species with altered charges (e.g., Hb_s or Hb_c) and glucose adducts that comigrate with HbA_1 species can interfere with this assay. These problems may become more apparent with different storage conditions, indicating stringent requirements for sample handling and a need for closed systems that are not affected by temperature fluctuations.

In recent years, boronic affinity chromatography has gained popularity *(182)*. This method involves the use of minicolumns of crosslinked agarose, with boronic acid as ligand, that has a high binding affinity for glycohemoglobin. This method is not affected by hemoglobin variants, labile Schiff base intermediates, or slight temperature changes. However, the precision is not as good as that obtained by ion-exchange HPLC, and the procedure is labor-intensive. If ion-exchange HPLC is combined with affinity columns, precision and specificity improve significantly. Automatic versions of this technique have recently been introduced *(183)*. Also, recently a simple automated procedure that uses the immunoassay instrument (IMX) (Abbott Diagnostics) and ion-capture technology has been introduced.

The diversity of methods used for glycohemoglobin AI_c analysis has made comparisons between different laboratories difficult. For patient management, results from one laboratory cannot necessarily be used in conjunction with or interpreted in light of those from another. Occasionally, therapeutic changes based on discrepant results from different laboratories may place patients at a significant risk, so standardizing these assays is critical. The $HBA1_c$ results are conventionally expressed as a percentage of total hemoglobin, which may account for the variability between methods. This issue has recently been addressed, and the calibration of most glycohemoglobin $A1_c$ assays using a single reference calibrator has been attempted. In a comparison of seven different methods, when a common reference calibrator was used, decreased between-method variability and improved interassay precision were observed, suggesting that such an approach to standardization may allow results from different laboratories to be compared directly *(184)*. Such standardization should further enhance the utility of glycohemoglobin $A1_c$ measurement to control tightly glucose concentrations in diabetic patients.

Fructosamine Assay

Like glycohemoglobin, glucose molecules are joined to protein molecules through a nonenzymatic glycation mechanism to form stable ketoamines termed "fructosamines." All serum proteins can be glycated, so all glycated proteins are fructosamines. Albumin is the most abundant serum protein, and it contains multiple lysine residues, all of which can be glycated. Therefore, fructosamine measurements primarily reflect glycoalbumin concentrations. Fructosamine measurements may be used in a manner analogous to glycohemoglobin, as an index of the mean concentration of glucose in the blood during the preceding several weeks. However, because serum proteins turn over relatively rapidly compared to hemoglobin, the fructosamine level reflects glucose control over a shorter period of 2–3 wk rather than 6–10 wk for glycohemoglobin. Because of this time difference, whether the fructosamine test is more clinically useful than the $HbA1_c$ assay remains debatable.

The fructosamine assay was first introduced in 1983 by Johnson et al. *(185)*, and is a colorimetric procedure based on the ability of ketoamines to reduce nitroblue tetrazolium (NBT) to produce a compound that is detected by absorption at 525 nm. The assay is commonly known as the NBT assay and has been adapted for many automated chemistry analyzers, including the Hitachi (405,705), Kobas (Bio Mira), Abbott, (ABA-100) Technicon (RA1000), and Centrichem (300 and 400). Other analytical approaches for fructosamine are affinity chromatography with *m*-aminophenylboronic acid, thiobarbituric acid (TBA), and other colorimetric procedures *(186)*. Among these methods, the affinity-chromatography and NBT assays are more practical, because they are fast, economical, and accurate. Since these assays detect glycoproteins, total protein concentration is likely to influence fructosamine results. Total protein or albumin concentrations seem to correlate with fructosamine levels. It is accepted that a significant change in albumin will result in a similar change in fructosamine levels. The current recommendation, therefore, is to normalize fructosamine results to a given serum albumin or total protein concentration. Also, being a colorimetric analysis, bilirubin, hemolysis, and lipemia will likely interfere in the measurement.

Measuring of fructosamine provides a number of clinical advantages over measuring glycohemoglobin $A1_c$. The fructosamine levels respond more quickly to changes in glycemic control than does glycohemoglobin $A1_c$, therefore allowing patients to achieve better control than has been possible in the past. Second, the measurement is simpler and more economical than the glycohemoglobin $A1_c$ assays. However, fructosamine assays are used currently only to complement glycohemoglobin $A1_c$ assays to manage diabetic patients when the detection of short-term metabolic changes is required.

Detection of Advanced Glycosylation End Products (AGEs)

Accumulation of glycated proteins (the so-called Amadori adducts) formed by the nonenzymatic glycation process is also converted in the circulation to AGEs through a series of chemical rearrangements. These AGEs continue to accumulate on long-lived proteins, and accumulation is rather rapid in tissues and in the circulation of patients with diabetes *(187)*. They are important risk factors in the pathogenesis of diabetic complications, because they can crosslink with other proteins. This subject has been extensively covered in a recent review *(188)*. Specific binding sites or receptors for AGEs have been identified on both murine and human macrophages *(189)*. These receptors are distinct from the binding that occurs on macrophages during the clearance of AGE-modified proteins.

Nonenzymatic glycation changes the function of some proteins. For example, if the glycation site is located in the active receptor binding site, some alteration in the binding activity can occur; for example, glycated low-density lipoprotein receptors have less internalization and degradation by human fibroblasts than do normal receptors *(188)*. This process can also change the immunogenicity of proteins. Data suggest that AGEs prepared in vitro have a common immunological epitope like the AGE formed in tissues in vivo. The antibody raised against the AGE epitope made in vitro after incubation of glucose with ribonuclease crossreacts with AGEs formed in vivo and is suitable for detecting AGEs in vivo *(190)*.

Lack of precise and specific methods to measure AGEs has been a hindrance in defining their role in diabetic complications. Nonspecific methods have been used, such as detection of AGE-dependent relative fluorescence. A competitive whole-cell radioreceptor assay for AGE using AGE receptors on a macrophage-like cell line (RAW 264.7) has been described *(191)*. This study found that AGEs increased significantly in the circulation of patients with diabetes, and the increase paralleled the severity of renal function impairment in diabetic nephropathy. However, the complex nature of this assay has hampered its use in routine clinical practice. Alternative assays include molecular sieving HPLC and PAGE. However, at present, no simple commercial procedures are available to assay AGE, limiting its use in most clinical laboratories.

Hypoglycemia

Unlike the hyperglycemia of diabetes, hypoglycemia, except when produced as a consequence of diabetic treatment, is not common. In healthy individuals, hypoglycemia occurs at plasma glucose concentration of about <50 mg/dL, and the associated symptoms are relieved by administration of carbohydrates. It is generally associated with an aberration in one or more of the mechanisms involved in glucose homeostasis. The symptoms of hypoglycemia reveal the interdependence of neural and humoral regulatory systems, and can be related either to adrenergic discharge or to neuroglycopenia. However, they predominately reflect the effect of hypoglycemia on the central nervous system.

Pathogenesis and Classification

The neuroendocrine system protects against an abrupt loss of glucose supply to the brain and other tissues when excessive insulin is present. This system includes hormones that antagonize insulin action, such as glucagon, catecholamines, growth hormone, glucocorticoids, and thyroid hormones. They act in synergy to replenish glucose during fasting and hypoglycemia by augmenting the hepatic output of glucose (glycogenolysis and gluconeogenesis), and simultaneously decreasing glucose uptake by insulin-sensitive tissues and mobilizing fuel from alternative sources. The subject has been recently reviewed *(192)*. Abnormalities of this counterregulatory system can contribute to the development of hypoglycemia. Among these hormones, glucagon is more important than epinephrine as a regulator of hepatic glucose output in the postabsorptive phase after a meal. The blockade of both α- and β-adrenergic systems has little effect on either absorptive glucose or hepatic glucose release, but suppression of glucagon can decrease hepatic glucose-release by 35–50% *(193)*. However, a combined deficiency of glucagon and epinephrine seriously impairs the ability of an individual to respond to hypoglycemia.

Impaired glycogen synthesis or breakdown also predisposes individuals to fasting hypoglycemia. Cortisol and growth hormone deficiencies are frequently associated with decreased hepatic glycogen *(194)*. Cortisol also is required for glucagon- or epinephrine-mediated stimulation of glycogenesis. Replacing these hormones restores normal glycogen synthesis. In summary, glycogenolysis is the major source of glucose in the early postabsorptive state. Impaired glycogen breakdown or reduced synthesis results in the the development of hypoglycemia as occurs in adrenal insufficiency with decreased glycogen-degrading enzymes or in autonomous insulin secretion.

Based on the time and type of symptoms, hypoglycemia can be divided into three major categories: reactive, fasting, and surreptitious hypoglycemia *(195,196)*. Each of these is discussed below.

REACTIVE HYPOGLYCEMIA

Reactive hypoglycemia is a mild hypoglycemic disorder that occurs only postprandially. It is characterized by symptoms that reflect primarily adrenergic responses, such as nervousness, tremor, sweating, and pallor. It can be further subdivided into idiopathic functional, alimentary, prediabetic functional, and endocrine-deficient hypoglycemia. Idiopathic functional hypoglycemia has an elusive pathophysiology and has no specific symptoms. Characteristically, these patients have primarily adrenergic symptoms of hypoglycemia a few hours after a meal. Generally, the glucose tolerance test shows normal fasting levels with a normal peak response: however, at about 4 or 5 h after glucose loading, the glucose concentration is well below 50 mg/dL and spontaneously reverts to normal at 6 h.

Alimentary hypoglycemia is caused by excessively rapid gastric emptying and is associated with rapid postprandial carbohydrate absorption. It commonly occurs in patients with upper gastrointestinal surgery or vagotomy. These patients show a more rapid and higher-than-normal increase in glucose after a meal, and delayed insulin release and action. At the time the insulin peaks, the glucose is no longer elevated, and insulin decreases it further, leading to hypoglycemia and the onset of adrenergic symptoms. Feeding the patient quickly reverses these symptoms. The glucose tolerance test generally shows a peak level at 30–60 min, instead of the normal peak at 120–180 min and shows low glucose values 2–3 h after the glucose challenge *(195)*.

Prediabetic hypoglycemia is associated with a delayed, but excessive insulin release that occurs early in the course of IDDM. The onset of symptoms usually begins 4–5 h after a meal. The oral glucose tolerance test shows diabetic patterns with excessive and delayed peak plasma glucose levels, and then a significant drop at hours 4 and 5. This decrease is followed by a spontaneous increase to a normal level.

A deficiency in insulin counter–regulatory hormones may occasionally be responsible for postprandial hypoglycemia. This type of hypoglycemia has symptoms associated with adrenergic deficiency and neuroglycopenia. Therefore, this hypoglycemia has been classified either as reactive or as fasting hypoglycemia. Why the symptoms of either adrenergic deficiency or neuroglycopenia can occur is not known. As previously mentioned, glucocorticoids, growth hormone, glucagon, and catecholamines work in concert to oppose the insulin action in obesity and during fasting. Spontaneous pancreatic glucagon deficiency is an extremely rare cause of hypoglycemia in both adults and neonates. A blunted glucagon response to severe glucopenia has been observed in infants of diabetic mothers, and a transitory lack of glucagon has been identified as the cause. Hypoglycemia may also result from adrenal deficiency *(197)*. Catecholamines may provide a secondary line of defense against hypoglycemia, especially when glucagon secretion is deficient. Further, both epinephrine and norepinephrine inhibit insulin secretion in humans despite concurrent hyperglycemia *(15)*. Nonetheless, with adequate glucocorticoid replacement, such hypoglycemia is corrected.

Thyroid hormones are also involved in glucose homeostasis *(192)*. The cause of hypoglycemia in a thyroid hormone-deficient patient, however, is likely to be multifactorial. It may be the result of both reduction in a gluconeogenic precursor like lactate and a defect in the conversion to glucose in the liver. Thyroid hormone replacement corrects the hypoglycemia.

Fasting Hypoglycemia

Fasting hypoglycemia is a serious and potentially life-threatening disorder. If untreated, the patient may lose consciousness, convulse, and become comatose. Unfortunately, it is often undiagnosed or is misdiagnosed for a considerable time. It can result from several different clinical conditions that are characterized by hyperinsulinism during fasting and includes pancreatic β-cell tumors (insulinomas *[198]*) or non-islet-cell tumors *(199)*. Fasting hypoglycemia can also be seen in patients with renal disease, malnutrition, hepatic dysfunction, or alcoholism *(200)*. Symptoms of fasting hypoglycemia usually occur during the night, before breakfast, or typically when a meal is missed; it is predominantly caused by neuroglycopenia.

Pancreatic β-cell tumors that produce insulin are rare, but are among the most common of the functional islet-cell tumors. Insulinomas can occur at any age, and

70–80% of these tumors are single adenomas. The remaining tumors are multiple or malignant *(196)*. Hyperglycemic symptoms usually present episodically and irregularly, and may not necessarily always repeat with fasting, making diagnosis difficult. In most cases, diagnosis can be made after an overnight or prolonged fast, or after strenuous exercise by measuring glucose, insulin, C-peptide, or all in the same specimen collected when the patient is symptomatic. Most patients become symptomatic with 24 h of fasting, and virtually all become symptomatic within 72 h. Diagnosis in some patients may be elusive and may require an extensive diagnostic workup *(196)*. The laboratory tests for insulinoma diagnosis are discussed below.

Insulin, C-peptide, and Proinsulin Levels in Insulinoma. Measurement of plasma insulin in cases with hypoglycemia is extremely useful in making the diagnosis. However, interpretation of the insulin concentration can be difficult, especially if the insulin values are in the low-normal range. In some with hypoglycemia, the insulin concentration is inappropriately high. Therefore, ratios of insulin and glucose have been devised for assessing relative hyperinsulinemia when the insulin concentration is normal. The most widely used ratio is the amended ratio of Turner et al. *(201)* and is expressed as:

$$[\text{Insulin } (\mu U/mL)/\text{plasma glucose } (mg/dL) - 30 \text{ mg/dL}] \times 100 \qquad (1)$$

The 30 mg/dL figure is a correction factor that is based on the fact that plasma insulin is undetectable in normal individuals when the blood glucose level is 30 mg/dL or less. In normal individuals, the amended ratio is below 50 mg/dL, whereas patients with insulinoma have values above 50 mg/dL. This ratio decreases the number of false-negative results, but may increase the false-positives. Therefore, the glucose-to-insulin ratio is of limited value for the diagnosis of hyperinsulinemia.

As mentioned previously here, C-peptide measurement may be a better indicator of β-cell function and is certainly more useful than insulin in making the diagnosis of insulinoma. If human C-peptide cannot be suppressed during insulin-induced hypoglycemia, this is diagnostic of an insulin-secreting islet-cell tumor. However, the C-peptide assay failed to establish a diagnosis of insulinoma in three patients who had proinsulin as a primary secretory product of the tumor *(202)*. Therefore, proinsulin measurement may be valuable in the diagnosis of hypoglycemia in occasional patients. Normally, it represents <20% of the total immunoreactivity; however, in some patients with an islet-cell tumor, it may account for the majority of immunoreactivity.

The iv tolbutamide test for plasma glucose and insulin determinations has also been used for the diagnosis of insulinoma *(196)*. Generally, it is positive in roughly 75% of true-positive cases. Normal individuals show hyperinsulinemia within 1–3 min after injection of 1 g tolbutamide, and hypoglycemia occurs in 20–30 min. Peak insulin values in normal subjects are <150 µU/mL and normalize in 90 min. However, in patients with insulinoma, insulin concentrations rapidly exceed 150 µU/mL, and glucose falls to <35% of basal values, but does not normalize spontaneously. The test has significant risk for the development of profound and prolonged hypoglycemia, and should be performed under careful supervision. Other less frequently used tests for this purpose include administration of glucagon or leucine *(196)*.

FACTITIOUS HYPOGLYCEMIA

Factitious hypoglycemia constitutes the third major category of hypoglycemia and is among the differential diagnoses for insulinoma. It is commonly seen in health professionals, or people who may have access to insulin or sulfonylurea drugs. The causes of self-induced hypoglycemia may vary, and many patients may suffer from underlying psychiatric problems. Surreptitious insulin administration increases the plasma insulin concentration, resulting in hypoglycemia, which suppresses the endogenous insulin and C-peptide release. Therefore, the combination of high-insulin and low-C-peptide values during hypoglycemia is evidence for factitious hypoglycemia *(54,203)*. Insulin antibodies in a nondiabetic patient suggest that it is either factitious or autoimmune hypoglycemia. Therefore, insulin antibodies have also been used to assess the insulin intake. However, their absence does not preclude the diagnosis. Many patients are diabetics and are on insulin therapy. The demonstration of insulin antibodies is not helpful; a suppressed plasma C-peptide during hypoglycemia is the only laboratory evidence that hypoglycemia in a diabetic patient is a result of insulin administration. However, in such a patient, an elevated C-peptide level can occur, because proinsulin and insulin antibody complexes can interfere with the assay. Therefore, free C-peptide measurement after PEG precipitation of these complexes may be needed to assess suppressed C-peptide levels accurately *(55)*.

When sulfonylurea abuse is suspected in a patient as a cause of hypoglycemia, plasma or urine should be tested for its presence.

SUMMARY

Advances in immunologic and molecular biology techniques have increased both the understanding and diagnostic precision of endocrine disorders of the pancreas. Diabetes mellitus remains the most prevalent and heterogenous disorder of the pancreas. Today, IDDM is considered to be a chronic autoimmune disease with a well-defined genetic susceptibility. Mechanisms of autoimmune insult in IDDM are well studied. The detection of ICAs is a reliable marker for predicting the development of IDDM. Assays used in the past (ICA detection with immunofluorescence) were less sensitive than the newer recombinant antigen-specific assays now available for GAD65 and IA-2 antigens. Combined use of these assays provides an even higher predictive value for determining the risk for disease. These tests are simple enough to be used for screening purposes. In the future, automation of these assays is very likely. When combined with the development of new, simple, interventional modalities (oral antigen vaccination), they provide new hope for preventing β-cell loss and thus IDDM. The mechanisms of insulin resistance in NIDDM are better understood today. Several mutations on the insulin receptor gene and several other gene markers have been identified. Future studies may delineate further the role of new genes, such as the TNFα or OB gene product, in glucose homeostasis and NIDDM.

New immunometric assays that have good sensitivity and specificity for pancreatic hormones, insulin, C-peptide, and proinsulin further contribute to the accuracy and precision of their measurement. Measurement of other hormones, amylin, glucagon, and somatostatin, seems to contribute little to the diagnosis or management of IDDM or NIDDM. The glucose tolerance test and glycohemoglobin $A1_c$ remain the best tests for the diagnosis of hyperglycemia. Recent attempts to standardize and automate glycohemoglobin $A1_c$ testing may further enhance its use in managing diabetes. Other tests, like those for fructosamine and AGE, can potentially complement the current glycohemoglobin $A1_c$ assays if proven to have a high predictive value for the development of diabetic complications. In contrast to hyperglycemia, hypoglycemia is relatively uncommon, and the measurement of glucose, insulin, C-peptide, and in some cases, proinsulin, can reveal the cause.

REFERENCES

1. Von Mering J, Minkowski O (1889) Diabetes mellitus nach Pankreas Extirpation. Arch Exp Pathol Pharmacol 26:371–387.
2. Meinhofer J, Schnabel E, Bremer H, Brinhoff O, Zabel R, Sroka W, Klostermeyer H, Brandenburg D, Okuda T, Zahn H (1963) Synthese der Insulinketten und ihre Kombination zu insulinaktiven Praparaten. Z Naturforsch 18b:1120–1121.
3. Lane MA (1907) The cytological characters of the areas of Langerhans. Am J Anat 7:409–422.
4. Harris IM (1995) Summary. In: Diabetes in America, 2nd ed. Bethesda, MD, NIDDK NIH Publication, #95–1468, pp. 1–13.
5. Yalow RS, Berson SA (1960) Immunoassay of endogenous plasma insulin in man. J Clin Invest 39:1157–1175.
6. Ahren B, Taborsky GJ, Porte D (1986) Neuropeptidergic as cholinergic and adrenergic regulation of islet hormone secretion. Diabetologia 29:827–836.
7. Pearse A (1979) The cytochemistry and ultrastructure of polypeptide hormone-producing cells of the APUD series and the embryologic, physiologic, and pathologic implications of the concept. J Histochem Cytochem 17:303–313.
8. Schmechel D, Marangos PJ, Brightman M (1978) Neuron-specific enolase is a molecular marker for peripheral and central neuroendocrine cells. Nature 276:834–836.
9. Wiedenmann B, Franke WW, Kühn C, Moll R, Gould VE (1986) Synaptophysin: marker protein for neuroendocrine cells and neoplasms. Proc Natl Acad Sci USA 83:3500–3504.
10. Gilon P, Campistron G, Geffard M, et al. (1988) Immunocytochemical localization of GABA in endocrine cells of the rat entero-pancreatic system. Biol Cell 62:265–273.
11. Jamal HP, Jones PM, Byrne J, et al. (1991) Peptide contents of neuropeptides Y, vasoactive intestinal polypeptide and beta calcitonin-gene-related peptide and their messenger ribonucleic acids after hexamethasone treatment in isolated rat islets of Langerhans. Endocrinology 129:3372–3380.
12. Teitelman G, Joh TH, Reis DJ (1981) Transformation of catecholaminergic precursors into glucagon (A) cells in mouse embryonic pancreas. Proc Natl Acad Sci USA 78:5225–5229.
13. Baekkeskov S, Aanstoot HJ, Christgau S, et al. (1990) Identification of the 64k autoantigen in insulin-dependent diabetes as the GABA synthesizing enzyme glutamic acid decarboxylase. Nature 347:151–156.
14. Levin SR, Karam JH, Kane S, et al. (1971) Enhancement of arginine-induced insulin secretion in man by prior administraiton of glucose. Diabetes 20:171–176.
15. Beard JC, Wienberg C, Pfeifer MA (1982) Interaction of glucose and epinephrine in the regulation of insulin secretion. Diabetes 31:802–807.
16. Samols E, Marri G, Marks V (1966) Interrelationship of glucagon, insulin and glucose. the insulinogenic effect of glucagon. Diabetes 15:855–866.
17. Alberti KG, Christensen NJ, Christensen SE, et al. (1973) Inhibition of insulin secretion by somatostatin. Lancet 2:1299–1301.
18. Rubenstein AH, Pottenger LA, Mako M, et al. (1972) The metabolism of proinsulin and insulin by the liver. J Clin Invest 51:912–921.
19. Ferrannini E, Wahren J, Faber OK, et al. (1983) Splanchnic and renal metabolism of insulin in human subjects. A dose response study. Am J Physiol 244:E517–527.
20. Kaden M, Harding P, Field JB (1973) Effect of intraduodenal glucose administration on hepatic extraction of insulin in the anesthetized dog. J Clin Invest 52:2016–2028.

21. Rojdmark S, Bloom G, Chou MCY, et al. (1978) Hepatic extraction of exogenous insulin and glucagon in the dog. Endocrinology 102:806–813.
22. Mirmira RG, Nakagawa SH, Tager HS (1991) Importance of the character and configuration of residues B24, B25, and B26 in insulin-receptor interactions. J Biol Chem 266: 1428–1436.
23. Given BD, Cohen RM, Shoelson SE, Frank BH, Rubenstein AH, Tager HS (1983) Biochemical and clinical implications of proinsulin conversion intermediates. J Clin Invest 76:1396–1405.
24. Patzelt C, Labrecque AD, Duguid JR, et al. (1978) Detection and kinetic behavior of preproinsulin in pancreatic islets. Proc Natl Acad Sci USA 75:1260–1264.
25. Rubenstein AH, Melani F, Pilkis S, et al. (1969) Proinsulin: secretion, metabolism, immunological and biological properties. Postgrad Med J 45(Suppl):476–481.
26. Csorba TR (1991) Proinsulin: biosynthesis, conversion, assay methods, and clinical studies. Clin Biochem 24:447–454.
27. Morgan CR, Lazarow A (1968) Immunoassay of two insulin antibody systems. Diabetes 12:115,116.
28. Ceska M, Grossmuller F, Lundkvist U (1970) Solid-phase radioimmunoassay of insulin. Acta Endocrinol 64:111–125.
29. Desbuguois B, Aurbach GD (1971) Use of polyethylene glycol to separate free and antibody-bound peptide hormones in radioimmunoassays. J Clin Endocrinol Metab 33:732–738.
30. Ward WK, LaCava EC, Paquette TL, Beard JC, Wallum BJ, Porte D Jr. (1987) Disproportionate elevation of immunoreactive proinsulin in type 2 (non-insulin-dependent) diabetes mellitus and in experimental insulin resistance. Diabetologia;30:698–702.
31. Saad MF, Kahn SE, Nelson RG, et al. (1990) Disproportionately elevated proinsulin in Pima Indians with non-insulin dependent diabetes mellitus. J Clin Endocrinol Metab 70: 1247–1253.
32. Hunter FC, Greenwood WM (1962) Preparation of iodine-131 labeled growth hormone of high specificity. Nature (Lond) 194:495–496.
33. Freychet P, Roth J, Nivelle DM (1971) Monoiodoinsulin: demonstration of its biological activity and binding to fat cells and liver membranes. Biochem Biophys Res Commun 43:400–408.
34. Shinkai H, Sohma M, Takahashi Y, Kojima R, Hashimoto M, Ogawa N (1980) An enzyme immunoassay system for measurements of serum insulin. Mol Immunol 17:377–381.
35. Ruan K, Hashida S, Yoshitake S, Ishikawa E, Walkisaka O, Yamamoto Y, Ichioka T, Nakajima K (1986) A more sensitive and less time-consuming enzyme immunoassay for insulin in human serum with less serum interference. Ann Clin Biochem 23:54–58.
36. Schroer JA, Bender T, Feldman RJ, Kim KJ (1983) Mapping epitopes on the insulin molecule using monoclonal antibodies. Eur J Immunol 13:693–700.
37. Marks A, Yip C, Wilson S (1985) Characterization of two epitopes of insulin using monoclonal antibodies. Mol Immunol 22:285–290.
38. Rathjen DA and Underwood PA (1986) Identification of antigenic determinants on insulin recognized by monoclonal antibodies. Mol Immunol 23:441–450.
39. Tolvonen E, Hemmila I, Marniemi J, Jorgensen PN, Zeuthen J, Lovgren T (1986) Two-site time-resolved immunofluorometric assay of human insulin. Clin Chem 32:637–640.
40. Comitti R, Racchetti G, Gnocchi P, Morandi E, Galante YM (1987) A monoclonal-based, two-site enzyme immunoassay of human insulin. J Immunol Methods 99:25–37.
41. Gupta MK (1996) AIA 1200 DX (1996) In: Automated immunoassay analyzer in immunoassay automation. An updated guide to systems, Chan DW, ed., San Diego, CA, Academic, pp. 201–214.
42. Nakagawa S, Nakayama H, Sasaki T, et al. (1973) A simple method for the determination of serum free insulin levels in insulin-treated patients. Diabetes 22:590–600.

43. Bosner AM, Garcia-Webb P (1984) C-peptide measurement: Methods and clinical utility. Crit Rev Clin Lab Sci 19:297–352.
44. Melani F, Rubenstein AH, Oyer PE, Steiner DF (1970) Identification of proinsulin and C-peptide in human serum by a specific immunoassay. Proc Natl Acad Sci USA 67: 148–155.
45. Faber OK, Binder C, Markussen J. et al. (1978) Characterization of seven C-peptide antisera. Diabetes. 27(Suppl 1)170–179.
46. Kumar D, Miller LY (1973) Proinsulin specific antibodies in human sera. Diabetes 22: 361–366.
47. Heding LG, Ludvigsson J (1977) Human proinsulin in insulin-treated juvenile diabetics. Acta Paediatr Scand Suppl 270:48–52.
48. Kuzuya H, Blix PM, Horwitz DL, et al. (1977) Determination of free and total insulin and C-peptide in insulin-treated diabetics. Diabetes 26:22–29.
49. Kumar MS, Schumacher OP, Deodhar SD (1980) Measurement of serum C-peptide immunoreactivity by radioimmunoassay in insulin-dependent diabetics. Am J Clin Pathol 74:78–82.
50. Faber OK, Binder C, Markussen J, et al. (1978) Characterization seven C-peptide antisera. Diabetes 27(Suppl 1)170–177.
51. Binder C, Faber OK (1978) Residual beta-cell function and its metabolic consequences. Diabetes 27 Suppl 1:226–229.
52. Ludvigsson J (1983) Methodological aspects on C-peptide measurements. Acta Med Scand 671(Suppl):53–59.
53. Koskinen, P (1988) Nontransferability of C-peptide measurements with various commercial radioimmunoassay reagents. Clin Chem 34:1575–1578.
54. Stellon A, Townell NH (1979) C-peptide assay for factitious hyperinsulinism. Lancet 2: 148–149.
55. Meistas MT, Kumar MS, Schumacher OP (1981) Diagnosis of self-induced hyperinsulinism in an insulin-dependent diabetic patient by radioimmunoassay of free C-peptide. Clin Chem 27:184–186.
56. Meistas MT, Zadik Z, Margolis S, Kowarski AA (1981) Correlation of urinary excretion of C-peptide with integrated concentration and secretion rate of insulin. Diabetes 30:639–643.
57. Blix PM, Boddie-Willis C, Landau RL, Rochman H, Rubenstein AH (1981) Urinary C-peptide: an indicator of beta cell secretion under different metabolic conditions. J Clin Endocrinol Metab 54:574–580.
58. Hoogwerf BJ, Goetz FC (1983) Urinary C-peptide: a simple measure of integrated insulin production with emphasis on the effects of body size, diet, and corticosteroids. J Clin Endocrinol Metabol 56:60–67.
59. Roth J, Gorden P, Pastan I (1968) "Big insulin": a new component of plasma insulin detected by immunoassay. Proc Soc Natl Acad Sci USA 61:138–145.
60. Rubenstein AH, Steiner DF, Horwitz DL, et al. (1976) Clinical significance of circulating proinsulin and C-peptide. Recent Prog Horm Res 33:435–475.
61. Mako ME, Starr JI, Rubenstein AH (1977) Circulating proinsulin in patients with maturity onset diabetes. Am J Med 163:865–869.
62. Gordon P, Hendricks CM, Roth J (1974) Circulating proinsulin-like component in men: increased proportion in hypoproteinemic states. Diabetologia 10:469–474.
63. Jasper JB, Mako ME, Kuzuya H, Blix PM, Horwitz DL, Rubenstein AH (1977) Abnormalities in circulating beta cell peptides in chronic renal failure: comparison of C-peptide, proinsulin and insulin. J Clin Endocrinol Metab 45:441–446.
64. Linde S, Welinder BS, Nielsen (1993) Analysis of proinsulin and its conversion products by reverse-phase high-performance liquid chromatography. J Chromatogr 614:185–204.
65. Hartlinger SG, Dinesen B, Kappelgard AM, Faber OK, Binder C (1986) ELISA for human proinsulin. Clin Chem Acta 156:289–297.

66. Røder ME, Hartling SG, Binder C, Welinder BS, Binder C (1991) Separation and quantitation of serum proinsulin and proinsulin intermediates in humans. J Chromatography 548:371–380.
67. Kitabchi AE, Duckworth WC, Brush JS, Heinemann M (1971) Direct measurement of proinsulin in human plasma by the use of an insulin-degrading enzyme. J Clin Invest 50:1792–1799.
68. Starr JI, Juhn DS, Rubenstein AH, Kitabchi AE (1975) Degradation of insulin in serum by insulin-specific protease. J Lab Clin Med 86;631–637.
69. Ward KW, Paquette TL, Frank BH, Porte D (1986) A sensitive radioimmunoassay for human proinsulin, with sequential use of antisera to C-peptide and insulin. Clin Chem 32;726–733.
70. Cohen RH, Nakabayashi T, Blix PM, Rue PA, Schoelson SE, Root MA, Frank BH, Revers RR, Rubenstein AH (1985) A radioimmunoassay for circulating human proinsulin. Diabetes 34:84–91.
71. Cohen RM, Given BD, Licinio-Paixao J, et al. (1986) Proinsulin radioimmunoassay in the evaluation of insulinomas and familial hyperproinsulinemia. Metabolism 35:1137–1146.
72. Sopwith AM, Hales CN (1980) Micromodification of an immunoradiometric assay for proinsulin. Ann Clin Biochem 17:185–187.
73. Rainbow SJ, Woodhead JS, Yue DK, Luzio SD, Hales CN (1979) Measurement of human proinsulin by an indirect two-site immunoradiometric assay. Diabetologia 17:229–234.
74. Chevenne D, Ruiz J, Lohmann L, et al. (1994) Immunoradiometric assay of human intact proinsulin applied to patients with Type 2 diabetes, impaired glucose tolerance, and hyperandrogenism. Clin Chem 40:754–757.
75. Engling US, Missler U, Kerner W (1995) Time-resolved immunofluorometric assay for quantifying proinsulin in serum. Clin Chem 41:942–43.
76. Cooper GJS (1994) Amylin compared with calcitonin-related peptide: structure, biology, and relevance to metabolic disease. Endocrine Rev 15:163–201.
77. Cooper GJS, Willis AC, Clark A, et al. (1987) Purification and characterization of a peptide from amyloid-rich pancreases of Type 2 diabetic patients. Proc Natl Acad Sci USA 84:8628–8632.
78. Leighton B, Cooper GJS (1988) Pancreatic amylin and calcitonin gene-related peptide cause resistance to insulin in skeletal muscle *in vitro*. Nature 335:632–635.
79. Cooper GJS, Leighton B, Dimitriadis GD, et al. (1988) Amylin found in amyloid deposits in human type 2 diabetes mellitus may be a hormone that regulates glycogen metabolism in skeletal muscle. Proc Natl Acad Sci USA 85:7763–7766.
80. Leighton B, Cooper GJS (1990) The role of amylin in the insulin resistance of non-insulin-dependent diabetes mellitus. Trends Biochem Sci 15:295–299.
81. Nagamatsu S, Caroll RJ, Grodsky GM, Steiner DF (1990) Lack of islet amyloid polypeptide regulation of insulin biosynthesis or secretion in normal rat islets. Diabetologia 33:115–117.
82. Bretherton-Watt D, Gilbey SG, Ghatei MA, Beacham J, Bloom SR (1990) Failure to establish islet amyloid polypeptide (amylin) as a circulating beta cell-inhibiting hormone in man. Diabetologia 33:115–117.
83. Westermark P, Wernstedt C, Wilander E, Sletten K (1986) A novel peptide in the calcitonin gene-related peptide family as an amyloid fibril protein in the endocrine pancreas. Biochem Biophys Res Commun 140:827–831.
84. Nagamatsu S, Nishi M, Steiner DF (1991) Biosynthesis of islet amyloid polypeptide. J Biol Chem 266:13737–13741.
85. Nakazato M, Asai J, Kangawa K, Matsukura S, Matsuo H (1989) Establishment of raioimmunoassay for human islet polypeptide and its tissue content and plasma concentration. Biochem Biophys Res Commun 164:394–399.

86. Mitsukawa T, Takemura J, Asai J, et al. (1990) Islet amyloid polypeptide response to glucose, insulin, and somatostatin analogue administration. Diabetes 39:639–642.
87. Ludvik B, Lell B, Hartter E, Schnack C, Prager R (1991) Decrease of stimulated amylin release precedes impairment of insulin secretion in type II diabetes. Diabetes 40:1615–1619.
88. Percy AJ, Trainor DA, Rittenhouse J, Phelps J, Koda HE (1996) Development of sensitive immunoassays to detect amylin and amylin-like peptides in unextracted plasma. Clin Chem 42:576–585.
89. Unger RH, Orci L (1975) The essential role of glucagon in the pathogenesis of diabetes mellitus. Lancet 1:14–16.
90. Staub A, Sinn L, Behrens OK (1955) Purification and crystallization of glucagon. J Biol Chem 214:619–632.
91. Bromer WW, Boucher ME, Kofenberger JE, Jr (1971) Amino acid sequence of bovine glucagon. J Biol Chem 246:2822–2827.
92. England RD, Jones BN, Flanders KC, et al. (1982) Glucagon carboxyl-terminal derivatives: preparation, purification and characterization. Biochemistry 21:940–950.
93. Unson CG, MacDonald D, Ray K, et al. (1991) Position 9 replacement analogs of glucagon uncouple biological activity and receptor binding. J Biol Chem 266:2763–2766.
94. Philippe J (1991) Structure and pancreatic expression of insulin and glucagon genes. Endocr Rev 12:352–271.
95. Rigopoulou D, Vaverde I, Marco J, et al. (1970) Large glucagon immunoreactivity in extracts of pancreas. J Biol Chem 245:496–501.
96. Valverde I, Villanueva ML (1976) Heterogeneity of plasma immunoreactive glucagon. Metabolism 24(Suppl 1):1393–1395.
97. Warne GL, Alford FP, Chissholm DJ, Court J (1977) Glucagon and diabetes. II. Complete suppression of glucagon by insulin in human diabetes. Clin Endocrinol 6:277–284.
98. Raskin P, Pietri A, Unger R (1979) Changes in glucagon levels after four to five weeks of glucoregulation by portable insulin infusion pumps. Diabetes 28:1033–1035.
99. Arimura A, Sata H, Dupont A, et al. (1975) Somatostatin: abundance of immunoreactive hormone in rat stomach and pancreas. Science 189:1007–1009.
100. Reichlin S (1983) Somatostatin part I. N Engl J Med 309:1495–1501.
101. Reichlin S (1983) Somatostatin, part II. N Engl J Med 309:1556–1563.
102. Brown M, Rivert J, Vale W (1981) Somatostatin-28: selective action on the pancreatic b-cell and brain. Endocrinology 108:2391–2396.
103. Kronheim S, Borclowitz M, Pimstone BL (1978) The characterization of somatostatin-like immunoreactivity in human serum. Diabetes 27:523–529.
104. Mackes K, Itoh M, Greene K, Gerich J (1981) Radioimmunoassay of human plasma somatostatin. Diabetes 30:728–734.
105. Hirsch HJ, Gabbay KHL (1978) Radioimmunoassay of somatostatin-like immunoreactivity in human plasma [Abstract] Diabetes 27:441.
106. Parel YC, Wheatley T, Fitz-Patrick D, Brock G (1980) A sensitive radioimmunoassay for immunoreactive somatostatin in extracted plasma: measurement and characterization of portal and peripheral plasma in the rat. Endocrinology 107:306–313.
107. Wright J, Abolfathi A, Penman E, Marks V (1980) Pancreatic somatocarcinoma presenting with hypoglycemia. Clin Endocrinol (Oxford) 12:603–609.
108. Shoelson SE, Polonsky KS, Nakabayashi T, Jaspan JB, Tager HS (1986) Circulating forms of somatostatinlike immunoreactivity in human plasma. Am J Physiol 250 (4 pt 1):E428–434.
109. Schwartz TW (1983) Pancreatic polypeptide: A hormone under vagal control. Gastroenterology 85:1411–1425.
110. Koch MB, Go VL, DiMango EP (1985) Can plasma human pancreatic polypeptide be used to detected diseases of the exocrine pancreas? Mayo Clin Proc 60:259–265.

111. Schwartz TW, Ginerich RL, Tager HS (1980) Biosynthesis of pancreatic polypeptide: identification of a precursor and a co-synthesized product. J Biol Chcm 225:11,494–11,498.
112. Chance RE, Moon NE, Johnson MG (1979) Human pancreatic polypeptide (HPP) and bovine pancreatic polypeptide (BPP). In: Methods of hormone radioimmunoassay, 2nd ed., Jaffe BM, Behrman HR, eds., New York, Academic, 657–672.
113. Bach J-F (1994) Insulin-dependent diabetes mellitus as an autoimmune disease. Endocrine Rev 15:516–542.
114. Eisenbarth GS (1986) Type I diabetes mellitus. A chronic autoimmune disease. N Engl J Med 314:1360–1368.
115. Laupacis A, Gardell C, Dupre J, Stiller CR, Keown P, Wallace AC (1983) Cyclosporin prevents diabetes in BB Wistar rats. Lancet 1:10–12.
116. Harrison LC, Colman PG, Dean B, Baxter R, Martin FIR (1985) Increase in remission rate in newly diagnosed type I diabetic subjects treated with azathioprine. Diabetes 34:1306–1308.
117. Silverstein J, MacLaren N, Riley W, Spillar R, Radjenovic D, Johnson S (1988) Immunosuppression with azathioprine and prednisone in recent-onset-insulin dependent diabetes mellitus. N Engl J Med 319:599–604.
118. Stiller CR, Dupre J (1989) Immune interventional studies in type I diabetes mellitus: summary of the London (Canada) and Canadian-European experience. In: Immunotherapy of diabetes and selected autoimmune diseases, Eisenbarth GS ed., Boca Raton, FL, CRC, pp. 73–84.
119. Muir A, Peck A, Clare-Salazar M, Song YH, Cornelius J Peck A, Luchetta R, Krischer J, Maclaren N (1995) Insulin immunization of nonobese diabetic mice induces a protective insulinitis characterized by diminished intraislet interferon-gamma transcription. J Clin Invest 95:628–634.
120. Kaufman DL, Clare-Salzler M, Tian J, Forsthuber T, Ting GS, Robinson P, et al. (1993) Spontaneous loss of T-cell tolerance to glutamic acid decarboxylase in murine insulin-dependent diabetes. Nature 366:69–72
121. Rossini AA, Mordes JP, Like AA (1985) Immunology of insulin-dependent diabetes mellitus. Ann Rev Immmunol 3:289–320.
122. Trucco G, Fritsch R, Giorda R, et al (1989) Rapid detection of IDDM susceptibility with HLA-DQ β-alleles as markers. Diabetes 38:1617–1622.
123. Todd JA, Bell JI, McDevitt HO (1987) HLA-DQ-beta gene contributes to susceptibility and resistance to insulin-dependent diabetes mellitus. Nature 329:559-563.
124. Bottazzo GF, Dean DM, McNally JM, Mackay EH, Swift PG, Gamble RD (1985) In situ characterization of autoimmunity phenomena and expression of HLA molecules in the pancreas in diabetic insulitis. N Engl J Med 313:353–360.
125. Signore A, Pozzilli P, Gale EAM, Andreani D, Beverely PCL (1989) The natural history of lymphocyte subsets infiltrating the pancreas of NOD mice. Diabetologia 32:282–289.
126. Prud'homme GJ, Parfrey NA (1988) Biology of disease. Role of T helper lymphocytes in autoimmune diseases. Lab Invest 59:158–172.
127. Roep BO, Arden SI, de Vries RRP, Hutton JC (1990) T cell clones from a type 1 diabetes patient respond to insulin secretory granule proteins. Nature 345:632–634.
128. Rabin DU, Pleasic SM, Palmer-Crocker R, Shapiro JA (1992) Cloning and expression of IDDM-specific human autoantigens. Diabetes 41:183–186.
129. Robin DU, Pleasic SM, Shapiro JA, et al. (1994) Islet cell antigen 512 is a diabetes-specific autoantigen related to protein tyrosine phosphatases. J Immunol 152:3183–3188.
130. Bottazzo GF, florin-Christensen A, Doniach D (1974) Islet cell antibodies in diabetes mellitus with autoimmune polyendocrine deficiencies. Lancet 2:1279–1283.
131. Bottazzo GF, Gleichmann H (1986) Immunology and diabetes workshops report of the first international workshop on the standardization of cytoplasmic islet cell antibodies. Diabetologia. 29:125,126.

132. Gleichmann H, Bottazzo GF (1987) Progress toward standardization of cytoplasmic islet cell-antibody assay. Diabetes 36:578–584.
133. Vardi P, Dibella EE, Pasquarello TJ, Srikanta S (1987) Islet cell autoantibodies: pathobiology and clinical applications. Diabetes Care 10:645–656.
134. Eisenbarth GS, Morris MA, Scearce R (1981) Cytotoxic antibodies to cloned rat islet cells in serum of patients with diabetes mellitus. J Clin Invest 67:403–408.
135. Palmer JP, Asplin CM, Clemons P, Lyen K, Tatpati O, Raghu PK, Paquette TL (1983) Insulin antibodies in insulin-dependent diabetics before insulin treatment. Science 222:1337–1339.
136. Ziegler AG, Ziegler R, Vardi P, Jackson RA, Soeldner JS, Eisenbarth GS (1989) Life-table analysis of progression to diabetes of anti-insulin autoantibody-positive relatives of individuals with type I diabetes. Diabetes 38:1320–1325.
137. Zhang ZJ, Davidson L, Eisenbarth G, Weiner HL (1991) Suppression of diabetes in nonobese diabetic mice by oral administration of procine insulin. Proc Natl Acad Sci USA 88:10,252–10,256.
138. Keller RJ, Eisenbarth GS, Jackson RA (1993) Insulin prophylaxis in individuals at high risk of type I diabetes. Lancet 341:927–928.
139. Greenbaum CJ, Palmer JP, Kuglin B, Kolb, H, and Participating Laboratories (1992) Insulin autoantibodies measured by radioimmunoassay methodology are more related in insulin-dependent diabetes mellitus than those measured by enzyme-linked immunosorbent assay: results of the Fourth International Workshop on the Standardization of Insulin Antibody Measurement. J Clin Endocrinol Metab. 74:1040–1044.
140. Bu D-F, Erlander MG, et al. (1992) Two human glutamate decarboxylases, 65-kDa GAD and 67-kDa GAD, are each encoded by a single gene. Proc Natl Acad Sci USA 89:2115–2119.
141. Hagopian WA, Karlsen AE, Gottsater A, et al. (1993) Quantitative assay using recombinant human islet glutamic acid decarboxylase (GAD65) shows that 64K autoantibody positivity at onset predicts diabetes type. J Clin Invest 91:368–374.
142. Atkinson MA, Kaufman DL, Newman D, Tobin AJ, MacLaren NK (1993) Islet cell cytoplasmic-autoantibody reactivity to glutamate decarboxylase in insulin-dependent diabetes. J Clin Invest 91:350–356.
143. Thivolet CH, Tappaz M, Durand A, et al. (1992) Glutamic acid decarboxylase (GAD) autoantibodies are additional predictive markers of type 1 (insulin-dependent) diabetes mellitus in high-risk individuals. Diabetologia 35:570-576.
144. Schmidli RS, Colman PG, Bonifacio E, Bottazzo GF, Harrison LC (1994) High level of concordance between assays for glutamic acid decarboxylase antibodies: The First International Glutamic Acid Decarboxylase Antibody Workshop. Diabetes 43: 1005–1009.
145. Atkinson MA, Kaufman DL, Campbell L, Gibbs, KA, Shah SC, et al. (1992) Response of peripheral-blood mononuclear cells to glutamate decarboxylase in insulin-dependent diabetes. Lancet 339:458–459.
146. Grubin CE, Daniels T, Toivola B, et al. (1994) A novel radioligand-binding assay to determine diagnostic accuracy of isoform-specific glutamic acid decarboxylase antibodies in childhood IDDM. Diabetologia 32:344–350.
147. Peterson JS, Hejnaes, Moody A, et al. (1994) Detection of GAD65 antibodies in diabetes and other autoimmune diseases using a simple radioligand assay. Diabetes 43: 459–467.
148. Vandewalle CL, Falorni A, Svanholm S, et al. (1995) High diagnostic sensitivity of glutamate decarboxylase autoantibodies in insulin-dependent diabetes mellitus with clinical onset between age 20 and 40 years. J Clin Endocrinol Metab 80:846–851.
149. Harrison LC (1992) Islet cell autoantigens in insulin-dependent diabetes: Pandora's box revisited. Immunol Today 13:348–352.

150. Christie MR, Tun RYM, Lo SSS, et al. (1992) Antibodies to glutamic acid decarboxylase and tryptic fragments of islet 64 kDa antigen as distinct markers for the development of insulin-dependent diabetes. Studies with identical twins. Diabetes 41:782–787.
151. Payton MA, Hawkes CJ, Christie MR (1995) Relationship of the 37,000- and 40,000-Mr tryptic fragments of islet antigens in insulin-dependent diabetes to the protein tyrosine phosphatase-like molecule IA-2 (ICA512). J Clin Invest 96:1506–1511.
152. Bonifacio E, Lampasona V, Genovese S, Ferrari M, Bosi E (1995) Identification of protein tyrosine phosphatase-like IA2 (islet cell antigen 512) as the insulin-dependent diabetes-related 37/40K autoantigen and a target of islet-cell antibodies. J Immunol 155: 5419–5426.
153. Yoon JW, Ihm SH (1991) Role of viruses in the pathogenesis of IDDM. Ann Med 23:437–445.
154. Yoon JW, Austin M, Onodera T, Notkins AL (1979) Virus-induced diabetes mellitus. Isolation of a virus from the pancreas of a child with diabetic ketoacidosis. N Engl J Med 300:1173–1179
155. Kaufman DL, Erlander MG, Clare-Salzler M, Atkinson MA, MacLaren NK, Tobin AJ (1992) Autoimmunity to two forms of glutamate decarboxylase in insulin-dependent diabetes mellitus. J Clin Invest 89:283–292.
156. Karjalainen J, Martin JM, Knip M, et al. (1992) A bovine albumin peptide as a possible trigger of insulin-dependent diabetes mellitus. New Engl J Med 327:302–307.
157. Atkinson MA, Bowman MA, Kao KJ, et al. (1993) ack of immune responsiveness to bovine serum albumin in insulin-dependent diabetes. N Engl J Med 329:1853–1858.
158. Karam JH, Lewitt PA, Young CW, et al. (1980) Insulinopenic diabetes after rodenticide (Vacor) ingestion: a unique model of acquired diabetes in man. Diabetes 29:971–978.
159. Bouchard P, Sai P, Reach G, Caubarrere I, Ganeval D, Assan R (1982) Diabetes mellitus following pentamidine-induced hypoglycemia in humans. Diabetes 31:40–45.
160. Reaven GM (1988) Role of insulin resistance in human disease. Diabetes 37:1595–1607.
161. Hammon RF (1992) Genetic and environmental determinants of non-insulin-dependent diabetes mellitus (NIDDM). Diab Metab Rev 8:287–338.
162. Bergman RN, Finegood DT, Ader M (1985) Assessment of insulin sensitivity in vivo. Endocr Rev 6:45–86.
163. Moller DE, Flier JS (1991) Insulin resistance: mechanisms, syndromes, and implications. N Engl J Med 325:938–948.
164. Flier JS (1992) Syndromes of insulin resistance: from patient to gene and back again. Diabetes 41:1207–1219.
165. Bar RS, Muggeo M, Kahn CR, Gorden PH, Roth J (1980) Characterization of insulin receptors in patients with the syndromes of insulin resistance and acanthosis nigricans. Diabeteologia 18:209–216.
166. Garvey WT (1992) Glucose transport and NIDDM. Diabetes Care 15:396–417.
167. Garvey WT, Maianu L, Huecksteadt TP, Birmbaum MJ, Mohna JM, Ciaraldi TP (1991) Pretranslational suppression of a glucose transport protein causes insulin resistance in adipocytes from patients with non-insulin-dependent diabetes mellitus and obesity. J Clin Invest 87:1072–1081.
168. Garvey WT, Maianu L, Hancock JA, Golichowski AM, Baron A (1992) Gene expression of GLUT4 in skeletal muscle from insulin-resistant patients with obesity. IGT, GDM, and NIDDM. Diabetes 41:465–475.
169. Hotamisligil GS, Shargill NS, Spiegelman BM (1993) Adipose expression of tumor necrosis factor-α: direct role in obesity-linked insulin resistance. Science 259:87–91.
170. Hotamisligil GS, Arner P, Caro JF, Atkinson RL, Spiegelman BM (1995) Increased adipose tissue expression of tumor necrosis factor-α in human obesity and insulin resistance. J Clin Invest 95:2409–2415.

171. Hotamisligil GS, Peraldi P, Budavari A, Ellis R, White MF, Spiegelman BM (1996) IRS-1-mediated inhibition of insulin receptor tyrosine kinase activity in TNF-α-and obesity-induced insulin resistance. Science 271:665–668.
172. Leahy JL (1990) Natural history of beta-cell dysfunction in NIDDM. Diabetes Care 13: 992–1010.
173. Halaas JL, Gajiwala KS, Maffei M, et al. (1995) Weight-reducing effects of the plasma protein encoded by the obese gene. Science 269:543–546.
174. Saladin R, De Vos P, Guerre-Millo M, et al. (1995) Transient increase in obese gene expression after food intake or insulin administration. Nature 377:527–529.
175. National Diabetes Data Group (1979) Classification and diagnosis of diabetes melllitus and other categories of glucose intolerance. Diabetes 28:1039–1057.
176. Balkau B, Eschwege E (1991) Repeatibility of the oral glucose tolerance test for the diagnosis of impaired glucose tolerance and diabetes mellitus. Diabetologia 34:201–202.
177. Barrett EJ, Defronzo RA (1984) Diabetic ketoacidosis: Diagnosis and treatment. Hosp Pract (Hosp Ed). 89–104.
178. Schwartz JG (1995) The role of glycohemoglobin and other proteins in diabetes management. Diabetes Rev 3:269–287.
179. Bunn HF, Gabbay KH, Gallop MP (1978) The glycosylation of haemoglobin: relevance to diabetes mellitus. Science 200:21–27.
180. John WG, Bullock DG, MacKenzie F (1992) Methods for the analysis of glycated hemoglobins: what is being measured. Diabetic Med 9:15–19.
181. Javid J, Pettis PK, Koenig RJ, Cerami A (1978) Immunologic characterization and quantification of hemoglobin A1C. Br J Haematol 38:329–337.
182. Mallia AK, Hermanson GT, Krohn RI, Fujimoto EK, Smith PK (1981) Preparation and use of a boronic acid affinity support for separation and quantitation of glycosylated hemoglobins. Anal Lett 14:649–661.
183. Fletchner M, Ramp J, England B, et al. Affinity-binding assay of glycohemoglobin by two-dimensional centrifugation. Clin Chem 1992;38:2372–2379.
184. Little RR, Wiedmeyer H-M, England JD, et al. (1992) Interlaboratory standardization of measurements of glycohemoglobins. Clin Chem 38:2472–2478.
185. Johnson RN, Metcalf PA, Baker JR (1983) Fructosamine: a new approach to the estimation of serum glycosylprotein: an index of diabetic control. Clin Chem Acta 127:87–95.
186. Armbruster DA (1987) Fructosamine: structure, analysis, and clinical usefulness. Clin Chem 33:2153–2163.
187. Brownlee M, Cerami A, Vlassara H (1988) Advanced glycosylation end products in tissue and the biochemical basis of diabetic complications. N Engl J Med 318:1315–1321.
188. Bucala R, Vlassara H (1995) Advanced glycosylation end products in diabetic renal disease: clinical measurement. Pathophysiological significance and prospects for pharmacological inhibition. Blood Purification 13:160–170.
189. Bucula R, Vlassara H (1986) Novel macrophage receptor for glucose-modified protein is distinct from previously described scavenger receptors. J Exp Med 164:1301–1309.
190. Makita Z, Vlassara H. Cerami A, Bucala R (1992) Immunochemical detection of advanced glycosylation end products in vivo. J Biol Chem 267:5133–5138.
191. Makita Z, Radoff S, Rayfield EJ, et al. (1991) Advanced glycosylation end products in patients with diabetic nephropathy. N Engl J Med 325:836–842.
192. Butler PC, Rizza RA (1989) Regulation of carbohydrate metabolism and response to hypoglycemia. Endocrinol Metab Clin North Am 18:1–26.
193. Clark W, Santiago K, Thomas L, et al. (1979) Adrenergic mechanisms in recovery from hypoglycemia in man: adrenergic blockade. Am J Physiol 263:E147–E152.
194. Cahill GF (1971) Action of adrenal cortical steroids on carbohydrate metabolism. In: The human adrenal cortex, Christy NP, ed., New York, Harper and Row, pp. 205–240.

195. Field JB (1986) Hypoglycemia: A systemic approach to specific diagnosis. Hosp Pract (Office Edition). 21:187–194.
196. Field JB (1989) Hypoglycemia. Definition, clinical presentations, classification, and laboratory tests. Endocrinol Metabol Clin North Am 18:27–44.
197. Scully R (1984) Case records of the Massachusetts General Hospital. N Engl J Med 310:580–587.
198. Fajans SS, Vinik AI (1989) Insulin-producing islet cell tumors. Endocrinol Metabol Clin North Am 18:45–74.
199. Daughaday WH (1989) Hypoglycemia in patients with non-islet cell tumors. Endocrinol Metab Clin North Am 18:91–101
200. Arky RA (1989) Hypoglycemia associated with liver disease and ethanol. Endocrinol Metabol North Am 18:75–90.
201. Turner RC, Oakley NW, Nabarro JDN (1971) Control of basal insulin secretion, with special reference to the diagnosis of insulinomas. Br Med J 2:132–135.
202. Turner RC, Heding LG (1977) Plasma proinsulin, C-peptide and insulin in diagnostic suppression tests for insulinomas. Diabetologia 13:571–577.
203. Scarlett JA, Mako ME, Rubenstein AH, et al. (1977) Factitious hypoglycemia, diagnosis by measurement of serum C-peptide immunoreactivity and insulin-binding antibodies. N Engl J Med 297:1029–1032.

Index

A

Adenosquamous carcinoma, of pancreas, 152
Abdominal surgery, 61, 62
Alpha-1 protease inhibitors,
 and trypsin, 83
 as markers of disease severity, 99
  diagnostic accuracy, 100
 in fat necrosis, 112
Alpha-2 macroglobulin,
 and trypsin, 83
 as markers of disease severity, 99
  diagnostic accuracy, 100
 in fat necrosis, 112
Amylase,
 amylase:creatinine clearance ratio, 76
 isoenzymes, 76–79, 95
 isoforms, 79, 80
 lipase:amylase ratio, 81
  in peritoneal fluids, 101
  in pulmonary effusions, 108
 macroamylase, 76
 sensitivity and specificity, 76, 77
  diagnostic accuracy, 77–80
 as test for rejection, 12
 in urine, 12
Anionic trypsin, 16
Anti-rejection drugs, 4
 in pancreas transplantation, 13
Artificial pancreas, 17
Autoantibodies, 2
 against glutamic acid decarboxylase, 2
 against islet cells, 2
Autoimmune etiology of diabetes, 2
Azathioprine, 4

B

Benzoyl-L-arginine ethyl ester, 38
Bicarbonate loss in transplantation, 11
Body Mass Index,
 as markers of disease severity, 100
Brequinar sodium, 4

C

Carboxypeptidase A,
 measurement, 84
 specificity for acute pancreatitis, 84, 85
Cardiac,
 complications in acute pancreatitis, 110, 111
 electrocardiographic changes, 110
Cationic trypsin, 16
CD4+ T-cells, 2
CD8+ T-cells, 2, 8
Cell chimerism, 5
Cerulein, 40
Cholecystokinin, 27, 28, 56
Chronic pancreatitis, 54–61
 clinical presentation, 55, 56
 diagnosis, laboratory, 56, 57
 evaluation of pancreatic sufficiency, 57–59
 radiological studies, 60
 therapy, monitoring, 60, 61
CMV activation, 8
CMV infection, 8
 detection by molecular methods, 9
 effect of immunosuppression, 8
 tests for, 8

Complement,
    and anaphylatoxins, 97
        effects of, 97
    as markers of disease severity, 97
    in pulmonary complications, 108, 109
    in retinopathy, 113
    terminal complement complex, 97
C-Peptide, 16
C-Reactive protein,
    as markers of disease severity, 95
Cross-match testing, 7
CSA in blood, 5
    assay for, 5
Cyclosporin A, 4
Cyclosporin G, 4
Cystadenocarcinoma, pancreatic, 151, 152
Cystadenoma, pancreatic, 152
Cystic Fibrosis, 48–54
    CF transmembrane conductance regulator, 48
    diagnosis, laboratory, 50–52
        sweat test, 50, 51, 62
    evaluation of pancreatic sufficiency, 52–54
    molecular biology, 48, 49
    muconium ileus, 51, 52
    mutations, 49
    screening, 49, 50
        DNA testing, 50
Cystitis after transplantation, 11
Cytotoxic T-cells and diabetes, 2

D

15-Deoxyspergualine, 13
Deoxyspergualine, 4
Diabetes incidence, 1
    autoimmune etiology, 11
    in Finland, 1
    in Greece, 1
    risk factors and cow's milk, 3
    viral etiology, 3
Diabetes Mellitus, 180–196
    insulin dependent (IDDM), 180–187
        autoantibodies, 183
        glutamic acid decarboxylase (GAD), 184, 185
        insulin, 184
        islet cell, 183, 184
        tyrosine phosphatase (IA-2/ICA-512), 185, 186
    cellular immunity, 182, 183
    environmental factors, 186, 187
    HLA and genetic risk, 181, 182
    pathogenesis, 180, 181
    laboratory tests, 192–196
        advanced glycosylation end products, 196
        c-peptide, 170, 171
        fructosamine, 195, 196
        glucose tolerance test, 192
        glycohemoglobin, 194, 195
        insulin, 169, 170
        islet amyloid polypeptide, 175
        ketone, 193
        pancreatic polypeptide, 179
        somatostatin, 179
    noninsulin-dependent (NIDDM), 187
        pathogenesis, 188
        B-cell failure, 192
        insulin resistance, 188
            glucose transplant system, 190, 191
            insulin receptor, 189, 190
            tumor necrosis factor, 191, 192
        obesity, 192
Diabetes risk factors, 3
    bovine serum albumin, 3
    viruses, 3
Diabetic "honeymoon," 3
Diet, 30
Digestion, 29–31
DNA testing, 7
    genotype, 7
    in graft survival, 7

E

Elastase,
    as causes of hemorrhage, 102
    as markers of disease severity, 95
    effects of, 95

ELISA testing for HCV, 9
Encapsulated islets, 17
Endocrine pancreatic loss, 1
Exocrine pancreatic loss, 1

F

Fat necrosis, 111, 112
Fecal fat, 46
FK 506, 4
Flow cytometry, 6
    characterization of cells, 6
Free radicals and beta cell destruction, 3

G

GAD, 2
Gastrin, 28
Giant-cell carcinoma, of pancreas, 152
Glucose tolerance and rejection, 12
Glutamic acid decarboxylase, 22
    antibodies to, 22
Graft loss, 5
Graft survival, 8
Gycosylated hemoglobin, 1

H

HCV-positive organs, 9
    testing for, 10
    transplantation, 9
Hepatotrophic effects, 4
Hereditary pancreatitis, 62, 63
Histocompatibility complex, 2
HLA, 2, 6, 8
    antigens, 6
    compatibility testing, 6
    mismatch and transplantation, 8
    phenotype association with diabetes, 2
Hyperacute rejection, 7
Hypocalcemia,
    and magnesium, 104
    mechanisms of, 104, 105
Hyperchloremic acidosis, 11
Hypoglycemia, 196
    factitious, 199, 200
    fasting, 198, 199
    as marker of disease severity, 106
    mechanisms of in acute pancreatitis, 106
    reactive, 197, 198
Hypertriglyceridemia,
    as marker of disease severity, 105
    mechanisms of, 105, 106
    in pulmonary complications, 110

I

Immunoisolation techniques, 16
Immunomodulation of pancreatic islets, 12
Infection vs rejection, 5
Infrared spectroscopy, 46, 47
Inherited enzyme deficiencies, 62, 63
Insulin requirements after transplantation, 15
Interleukin-6,
    and acute phase response, 98
    and CRP, 98
    as markers of disease severity, 98
    and tumor necrosis factor, 98
Intestinal disease, 63–64
Islet cells, 2, 3, 13
    antibodies to, 2
    implantation, 3, 13
    isolation, 12
    purification, 12
    transplantation, 3, 12, 17

J

Johanson-Blizzard syndrome, 62

L

Leflunomide, 4
Lewis antigen, 130
Lipase,
    colipase, 80
    isoforms, 82
        in peritoneal fluid, 101
    lipase:amylase ratio, 81

M

Major histocompatibility complex, 2
Malabsorption, 64
Methemalbumin,
    and disease mortality, 101
    in hemorrhagic pancreatitis, 100
    as markers of disease severity, 101
Microcystic adenoma, of pancreas, 152, 153
Mizoribine, 4
Mofetil, 4
Molecular mimicry and diabetes, 3
Multiple endocrine neoplasia syndrome (MEN-1), 143
Mycophenolic acid, 4

N

Neocuprene occlusion techniques, 14
Neopterin, 16
Nephrotoxicity, 5
    of anti-rejection drugs, 5
New England Organ Bank, 10
N-substituted tyrosine esters, 39

O

Octreotide scanning, 143–244
Organ procurement protocol, 10

P

Pancreas transplantation, 3, 14
    complications of, 4
    cyclosporin A in treatment, 3
    glycemia in, 14
    testing for rejection, 16
Pancreatic abscess,
    as markers of disease severity, 103
    diagnosis of, 103
Pancreatic enzymes,
    activation of, 29
    amylase, 30, 34, 36, 56
    carboxyl ester hydrolase, 34, 35, 61
    carboxypeptidase, 29, 33
    chymotrypsin, 29, 32, 37, 53, 62
    colipase, 29, 34, 63
    elastase, 29, 33
    kallikrein, 33
    lipase, 34, 56, 57, 60, 63
    nucleases, 35
    phospholipase, 35
    precursor forms, 29, 30
    replacement of, 53, 60, 61
    trypsin, 29, 31, 32, 38
        immunoassay for, 36, 37, 49, 50, 56
        inhibitors, 29, 30, 36
Pancreatic fluid, 27–29, 41
    hormonal control of, 27
Pancreatic function tests, 25–47
    direct, 35–40
        enzyme measurements in serum, 35–38, 56, 57
        enzyme measurements in stool, 38–39, 53, 57, 62
    indirect, 40–47
        amino acids, plasma, 44, 45, 59, 62
        breath tests, 45, 59, 61
        lipids, stool, 46, 47, 57
        NBT-PABA test, 41–43, 53, 57–59, 62
        Pancreolauryl test, 43, 44, 53, 57
        Schilling test, 45, 46
    provocative, 39, 40
        Lundh meal, 39, 42
        secretin-CCK test, 40, 52
        secretin test, 39, 40
Pancreatic insufficiency, 43, 44, 52, 53, 56–58
Pancreatic neoplasms, 125–162
    exocrine neoplasms, 147–154
        diagnosis, 149–151
        epidemiology, 147–149
        histological classification, 151–153
        laboratory diagnosis, 126–139
        prognosis, 152–154
        treatment, 153, 154
    endocrine neoplasms, 139–147
        gastrinoma, 142–144
        glucagonoma, 145
        insulinoma, 140–142

Index 217

nonfunctioning islet cell tumors, 147
PPoma, 146, 147
somatostatinoma, 145, 146
VIPoma, 144, 145
Pancreaticoduodenectomy, 153
Pancreatic polypeptide, 57, 179, 180
   biosynthesis/biochemistry, 179
   measurement, 179, 180
Pancreatitis,
   anatomic abnormalities,
      pancreatitis divism, 91
   causes of,
      acetaldehyde, 90
      biliary obstruction, 81, 91, 92
         enzyme changes in, 82
      drugs and toxins, 85
      ERCP, 89
      ethanol, 81, 87, 90
      free radicals, 87, 89, 90
      HIV, 86
      hypercalcemia, 87–89, 104, 105
      hypertriglyceridemia, 87, 88
      postoperative, 88
   complications of, 101–113
   edematous, 107
   infection, 91
   ischemia, 90
   necrotizing, 108
   severity, 83
      markers of, 93–101
      scoring systems, 94
Pancreatitis-associated protein,
   and ethanol, 97
   as markers of disease severity, 96, 97
   synthesis, 96
Papillary neoplasms, of pancreas, 152
Peritoneal tap,
   amylase and lipase in, 101
   as markers of disease severity, 101
PCR testing for hepatitis C, 9
Phlegmon, 103
Phospholipase A,
   as markers of severity, 83, 100
   measurement, 84, 100
   in pulmonary complications, 108, 109

Predictors of diabetes in children, 2
Pseudocyst,
   complications of, 102, 103
   following surgery, 88
   formation of, 102
   hemorrhage, 102
Pulmonary,
   complications, 108–110
   effusions, 108
   hypoxemia, 108

R

Rampamycin, 4
Renal,
   complications in acute pancreatitis, 111
Retinopathy,
   mechanisms of in acute pancreatitis, 112, 113
   prognostic significance, 113
RIBA testing for HCV, 10
Ribonuclease,
   as markers of disease severity, 98, 99

S

Schwachman syndrome, 62
Secretin, 27, 39, 40
Shell vial assay for CMV, 9
Somatostatin, 178
   biosynthesis/biochemistry, 178, 179
   measurement, 179
Squamous cell carcinoma, of pancreas, 152
Steatorrhea, 46, 52, 57, 63, 64
Surgical techniques, 10, 11
   duct occlusion, 11
   ileal drainage, 11
   routing of pancreatic juice, 11

T

Tacrolimus, 4
T-cell cytotoxicity test, 6
Tests for rejection of pancreas, 16
Tumor markers, 128–139
   enzyme activities, serum, 137, 138

amylase, 137
elastase 1, 137
galactosyltransferase II (GTII), 137, 138
lipase, 137
ribonuclease, 138
hormonal and oncofetal products, 138
alpha-fetoprotein (AFP), 138
beta-2-microglobulin, 138
beta-human choriogonadotropin (beta-HCG), 138
tumor-related antigens, 128
CA19-9, 129–133
CA-50, 133, 134
CA-195, 133, 134
CA-242, 135
CA-494, 135, 136
CAM-43, 135
CAR-3, 134, 135
carcinoembryonic antigen (CEA), 128, 129
DU-PAN-2, 134
Span-1, 134
tumor-associated trypsin inhibitor (TATI), 136
tissue polypeptide antigen (TPA), 136
tissue polypeptide specific antigen (TPSA), 136
Tumor necrosis factor,
as markers of disease severity, 98
Trypsin,
protease inhibitors, 83
trypsinogen activation peptide, 83
in coagulation disorders, 107
Trypsinogen activation peptide,
as markers of disease severity, 96

U

Urine drainage of pancreatic fluid, 10

V

Verner-Morrison syndrome, 144, 145
Viral etiology of diabetes, 2

X

Xenogeneic transplants, 17

Z

Zollinger-Ellison syndrome, 142–144